Individualized Drug Therapy for Patients

Individualized Drug Therapy for Patients

Basic Foundations, Relevant Software, and Clinical Applications

Edited by

Roger W. Jelliffe, MD, FCP, FAAPS

Professor of Medicine Emeritus;
Founder and Director Emeritus,
Laboratory of Applied Pharmacokinetics and Bioinformatics,
University of Southern California Keck School of Medicine,
Los Angeles, CA, United States

Consultant in Infectious Diseases, Division of Pediatric Infectious Diseases,
Children's Hospital Los Angeles, Los Angeles, CA, United States

Michael Neely, MD, MSc, FCP

Director, Laboratory of Applied Pharmacokinetics and Bioinformatics,
The Saban Research Institute, Children's Hospital Los Angeles,
Los Angeles, CA, United States

Associate Professor and Clinical Scholar, Division of Infectious Diseases,
Department of Pediatrics, Keck School of Medicine,
University of Southern California Keck School of Medicine,
Los Angeles, CA, United States

AMSTERDAM • BOSTON • HEIDELBERG • LONDON
NEW YORK • OXFORD • PARIS • SAN DIEGO
SAN FRANCISCO • SINGAPORE • SYDNEY • TOKYO

Academic Press is an imprint of Elsevier

Academic Press is an imprint of Elsevier
125 London Wall, London EC2Y 5AS, United Kingdom
525 B Street, Suite 1800, San Diego, CA 92101-4495, United States
50 Hampshire Street, 5th Floor, Cambridge, MA 02139, United States
The Boulevard, Langford Lane, Kidlington, Oxford OX5 1GB, United Kingdom

Notices
Knowledge and best practice in this field are constantly changing. As new research and experience broaden our understanding, changes in research methods, professional practices, or medical treatment may become necessary.

Practitioners and researchers must always rely on their own experience and knowledge in evaluating and using any information, methods, compounds, or experiments described herein. In using such information or methods they should be mindful of their own safety and the safety of others, including parties for whom they have a professional responsibility.

To the fullest extent of the law, neither the Publisher nor the authors, contributors, or editors, assume any liability for any injury and/or damage to persons or property as a matter of products liability, negligence or otherwise, or from any use or operation of any methods, products, instructions, or ideas contained in the material herein.

British Library Cataloguing-in-Publication Data
A catalogue record for this book is available from the British Library

Library of Congress Cataloging-in-Publication Data
A catalog record for this book is available from the Library of Congress

ISBN: 978-0-12-803348-7

For information on all Academic Press publications
visit our website at https://www.elsevier.com

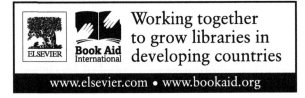

Working together
to grow libraries in
developing countries

www.elsevier.com • www.bookaid.org

Publisher: Mica Haley
Acquisition Editor: Kristine Jones
Editorial Project Manager: Molly McLaughlin
Production Project Manager: Julia Haynes
Designer: Mark Rogers

Typeset by MPS Limited, Chennai, India

Dedication

To Joyce, who stood by me through everything while she was able, and who still does

To Richard Eckstein, who taught me cardiovascular physiology like I never had it in medical school

To the Oak Ridge Institute of Nuclear Studies, who in 1966 showed me the beginnings of what has become pharmacokinetics

To Richard Bellman, who showed me the idea of adaptive control

And especially, to all our team, over all the years!

Roger W. Jelliffe

I dedicate this book to my wife, Lisa, and son, Jake, who remind me daily what is important rather than what is urgent. I thank my parents for the loving and stable home that gave me such a good example for my own home. I also dedicate this book to my co-editor, Roger Jelliffe, who has been a friend and mentor for over a decade now. I wouldn't be where I am today without his inspiration and undying passion to treat patients better. Finally, I thank all the patients in this book whom I've treated, and many more who aren't in this book, but who are part of me. Thank you for sharing your trust. It has been a privilege to care for you.

Michael Neely

Contents

SECTION I BASIC TECHNIQUES FOR INDIVIDUALIZED THERAPY

SECTION II THE CLINICAL SOFTWARE

List of Contributors

A. Aldaz
Clinica Universidad de Navarra, Pamplona, Spain

A. Åsberg
University of Oslo, Oslo, Norway; Oslo University Hospital — Rikshospitalet, Oslo, Norway

D. Bayard
Children's Hospital Los Angeles, Los Angeles, CA, United States

N. Bleyzao
Institute of Pediatric Hematology and Oncology, Lyon, France; Hospices Civils de Lyon, Lyon, France; Université Lyon 1, Lyon, France

I. Bondareva
Research Institute of Physical Chemical Medicine, Moscow, Russia

L. Bourguignon
Université Lyon I, Lyon, France; Geriatric Hospital Antoine Charial, Francheville, France

G.L. Drusano
University of Florida, Gainesville, FL, United States

M. Ducher
Geriatric Hospital Antoine Charial, Francheville, France

S. Goutelle
Hospices Civils de Lyon, Lyon, France; Université Lyon 1, Lyon, France; Geriatric Hospital Antoine Charial, Francheville, France

R.W. Jelliffe
University of Southern California, Los Angeles, CA, United States; Children's Hospital Los Angeles, CA, United States

P. Maire
Hospices Civils de Lyon, Lyon, France; Université Lyon 1, Lyon, France; Geriatric Hospital Antoine Charial, Francheville, France

P. Marquet
University Limoges, Limoges, France; INSERM, U850, Limoges, France; CHU Limoges, Limoges, France

M. Neely
Children's Hospital Los Angeles, Los Angeles, CA, United States; University of Southern California, Los Angeles, CA, United States

M. Philippe
University of Southern California Children's Hospital Los Angeles, Los Angeles, CA, United States; Institute of Pediatric Hematology and Oncology, Lyon, France; Hospices Civils de Lyon, Lyon, France; Université Lyon 1, Lyon, France

N.Y. Rakhmanina
Children's National Health System, Washington, DC, United States; George Washington University, Washington, DC, United States; Elizabeth Glaser Pediatric AIDS Foundation, Washington, DC, United States

P. Schaiquevich
Hospital de Pediatria JP Garrahan, Buenos Aires, Argentina

A. Schumitzky
University of Southern California, Los Angeles, CA, United States

Preface

Quantitative approaches
to optimally precise individualized drug therapy
are more useful,
scientifically, medically, and socially,
than all the memorized words and facts
about categorized and classified experiences
can ever be.

Our purpose with this book is to introduce the interested clinician and the curious reader to the quantitative tools for dosage individualization in the most logical and least mathematical way possible, along with their embodiment in clinical software and their current applications in several relevant clinical areas. In the distant past, clinicians worked using only their personal capabilities and senses to listen to a patient's history, to use their personal senses of sight, hearing, and touch to gather more information from the physical examination, and then to develop a clinical impression, a differential diagnosis, and a plan, out of their experience and their powers of intuitive reasoning.

In the last century, however, we have supplemented our senses with many other tools to gather still more information with laboratory tests, X-rays, electrocardiograms, and more recently, a whole new armamentarium of computerized imaging techniques. We have used our experience and reasoning to consider what drugs may be appropriate to use for therapy, and we have been taught to use our intuitive judgment to consider what the appropriate doses of these drugs should be.

The pharmaceutical industry develops drugs and performs studies to determine the "appropriate" dosage of each drug. This information is then incorporated into the package insert. Clinicians use the inserts directly (or, more often, indirectly) through guidelines and references from authoritative bodies to determine the correct doses for the patient. For each drug, the dose is usually the same for all patients—one-size-fits-all—particularly for adults. If the drug has significant renal excretion, the dose may be categorized according to various ranges of renal function. All these facts are carefully memorized.

However, some drugs have narrow margins of safety. It has become customary to measure their serum concentrations from time to time to check what we have done. We are told to interpret the "meaning" of these concentrations, and so we have classified them into various ranges such as subtherapeutic, therapeutic, and toxic. Our entire approach has been to classify our often quantitative experiences. Committees meet and develop guidelines as to what these acceptable drug concentration ranges are. We commit these to memory and intuitively adjust doses to try to achieve concentrations within these ranges.

Measuring serum drug concentrations in this way is called *therapeutic drug monitoring (TDM)*. TDM is usually done on an ad hoc basis, without careful planning in advance to optimize the process by employing any other quantitative tools. We are always supposed to do this by careful thinking, whatever that means. A good clinician is somehow supposed to have those intuitive powers of clinical reasoning.

However, instead of simply checking what we have done, we can do better by planning therapy in advance and using quantitative techniques to optimize the entire process of planning, monitoring, and adjusting drug dosage regimens for each individual patient. First, we can use quantitative methods to describe the behavior of drugs in patients, with pharmacokinetic (PK) models. Models are mathematical constructs that more formally and precisely describe past experience with a drug or other medical intervention than our own memories or experience are able to do. Second, we can use these models to calculate (compute) the initial dosage regimen to achieve a specific selected target goal for each patient (not just a guideline set up by a committee who never saw the patient). Third, we can couple this with an approach, again optimally planned in advance, to learn most rapidly and precisely just how the drug is behaving in the patient. Fourth, we can follow this with an adjusted maximally precise dosage regimen to hit the current target, or any new selected target.

Just as we use X-rays and other computerized imaging techniques to supplement what we can see, hear, and feel, we can now also use quantitative tools implemented in computer software to enhance our ability to develop the best and most precise dosage regimen for each patient. This is another useful tool for a clinician to use, just like a stethoscope. This new change in thinking is therapeutic drug *management* (also called TDM). Clinical software now enables us to plan the optimally precise therapy for each patient. Just as one used to use eye-hand coordination to aim guns to shoot down enemy aircraft 50 years ago, we now use radar and computers to track the targets to calculate where they are, and also to aim the guns to hit most precisely the calculated place where the targets are predicted to be in the near future.

This is what this book is about: optimizing drug therapy. It is not a textbook on PK. It uses PK only for optimal descriptions of drug behavior in patients. We want to optimize the process of learning about the behavior of the drug in each individual patient while treating him or her at the same time. Then, we want to optimize the adjustment of the dosage regimen in each patient to most precisely hit a specific clinically desired target concentration of the drug in the serum or at an effect site, or to optimize its effect in a particular way.

To do this, the approach taken in this book borrows heavily from methods and techniques used in the aerospace community to control the flight of aircraft and spacecraft—to *control* the trajectory of drug concentrations in the body, or of the effect itself, in a specific, desired way.

Some of these modeling techniques have been used in connection with drug development and various clinical applications. To date, most applications have been in the area of infectious diseases, transplants, and oncology. However, the use of the models that they have made has usually not been optimal.

The wider medical community remains largely unaware of these tools and has even actively resisted them. For example, one of us taught a course in individualized drug therapy as an elective for third- and fourth-year medical students at the University of Southern California (USC) School of Medicine. It lasted for about 5 years, and then was dropped by the curriculum committee because of negative feedback from the students, who felt that it was "too hard," "not worth the work," and "more suited for pharmacists." Is a physician *not* a therapist? In our experience, there is still not a single medical school we know of that teaches its students quantitative tools to optimize drug therapy in any clinically meaningful way. One cannot memorize such quantitative approaches or do them with pencil-and-paper arithmetic. Computer software is required, and it now can be easily used by clinicians on laptops.

As a result, the medical community has learned about the dosing of drugs mainly from the drug companies. This material provided by them is usually restricted to the package insert, with specific indications for its use, and the specific dosage regimens to be given, usually regardless of body weight in adults or any other factor or covariate—one dose fits all. Since some drugs are renally excreted, dosage alterations may be recommended for various categories of renal function, such as that of a creatinine clearance of over 80, less than 50, or less than 30 mL/min, for example.

In general, this appears to be sufficient for what the medical community thinks it needs. It happily but passively receives its instructions from the drug industry, seemingly without any significant curiosity about what is really going on, following their instructions by simple rote memory. The information from the drug industry is geared to what can be easily remembered by a clinician. It carefully omits any mention of what the real goals of therapy are, or of the many software tools that have been available for *decades* to quantify and optimize the planning, monitoring, and individualizing of dosage regimens to suit each patient's clinical situation and needs. If you just use the package insert, you are a good person. If you make any changes, you are departing from the "standard of practice," and you do so at your peril. This is the main content of the package insert of any drug, and, sad to say, of several experiences with the Food and Drug Administration (FDA). Almost the entire medical culture seeks to do no more than that.

Much of the thought patterns of the medical community appear to come from those of Linnaeus, who classified the various plants and animals. Much of the biomedical culture also is derived from that approach, which has classified and categorized its experiences (criteria for hypertension, diabetes, or hypothyroidism, for example) rather than by using quantitative tools when they become relevant. It has simply recorded these experiences as if these quantitative relationships were facts to be memorized. That is what "criteria," or breakpoints, are for. A good example is that "hypokalemia aggravates digitalis toxicity." This "fact" has been passed down over generations, without anyone ever seeking to know the quantitative aspects of this relationship. For those who might be interested, it appears that when a patient's serum potassium is about 3.0 mEq/L, only about half as much digoxin in a patient's body may be required to produce toxicity as when the serum potassium is 5.0 mEq/L [1].

Despite all this, it has become obvious that many drugs have narrow margins of safety and need to have their concentrations in blood or serum checked and some sort of individualized dosage adjustment made. The International Association for Therapeutic Drug Monitoring and Clinical Toxicology (IATDM-CT) has played an especially notable role here and has been working hard to overcome the passive resistance of the medical community and the silent but strong opposition of the pharmaceutical industry.

The greatest response to the need for dosage individualization has been in the areas of infectious diseases and transplants, and some in oncology and epilepsy as well. Despite this fact, only a very few hospitals, even those with significant transplant services, have incorporated any individualized dosing service as part of their departments. The single exception has been that for anticoagulant therapy with coumadin, in which the dosage adjustment has usually been done intuitively, based on the international normalized ratio (INR), without much explicit use of quantitative tools. However, it is at least being done.

Again, this is a book on how to develop individualized dosage regimens of drugs for patients— to help physicians and clinical pharmacists be, and to regard themselves as, *therapists.* To address the lack of training and the resistance of the general medical community, our goal with this book, once again, is to introduce the interested clinician and the curious reader to the quantitative tools for dosage individualization, their embodiment in clinical software and their current applications in several relevant clinical areas. It is hoped that the concepts and approaches described here may find their way into curricula for medical and pharmacy students, as well as into information and already-available software tools for physicians and pharmacists, to form a seed for further improvements in the future. Optimal drug dosage *controls* the patient's pharmacokinetic drug *system* optimally for each patient. It is a procedure of stochastic adaptive control.

Roger W. Jelliffe, MD, FCP, FAAPS
Michael Neely, MD, MSc, FCP

REFERENCE

[1] Jelliffe RW. Effect of Serum Potassium Level Upon Risk of Digitalis Toxicity American College of Physicians, Chicago, Illinois, April 9–13, 1973 Ann Int Med 1973;78(5):821.

Acknowledgments

The work leading up to this book has been supported in part by NIH grants GM068968, EB005803, GM65619, LM05401, HD070886, and RR11526, and by the Stella Slutzky Kunin Fund.

Introduction: Don't Just Dose—Choose a Specific Target Goal, Suited to the Patient's Need, and Dose to Hit It Most Precisely

1 WAYS OF THINKING—QUALITATIVE AND QUANTITATIVE

Linnaeus set the scientific pattern to classify and categorize the plants and animals that we see in the world. In my opinion, we have continued to apply these same thought processes to the organization of much of our medical knowledge. This is true even though a significant amount of what we see consists of quantitative disturbances rather than qualitative ones.

When I was a resident in medicine, it was common to ask if a patient's nausea, vomiting, or arrhythmia were "due to digitalis or not." Often in our culture, something is felt to be either this or that, true or false, yes or no.

I finally came to the conclusion that if a patient was on digitalis, his or her behavior was *always* due to the drug—to some degree—as well as to all the other environmental factors that surround the myocardial cells (the cells of the sino-atrial node, the atrial conducting system, the atrioventricular node, and the Purkinje cells and their branches and the ventricular myocardial cells themselves) such as the concentrations of sodium, potassium, calcium, and magnesium and the oxygen and CO_2 tensions. All of these play significant roles in determining the behavior of those cells. If a patient has an atrial tachycardia, for example, and his or her serum digoxin concentration is high, one usually sees a significant clinical improvement when the drug is stopped or dosage reduced. If the serum concentration is not so high, there is usually a less dramatic response. Finally, when there is no digoxin in the serum, one does not expect to see any change, as there is nothing to stop. Much behavior of this type is multifactorial and quantitatively determined, and it is not appropriate to ask a yes/no question and expect a yes/no answer that will work.

We still commonly tend to classify our experiences this way. Serum drug concentrations are classified as subtherapeutic, therapeutic, or toxic simply if they are within certain general ranges, regardless of the actual behavior of any individual patient at that time.

Many clinical trials of drugs describe quite variable degrees of responses and clinical outcomes, but neglect to quantify the input to the study—the relationship of dose given not only to body weight or surface area, but also to the especially important quantification of the degree of exposure of each patient to the drug, such as serum concentrations or area under the serum concentration curve (AUC). A subject is simply described as being on the drug or not, or as being given this drug or that one. There are carefully randomized clinical trials, often involving thousands of patients, to obtain statistical power with regard to the extremely wide spectrum of final responses and outcomes, comparing one drug with another at a certain fixed dose of each. An intermediate effect may be measured and related to outcome, but usually relating only the mean effect of each drug with the overall incidences of the various outcomes. What is usually not described is a quantitative relationship between dose, serum concentration, intermediate effect and the outcome in each individual patient, so that one can see the relationship between good responders and their effects, poor responders and theirs, and an effect that is associated with overall best outcome and least toxicity, which then can provide a target for individualized initial and subsequent dosing. Without such information and individualized dosing, neither the physician nor the patient have any idea where he or she has been placed in the all-too-often very broad spectrum of overall responses to drugs.

2 GRAPHICAL PLOTS AND OPTICAL ILLUSIONS

In 1966, Dr. Richard Bellman, in the Department of Mathematics and Biomedical Engineering at the University of Southern California, used to hold seminars every Wednesday afternoon. On one of these occasions, there was a Russian mathematician (whose name I unfortunately did not learn, so there is no way to give him proper credit). Dr. Bellman's Russian guest was especially interested in just where people looked when they were asked to view a simple geometrical form or figure. Fig. 1 was the focus of his talk. He put mirrors on his subjects' corneas to record the exact place their eyeballs fixed. He showed that if someone were asked to look at an acute angle, the eyeball fixed within the image (the cross inside the acute angle in Fig. 1). In this location, he said, one could place the area of macular vision to "rub it up" against the figure to extract the most information possible from it. If the angle widened and became obtuse, as in the top right of Fig. 1, the eyeball fix moved farther in, once again to extract the most visual information. Next, if subjects were asked to look at the end of a line, the interesting thing was that they did not do that—rather, they looked just inside the end, once again, to best locate the end of the line.

Then came the bombshell. He then said that he had the explanation for the common optical illusion shown in the two figures at the bottom of Fig. 1. He said that people look inside the ends (inside the angles) of the line for the upper of the two figures at the bottom, but outside the ends of

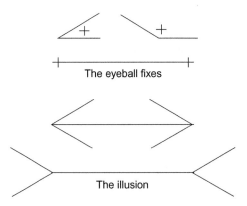

FIGURE 1

A common optical illusion. Which horizontal line of the two at the bottom appears to be longer? The crosses represent the points of eyeball fixes when subjects were asked to look at the angle figures at the top, and inside each end of the top horizontal line. In the upper of the two bottom figures, the eyeball fix is inside the ends of the horizontal line, and also within its angles at each end. However, in the very bottom line, the eye fixes outside the end of the horizontal line, but still inside each angle.

the line (yet still inside the angles) for the very bottom figure, and yet within the angles at the end of each bottom line. He said that people use the proprioceptive information from their eyeball fixes as the initial estimate of the length of each line. This, he said, is the explanation for this very common optical illusion, in which the bottom line appears longer. It seems to me that he was quite right, and that this feature of perception also applies to several other graphical situations as well, some of which are relevant to our subject, and are discussed next.

3 OTHER ILLUSIONS SHARING THIS FEATURE OF PERCEPTION

I would suggest that several important concepts also appear to be examples of such eyeball fixes, with similar illusions. When one looks at graphical data, one is inclined to classify what is seen based on where one looks. In the following discussion, do not be concerned for now with the mechanism of the relationship—just with the visual impression that you get from what you see.

3.1 THE CONCEPT OF "HALF-TIME"

Fig. 2 is a plot of the usual manner of excretion or elimination of most (but not all) drugs from the body. In this case, the more drug in the body, or the higher the serum concentration, the more drug is eliminated in a certain period of time. One eliminates half the drug in a certain time, then half of the

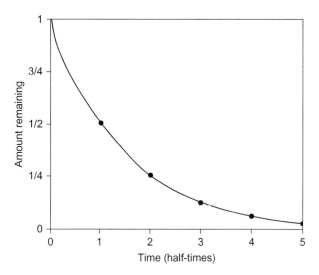

FIGURE 2

The exponential disappearance of a drug over time. The eye is drawn to a point approximately halfway down the disappearance curve when the disappearance is plotted on a linear scale. One can see that the same fraction of the drug is eliminated during each successive time period. Half is a simpler fraction than any other with which to see this behavior, although any other fraction (1/10, for example) provides an equally valid reference. The halfway point provides an easy and convenient visual point of reference along this plot.

remaining drug in the same time, and so on. One can see that in theory, at least, one never eliminates the very last molecule of a drug, but that after 5 half-times, only 1/32 of the drug (not very much) remains.

In Fig. 2, there is a gentle curve with a clear bend in the general region where about half the drug has disappeared, thus drawing the eye (and one's mind) to that region. I believe this feature of visual perception makes it easy to visualize and "understand" the concept of "half-time" compared to 1/3 or 1/4 or 1/10 time, for example. Half-time is a simple and easy concept, which is strongly reinforced visually by the plot in Fig. 2.

3.2 THE SAYING THAT "ONE HAS TO LOSE TWO-THIRDS TO THREE-QUARTERS OF ONE'S RENAL FUNCTION BEFORE THE SERUM CREATININE BEGINS TO RISE SIGNIFICANTLY"

Fig. 3 shows the basically hyperbolic relationship between serum creatinine and creatinine clearance from a representative patient based on general information incorporated into the BestDose clinical software [1] for estimating creatinine clearance based on data of serum creatinine and a patient's age, gender, height, and weight [2]. Here too, without any consideration of the mechanisms involved, the eye is drawn to the main bend in the line in the plot of the relationship between creatinine clearance and serum creatinine. I can think of no other reason for making such a statement, which is actually not very useful. I would suggest that for any patient, any loss of renal function is significant. However, where the eyeball fixes, the brain often acts and classifies. An interesting example of this can be found in the first page of [5], concerning data presented in the abstract of [6].

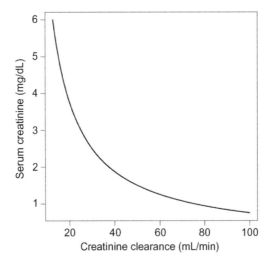

FIGURE 3

Plot of the relationship between creatinine clearance (horizontal) and serum creatinine (vertical). The eye is drawn to the bend in the line, where the brain, which has been trained to classify based on what the eye sees, makes a judgment.

3.3 THE SAYING "GET A 'PEAK' AMINOGLYCOSIDE SERUM SAMPLE HALF AN HOUR AFTER THE END OF THE INFUSION"

If one takes the data of the exponential disappearance of a drug with a half-time and plots it on a semilogarithmic scale instead of a linear scale, the plot becomes a straight line. This has been a major means in the past for determining the half-time of elimination of a drug by first converting the data from a linear to a semilogarithmic scale to describe the behavior of a drug that is eliminated from only a single compartment in the body. This was especially useful before the computer age.

However, one can also see that if the disappearance of a drug has two phases, at least two compartments are involved. In such a plot, the more rapid phase consists of distribution from the serum out to the other tissue compartments of the body in addition to elimination. After the drug has equilibrated into the other body compartments, the slower phase elimination occurs. This is shown graphically in Fig. 4. The idea that one should draw a so-called peak serum sample for monitoring aminoglycoside concentrations a half-hour after the end of the intravenous infusion instead of at the true peak at the end of the infusion has been widely employed for decades. Moreover, this has been done without any scientific validation that I can find, simply by people looking at the plots such as Fig. 4. When the question comes up, the rationale usually offered for this approach is that this bend in the line represents the time when the disappearance profile of serum concentrations (note that the bend exists only when plotted on a semilogarithmic scale) "shifts" from the early phase primarily of distribution from the vascular compartment to other body compartments to the next phase primarily of elimination after such equilibration. It is said that one will perceive the elimination phase of the drug best by getting a first sample at this particular bend in the line, followed by another sample at the end of the dose interval.

However, this is incorrect. The true peak is always at the exact end of the intravenous infusion, not later. The bend in the line shown in Fig. 4 occurs only when the serum concentrations are

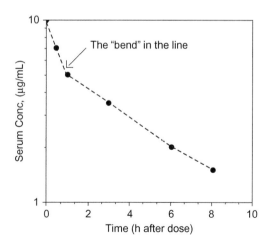

FIGURE 4

Graph of the disappearance of gentamicin after an intravenous infusion. Vertical axis—serum gentamicin on a semilog scale. Horizontal—time after end of infusion of the dose.

transformed and plotted on a semilog scale, and only when the two rates of disappearance are different enough from each other (usually by a factor of about 3) to be visible on that type of plot.

As we will see in later chapters of this book, this visual impression has led to a widespread but suboptimal approach to therapeutic drug monitoring and PK analysis, and yet this incorrect procedure is still being taught in many courses in "basic pharmacokinetics" in pharmacy schools. Be careful when you look at something, not to be caught by an illusion. Many books have been written on how to lie with figures.

3.4 "THERAPEUTIC RANGES" OF SERUM DRUG CONCENTRATIONS

Therapeutic ranges of serum drug concentrations appear to be similarly classified by eyeball fixes to plots of quantitative data rather than by anything more scientific. I am not aware of any other really scientific approach to setting such ranges.

The concept of a general "therapeutic range" of serum drug concentrations is only a generalization. However, such guidelines create heavy social pressure in the biomedical community to conform. The therapeutic range is a general region in which most patients, but certainly not all, do well. As shown in Fig. 5, the eye is again drawn to the bends in the lines as they are plotted, and

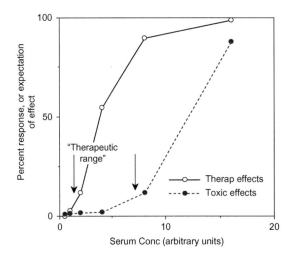

FIGURE 5

General relationships usually found between serum drug concentrations and the incidence of events that are then classified as subtherapeutic, therapeutic, or toxic. The eye is drawn to the bends in the curves, and the therapeutic range is usually classified in relation to these bends. This qualitative procedure of classification, without further thought of the real meaning of the word *significance*, discards the important quantitative relationships of the incidence of therapeutic and toxic effects versus serum concentration.

Reproduced with permission from Jelliffe R, Schumitzky A, Leary R, Botnen A, Gandhi A, Maire P, Barbaut X, Bleyzac N, and Bondareva I: Optimizing Individualized Dosage Regimens of Potentially Toxic Drugs, in Pharmacokinetic Applications in Drug Development, ed by Rajesh Krishna, Ph.D., Kluwer Academic/Plenum Publishers, pp 477–528, 2003.

the limits of a general therapeutic range are again classified as subtherapeutic, therapeutic, or toxic based on the eyeball fixes. I believe this is done without further thought about just when the incidence of something actually becomes clinically significant. It could just as well be set at any other point on the graph, depending on the importance or actual significance of what is being considered.

As shown in Fig. 5, the onset of a therapeutic range is usually set at the first bend in the line—the left arrow—where the rate of increase in the incidence of therapeutic events becomes visibly greater than before. In a similar way, its upper bound (right arrow) is usually taken at the bend of the line representing the relationship between serum concentration and the rate of increase in incidence of toxicity is similarly viewed.

Fig. 6 shows the data of serum digoxin concentrations described by Doherty [3]. Two things are immediately apparent. The first is that patients actually tolerate an extremely wide range of serum digoxin concentrations. One patient in Doherty's study tolerated a concentration of 6.5 ng/mL, while another patient exhibited toxic behavior at a concentration as low as 1.4 ng/mL. I have seen

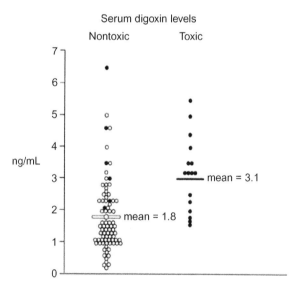

FIGURE 6

Serum digoxin concentrations in toxic and nontoxic patients found by Doherty [3], (reprinted with the permission of American College of Physicians, Inc.). Great variation in sensitivity of patients to serum digoxin concentrations can be seen. Note the great overlap in concentrations between nontoxic and toxic patients, and that the incidence of toxicity rises from essentially 0% at concentrations below 1.0 ng/mL, to 11% from 1–2 ng/mL, to 14% from 2–3 ng/mL, and to 63% from 3–7 ng/mL. The highest serum concentration shown here actually belongs to a nontoxic patient. The clinician must evaluate each patient and decide on a specific target goal based on the patient's current status and his/her clinical need for the drug, balanced against the risk of toxicity that appears to be acceptable in order to obtain the anticipated benefit from the drug. One can then develop a dosage regimen to achieve and maintain such a thoughtfully selected target goal with the maximum precision possible.

Reproduced with permission from Doherty J: Digitalis Glycosides: Pharmacokinetics and their Clinical 396 Implications.

Ann. Int. Med. 79: 229–238, 1973.

data concerning a patient who required a huge maintenance dose of 0.5 mg of digoxin three times daily in order to control his ventricular rate adequately with his atrial fibrillation (AF). He did not have impaired oral absorption of the drug, as his serum digoxin concentration was 8.0 ng/mL. He was never toxic. He was then switched to digitoxin, and again required a very large maintenance dose of 0.4 mg/day for similar rate control. He again was never toxic. His serum digitoxin concentration was 110.0 ng/mL. A colleague in Albuquerque has told me of a similar patient who required a serum digoxin concentration of 6.0 ng/mL to achieve proper control of his ventricular rate with his AF [4].

Clearly, there is great variation in the sensitivity of patients to digitalis glycosides, perhaps due to variations in the binding constants of these drugs to their Na-K ATPase receptors. The entire issue of the sensitivity of any patient to digoxin (or any other drug) has been almost totally ignored since it became fashionable to measure serum concentrations and to constrain therapy to place patients within general guidelines, without much further thought. The important thing, however, is to achieve, and then to maintain, a serum concentration that is best for each individual patient, whatever that is.

How can one use such raw data best? Again, if one has been trained primarily to classify one's experiences in order to summarize them, one might look at Figure 6 and say, as most of the biomedical community has done, that most patients with digoxin toxicity have serum concentrations at or above a concentration of 2.0 ng/mL, and that this cutoff point therefore defines the "upper bound of the therapeutic range." This is the case despite the fact that an equal number of Doherty's patients (count the points in Fig. 6) tolerated serum concentrations above 3.0 ng/mL as those who were toxic, and the nontoxic patients apparently received benefit from that level or they probably would not have been dosed to that degree.

Because of the culture that encourages categorizing and classifying plots of data around visual breakpoints that are often bends in lines, many drugs have had "therapeutic ranges" of their serum concentrations defined in this way. This is how, I believe, serum drug concentrations are classified into general ranges such as "subtherapeutic," "therapeutic," and "toxic," without consideration of any individual patient's actual behavior at those concentrations. Fig. 5 illustrates this point. Even for so-called individualized therapy, many hospitals and laboratories simply monitor serum concentrations, never see the patient, and yet empirically adjust the dose to keep the patient's serum drug concentrations in a general, socially acceptable "therapeutic" range. That approach may be reasonable for initial dosing, but it ignores the extremely wide variation in individual patient sensitivity and response to those serum concentrations, and only seeks to place the patient in a general group where the serum concentrations are felt to be socially acceptable.

We will see later on that it is quite possible to develop a dosage regimen of any drug that will do that task optimally—which specifically can maximize the probability of a patient's serum concentrations being within a specific range. However, there is a significant problem with this approach, as discussed next.

Decision analysis is a subject hardly ever taught to medical students. In this clinically very significant area, one is often asked to estimate the probability of various courses of action, and then to quantify their relative importance or significance, to arrive at an expected value of such a course of action.

The expression of (Probability × Importance) provides a good means to evaluate and compare the overall value of common outcomes of courses of action having modest risk or benefit versus uncommon or rare outcomes that can be much worse or better. One may object that it is very difficult to determine a number that reflects the relative importance of various outcomes. However, I have found it useful here to use a reference number of −100 to reflect an outcome of death, and then to relate other outcomes to this, with a plus sign to signify benefit and minus sign to signify harm. After a few tries, one gets used to this and can settle on some numbers that seem reasonable. This trial-and-error process may be called *sensitivity analysis*. After several tries, and often with considerable effort and some mental pain, one often has acquired much deeper insight into a particular clinical problem, comparing various courses of action in this way, than before doing such an analysis.

In addition, within a so-called therapeutic range, there is no zone of neutrality. With increasing serum concentration, there is a greater incidence and magnitude of desired effects, and the same applies for the undesired (toxic) effects. At the bottom of the therapeutic range, the risks are usually associated with lack of effect, whereas at the top, they are more likely to be those of toxicity. These outcomes have consequences of very different magnitudes. Overall data about the incidence, manifestations, and importance of such outcomes are usually lacking. Because of this, it is usually not possible to develop a plan of therapy that carries with it the greatest expected value for a given patient when one plans dosage regimens using the concept of a "therapeutic window."

However, if one considers quantitatively each patient's need for the drug in question, and balances that against the risks associated with a given serum concentration, one can do at least as well using conventional clinical judgment to select a specific target serum concentration goal associated with a risk of toxicity that one finds acceptable in order to obtain the anticipated benefit of the drug for that individual patient. Then one can strive to hit that specific target goal most precisely.

In this case, the risk of achieving a serum concentration slightly less that the target goal is hardly different than of having one just a little bit higher. This risk approaches an infinitesimal (like an infinitesimal in calculus) if one selects a specific target goal. Because of this, one can set a specific target goal to be achieved for a given patient, such as a desired serum concentration at a desired time, and then work to hit that target goal most precisely. This is the rationale for the specific target-oriented approach taken in this book.

One must always check each individual patient and ask if he or she is doing not only well, but optimally, on clinical grounds, regardless of what the serum concentration actually is. This approach is quite different from much current, guideline-oriented clinical teaching, but it still is similar to what many clinicians may still consider—"Look at the patient, not just at the serum concentration." Who is best qualified to make such a decision? A faraway committee setting guidelines, or the clinician at the patient's bedside, who knows those guidelines, and also knows that individual patient as well?

---

4 GENERAL REMARKS ABOUT DOSING

It is also said in drug package inserts, for example, that one should individualize dosage to body weight and renal function, for example. But again, to what specific end—what specific goal? The answer to this question is usually not explicitly stated. This lack of information is typical of drug package inserts, which mention only a dose, "one-size-fits-all," not the need to hit a specific, individualized target goal.

For good patient care, we should carefully individualize drug dosage for each patient to achieve some desired target goal, such as a serum concentration, or an effect, such as bacterial kill and a tolerable degree of toxic leucopenia, or its profile over time. We must then observe the patient, and often we should monitor serum concentrations or other responses at appropriate and optimally informative times, and adjust the dose as needed.

Optimal times to make such observations can also be calculated (see Chapter 8), to maximize the information contained in the data, to optimize the process and minimize the costs of learning about each individual patient while we have to treat him or her at the same time. We then follow this up with optimal dosage adjustments to most precisely achieve our selected target goal for that patient. These issues will be specifically discussed in this book. Of course, we may also change the patient's target goal as we learn more about each patient's sensitivity to, and need for, the drug being given.

In the area of infectious disease, we specifically consider the minimum inhibitory concentration (MIC) of an organism that we wish to kill. We need to do the same when we think about our patients. Their sensitivity to various drugs varies greatly, probably at least as much as that of the individual organisms and their MICs.

The expected incidence of toxicity to be accepted for any individual patient should be no greater than what is felt to be appropriate for that patient's clinical need for the drug. In many cases, if the need for the drug is not great or not acute, the target goal should first carry a low incidence or risk of toxicity, leading to a gentle dosage regimen. Based on the patient's response, the target goal can then be revised upward as needed and a higher dosage given to achieve it, even if the target is outside some general therapeutic range.

Examples of this approach are the acceptance of a certain risk of toxicity with transplant or cancer chemotherapy, therapy for AIDS, and the use of digoxin, aminoglycosides, vancomycin, and voriconazole therapy, where one has the opportunity to select a target goal for each patient and then to design a dosage regimen that will hit it most precisely. The remainder of this book deals with the various techniques to do this, relevant software to implement these approaches, and the clinical areas where individualized approaches have been found to be useful.

In this way, the eternal bond between clinician and patient, which clearly passes all understanding, can be forged even now by giving a medicine that represents our very best scientific efforts today, and giving it in a dose carefully planned to make things go best for each and every patient.

Roger W. Jelliffe

REFERENCES

[1] The BestDose clinical software is available for evaluation and download at <www.lapk.org>.

[2] Jelliffe R. Estimation of creatinine clearance in patients with unstable renal function, without a urine specimen. Am J Nephrol 2002;22:320—4.

[3] Doherty J. Digitalis glycosides: pharmacokinetics and their clinical implications. Ann Int Med 1973;79: 229—38.

[4] Lueker R. Personal communication.

[5] Sunder S, Jayaraman R, Kahapatra HS, Sathi S, Ramanan V, Kanchi P, et al. Estimation of renal function in the intensive care unit: the covert concepts brought to light. J. Intensive Care 2014;2:31 http://www.jintensivecare.com/content/2/1/31

[6] Tomlanovich S, Golbetz H, Perlroth M, Stinson E, Myers B. Limitations of Creatinine in Quantitying the Severity of Cyclosporine — Induced Chronic Nephropathy. Am. J. Kidney Diseases 1986;8:332—7 http://dx.doi.org/10.1016/S0272-6386(86)80107-X.

BASIC TECHNIQUES FOR INDIVIDUALIZED THERAPY

BASIC PHARMACOKINETICS AND DYNAMICS FOR CLINICIANS

R. Jelliffe and M. Neely

CHAPTER OUTLINE

Many pharmacokinetic/dynamic (PK/PD) textbooks are available that go into great detail. These may be needed to become really fluent in the subject. Here are two suggestions [1,2]. However, such books get very mathematical very quickly and are not as clinically oriented as they might be. They also concentrate on parametric approaches to modeling without any mention of nonparametric ones, which have been around since the 1980s and which are more useful in general (see Chapter 2: Describing Drug Behavior in Groups of Patients). We would like instead to concentrate in this chapter on the basic logic behind PK and PD, in order to present a brief and general description of how drugs behave in patients, primarily for clinical purposes.

Individualized Drug Therapy for Patients. DOI: http://dx.doi.org/10.1016/B978-0-12-803348-7.00001-0

In other chapters, we will deal with various related issues, but step by step. We also want to avoid going incrementally from so-called traditional basic, often obsolete, issues to more advanced topics. Instead, we wish to cut to the chase and concentrate on those topics having the greatest direct clinical relevance today, whatever their level. Some are basic, and some quite advanced. But all are easily understood through words and pictures. We want to present those concepts and techniques that have the greatest bearing on how best to describe drug behavior, and how best to permit individualized drug therapy to be done in clinical settings with the *greatest precision* throughout for each individual patient.

1.1 EXCRETION IS USUALLY PROPORTIONAL TO AMOUNT OR CONCENTRATION

Interestingly, the equations that describe the behavior of the great majority of drugs are also those that describe radioactive decay and many other processes. For most drugs, it is generally true that the more you take, the more you have in your body, and the more you excrete, during some stated time period. These processes take place at certain rates: a dosage *rate* (mg/day, for example) and a rate of excretion.

For our present purposes, an oral dose of a drug can be regarded as being instantaneously placed into a single compartment that represents the patient's entire body. Then, if there is a certain total amount of drug in the body, the drug will be excreted at some rate that is usually linearly proportional to the amount present in the body at any given moment. There is a rate constant, usually called k, which quantitatively describes this rate per unit time, which is often described in units of h^{-1}, but which can be in any other unit of 1/time one wishes to use. A closely related measure of drug elimination is the half-time of the drug, with units of time such as hours.

If a dose is instantaneously given so there is a certain amount A of drug suddenly placed in the body, the subsequent rate of loss of drug from the body is usually written as dA/dt (for the instantaneous rate of change in A per change in time). Since the amount of drug in the body is decreasing as the drug is lost, this is a decreasing process. It is like compound interest in the bank, only in reverse. One loses a fraction of something per unit time rather than gaining it. So we can say that

$$\frac{dA}{dt} = -kA \qquad (1.1)$$

Suppose that $k = -0.1\,h^{-1}$, meaning that about 10% of the drug is lost per hour. Then, after 1 h, 90.48% of the drug actually remains in the body. After 2 h, $-0.1 \times 2 = -0.2$, and 81.87% remains. Table 1.1 is a general table of an amount, a rate constant, which can be either positive (for a gain, as in compound interest at the bank), or negative, for a compound loss, as with excretion of a drug from the body.

Table 1.1 shows this for the first 6.9315 h of loss or gain. In this table, e is the base of the natural logarithms and is the number 2.71828, and e^{-kt} or e^{kt} is the decimal fraction or percent lost or gained over a certain period of time.

Table 1.1 shows that if one loses 10% of a drug from the body in 1 h, one loses half the drug in 6.9315 h. In the same way, if one gained 10% per hour on some money in a bank account (a pretty good deal!), one would double one's money in that same time, 6.9315 h. So the usual way drugs are excreted from the body is like compound interest in reverse.

Table 1.1 Relationship Between Exponential (or Compound) Loss, as of a Drug From the Body, or the Reverse, Exponential (or Compound) Gain, as at the Bank

Amount	k (h^{-1})	t (h)	Compound Loss		Compound Gain	
			$-kt$	e^{-kt}	kt	e^{kt}
1	0.1	1	−0.1	0.9048	0.1	1.1052
		2	−0.2	0.8187	0.2	1.2214
		3	−0.3	0.7408	0.3	1.3498
		4	−0.4	0.6703	0.4	1.4918
		5	−0.5	0.6065	0.5	1.6488
		6	−0.6	0.5488	0.6	1.8221
		6.9315	−0.69315	0.5	0.69315	2.0000

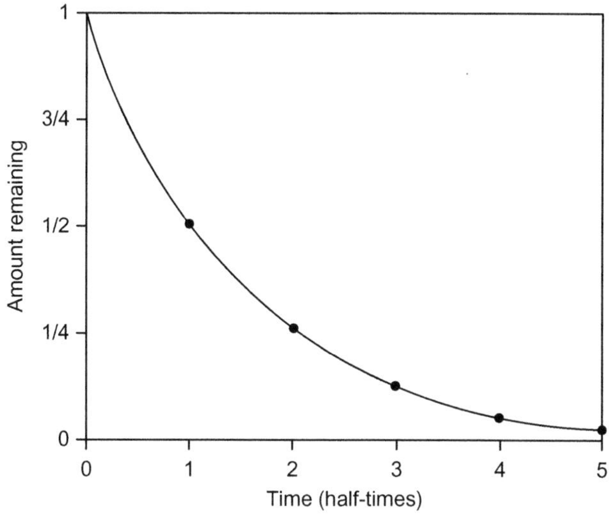

FIGURE 1.1

Graph of the elimination of most drugs from the body, with the process of compound or exponential loss. After 1 half-time, half is gone, and after 2, half the remaining, and so on, until after 5 half-times, only 1/32 of the drug remains in the body, and the patient has proceeded 31/32 of the way from having the drug in him to not having any drug aboard.

Fig. 1.1 shows this process graphically, in which the drug is eliminated from the body, but now in units of half-time. One might also say that if the rate constant for elimination is 0.69315 h^{-1}, then the half-time of that drug is 1 h. The rate constant for elimination is related to the half-time ($T\frac{1}{2}$) by

$$T\frac{1}{2} = \ln{(0.5)}/-k \tag{1.2}$$

where ln (0.5) is the natural log of the number 0.5 (which is -0.69315) and k is the rate constant for elimination. k is negative because the drug is being lost from the body. If we were talking about compound interest, then we might say that the

$$\text{Doubling time} = \ln(2)/k \qquad (1.3)$$

where ln(2) is 0.69315, a positive number, and k is positive, as the process is one of growth instead of loss.

Not only is the drug eliminated with a half-time, but the patient proceeds from an *initial condition* of having the drug aboard, at a stated time, to a *final condition* of not having the drug in the body any more. That is another important thing to keep in mind—the transition from an initial condition to a new final condition or steady state—as we will see next.

1.2 ACCUMULATION TAKES PLACE BY THE MIRROR IMAGE OF ELIMINATION

Let us now begin to give a drug to a patient intravenously at a fixed rate R, and let us describe it also in units per hour (eg, mg/h). So the rate of input of drug in the body is R. We can also say that the input is

$$\frac{dA}{dt} = R \qquad (1.4)$$

However, since the drug also begins to be eliminated as soon as the infusion starts, we must revise this to say that

$$\frac{dA}{dt} = R - kA \qquad (1.5)$$

Eq. (1.5) now describes the accumulation of drug in the body on a fixed-rate infusion. Since drug elimination is linearly proportional to the amount of drug present in the body, Eq. (1.5) describes the trajectory of the amount of drug in the body over time, and the approach to equilibrium and a steady state at this infusion rate. The amount of drug in the body will increase until the rate of elimination equals the rate of infusion R, when it will reach a final plateau, as shown in Fig. 1.2. Fig. 1.2 also shows that a drug accumulates in the body by the mirror image of its

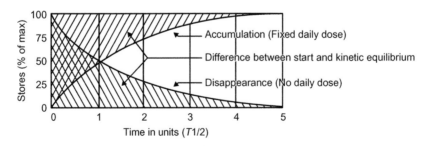

FIGURE 1.2

Accumulation of a drug in the body takes place by the mirror image of excretion.

eliminations. All drugs accumulate in the body. Some do it hardly at all, but others do it to a significant degree. It all depends on how much drug is present in the body when the next dose is given.

When the infusion is stopped, the drug will then disappear as shown in Fig. 1.1, and R becomes zero.

1.3 SUITING LOADING AND MAINTENANCE DOSES TO EACH OTHER

Fig. 1.3 describes the behavior of a drug having a half-time of 1 day. If we begin by giving a dose of 1 mg/day, as shown by X in the figure, we see that the drug accumulates in the body incrementally with each dose, and also by the mirror image of elimination. After 1 day, half the drug remains in the body. The next dose raises the total amount in the body to 1 1/2 mg, and half of this is lost over the second day, down to 3/4 mg. The next dose then raises that amount to 1 3/4 mg, and half of this is lost, down to 7/8 mg after 3 half-times. The next dose raises the total amount to 1 7/8 mg, and half of this is lost, down to 15/16 mg, and so on. This repeats the time course of the excretion of the drug shown in Fig. 1.1, and the accumulation of drug shown in Fig. 1.2, except that now this all happens in increments. At a final steady state, a limit is reached at which the total

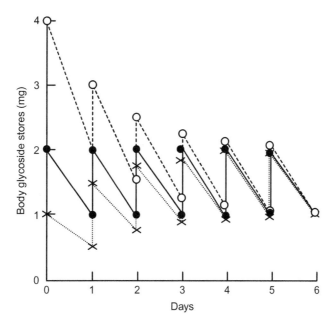

FIGURE 1.3

Behavior of a drug having a half-time of 1 day. X represents the trajectory of drug amount in the body when a dose of 1 mg of this drug is given every day. Filled circles: the trajectory when a loading dose of 2 mg is given on Day 1, followed by a maintenance dose of 1 mg/day thereafter. Open circles: the trajectory when a loading dose of 4 mg is given, followed by a maintenance dose of 1 mg/day thereafter.

amount of drug in the body is 2 mg just after taking the dose, and one loses half of this each day down to 1 mg just before taking the next dose.

On the other hand, if a very large loading dose is given, 4 mg for example, again half the drug is lost the first day down to 2 mg. The subsequent daily dose of 1 mg raises the amount to 3 mg, and half of this is lost, down to 1 1/2 mg after 2 days. Then the amount is increased to 2 1/2 mg on Day 3, and half of this is lost, down to 1 1/4 mg, and so on. Once again, after a steady state is reached, the maximum amount of drug in the body is 2 mg, falling to 1 mg just before the next dose.

Now, if one wishes to achieve and maintain a target peak goal of a total amount of 2 mg of drug every day in such a patient, what is the correct loading and maintenance dosage regimen? It will be a "loading" dose of 2 mg on the first day, followed by a "maintenance" dose of 1 mg/day thereafter. The words "loading dose" and "maintenance dose" actually *mean something quantitative,* something more than merely something given vaguely to "load" and something given vaguely to "maintain," as the terms are usually employed. They really should have the correct quantitative relationship to each other.

We see that if one loses half the drug from the body each day, one can never have more than 2 mg in the body just after taking the 1 mg daily maintenance dose, and this amount will fall to 1 mg just before taking the next dose.

And now, in general, we see that if someone loses 1 Nth of the drug from the body during each dose interval, one can never maintain more than N doses in the body in the final steady state. A clinical correlate of this is that when renal function is normal, about one-third of the total amount of digoxin in the body is excreted each day, and so one can never have more than 3 doses in the body (Table 1.2).

A 70 kg patient with normal renal function taking 250 mcg of digoxin daily will eventually (in more than 5 half-times) reach a maximum of about 3 doses in the body, or about 750 mcg. Furthermore, if creatinine clearance (CCr) is 100 mL/min/1.73 M^2, the correct maintenance dose is 1/3 of the total amount of digoxin you wish the patient to have in the body, decreasing to 1/7 when someone is anuric, with a CCr of zero, at which point one will sustain about 7 doses in the body. Similarly, if CCr is 75, the dose is probably about 1/4 of what is in the body, or 3/4 of the usual dose when CCr is 100. If CCr is 50, the dose is about 3/5 of the usual; if CCr is 25, about 3/6 (or 1/2) of the usual; and if zero, about 3/7 of the usual given for a CCr of 100.

Table 1.2 Approximate Relationship Between Creatinine Clearance (CCr), Digoxin Half-Time ($T1/2$), Daily Fraction Lost $F = 1/N$, Total Doses (N) Sustained in the Body in a Steady State Just After Taking the Dose, and ($N-1$), Total Doses Present in the Steady State Just Before Taking the Next Daily Dose

CCr	T1/2	F = 1/N	N	N − 1
100	1.4 days	1/3	3	2
75	2.0	1/4	4	3
50	2.5	1/5	5	4
25	3.0	1/6	6	5
0	4.5	1/7	7	6

Since the usual oral bioavailability of digoxin is about 65%, adjust accordingly, and also adjust for body weight to estimate the total concentration of drug in the body.

1.4 THE BASIC IDEA—DOSE AND HALF-TIME—THEY LET YOU CONTROL THE TOTAL AMOUNT OF DRUG YOU PERMIT THE PATIENT TO HAVE IN THE BODY AT ANY TIME

To oversimplify things for purposes of the present discussion, if we give a certain dose of drug to a patient, that amount of drug is somewhere in the patient's body or gut. Since it is eliminated with a certain half-time, we now have the tool to control the total amount of drug we permit a patient to have in the body.

This is a powerful thing. Now you are no longer limited by the ritualistic package insert in which the company tells you only about the standard dose, and does not want you to think about the events that take actually place after a dose is given. Now the clinician is in control again. One is no longer blindly just giving a dose. Our eyes are open. Knowing the dose and knowing the half-time of the drug, the clinician can now *control* the total amount of drug in a patient's body, and therefore can control everything else: the serum concentration, the concentration in a peripheral nonserum compartment, and the degree of clinical effect.

You can also look at the patient, not just the serum concentration. The patient, by his clinical behavior, will tell you specifically if he is doing well or not on the drug at that time. You can compare his behavior with his individual PK/PD model and serum concentration, and then you can select the target concentration in the appropriate target compartment, according to that patient's clinical need for the drug.

You are in the driver's seat. You can now develop the individualized dosage regimen to achieve your target goal for that particular patient most precisely. Do not just do something blindly and then check yourself later. Plan ahead, and make it happen the way you want it to go for the patient-each individual patient.

That is what this book is about. It starts with this very simple idea: the relation between the drug half-time, the dosage regimen, and the resulting total amount of drug in the patient's body, which can now be controlled if you know the half-time of the drug. You can give doses at chosen dose intervals, and the total amount of drug in the body can easily be *controlled* by giving the right doses at the right dose intervals.

1.5 EVENTS FOLLOWING A CHANGE IN DAILY MAINTENANCE DOSE

Just as Fig. 1.3 described the events following various combinations of loading and maintenance doses, Fig. 1.4 shows the results with the same drug of doubling the daily dose from 1 to 2 mg/day. One still loses half the drug each day, but now the dose is doubled. The patient again proceeds, and at the same rate, from the initial steady state at the left, from that of having 2 mg aboard just after to 1 mg aboard just before each dose, but the dose is now doubled. The patient proceeds with the same half-time as before, but the first double dose now puts a total amount in the body of:

3 mg aboard after the first new dose, falling to 1.5 mg at the end of the first day. The next 2 mg dose takes the patient to
3.5 mg on Day 2, falling to 1.75 mg. The next dose takes the total to

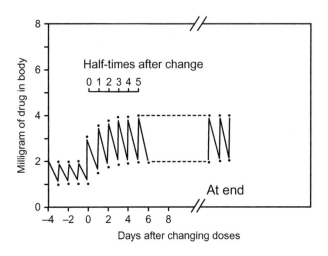

FIGURE 1.4

Effect of doubling the daily dose. The patient progresses from having 2 doses of 1 mg aboard just after the dose to having 2 doses of 2 mg aboard once the new steady state is reached. The half-time of the drug remains the same, 1 day.

> 3.75 mg on Day 3, falling to 1.875 mg. The next dose raises this to
> 3.875 mg on Day 4, falling to 1.9375 mg. The next dose takes this to
> 3.9375 mg on Day 5, falling to 1.96875 mg, and so on.

The patient reaches a final steady state of having 4 mg aboard just after each daily dose, losing half of that down to 2 mg just before the next daily dose. He again has 2 doses aboard at peak and 1 dose aboard at trough. It is just that everything has doubled since Day 1.

1.6 EVENTS FOLLOWING A CHANGE IN EXCRETION RATE

On the other hand, if the rate of excretion (the daily fraction lost) changes, the amount of drug in the body will also change, but with a different half-time determined by the new rate of excretion. Suppose the fraction lost per day changes from ½ to ¼. Then, on the same dose of 1 mg daily, the drug will now start to accumulate until a total of 4 doses in the body is reached, with 3 doses remaining just before the next dose. This will take place with a longer half-time, due to the slower rate of loss, as shown in Fig. 1.5.

On the first day of the change, the total amount of drug in the body will fall from 2 to only $2 \times 0.75 = 1.5$ mg on the first day. The dose on Day 2 will raise the total amount to:

> 2.5 mg on Day 2, falling to 1.875 mg. The next day's dose takes this to
> 2.875 mg on Day 3, falling to 2.15625 mg. The next day's dose takes this to
> 3.15625, on Day 4, falling to 2.3671875 mg. The next day's dose takes this to
> 3.3671875 on Day 5, falling to 2.52539 mg. The next day's dose takes this to

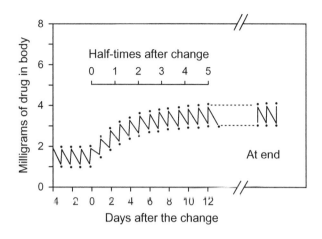

FIGURE 1.5

If the daily fraction lost changes from ½ to ¼, for example, the half-time is longer, and it takes five of the longer half-times to reach the new steady state of 4 mg just after, and now 3 mg just before, the next dose.

3.52539 on Day 6, falling to 2.644 mg. The next day's dose takes this to 3.644 on Day 7, falling to 2.733 mg. The next day's dose takes this to 3.733 on Day 8, falling to 2.79975 mg. The next day's dose takes this to 3.79975 on Day 9, falling to 2.8498 mg. The next day's dose takes this to 3.8498 on Day 10, falling to 2.8874 mg. The next day's dose takes this to 3.8874 on Day 11, falling to 2.91555 mg. The next day's dose takes this to 3.91555 on Day 12, falling to 2.9363 mg. The next day's dose takes this to 3.9363 mg on Day 13, falling to 2.9525 mg, and so on. Eventually, at the limit, the amount after the dose of 1 mg/day reaches 4.0 mg. It then falls to 3.0 mg after that day, just before the next daily dose.

1.7 SEPARATING ELIMINATION INTO RENAL AND NONRENAL COMPONENTS

One can separate elimination into renal and nonrenal losses, simply by having a separate rate constant for each process, such as a renal k_r and a nonrenal k_{nr}. Then one can relate k_r to renal function by describing it per unit of creatinine clearance (CCr). Call this k_{slope}. Then $k_r = k_{slope} \times CCr$. The sum of the two routes of loss is the total elimination rate constant k_e, where $k_e = k_r + k_{nr}$ (Fig. 1.6).

1.8 ADDING MORE COMPARTMENTS FOR A MORE REALISTIC PHARMACOKINETIC MODEL

Fig. 1.7 shows a more realistic model in which there are separate oral, serum, and nonserum compartments.

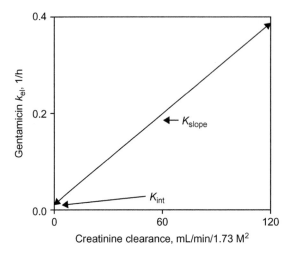

FIGURE 1.6

Partitioning the elimination rate constant (k_{el}) for gentamicin into nonrenal (k_{nr} or k_{int}) and renal (k_{slope}) components, with the k_{slope} linked to creatinine clearance (CCr).

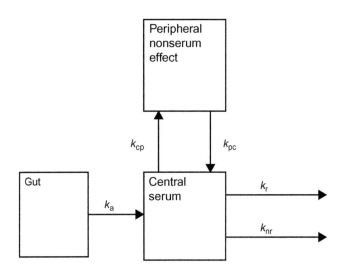

FIGURE 1.7

Adding more compartments to make a very common model having (1) a separate gut compartment A_1, (2) a central serum compartment A_2, and (3) a peripheral (perhaps an effect) compartment A_3, where A_1, A_2, and A_3 represent the amount of drug in each compartment.

In this case, we can write the differential equations for each compartment as

$$\frac{dA_1}{dt} = \text{an instantaneous oral dose } A_1 - k_a A_1 \tag{1.6}$$

$$\frac{dA_2}{dt} = R, \text{ if infused, } + k_a A_1 - (k_{slope} \times CCr)A_2 - k_{nr}A_2 - k_{cp}A_2 + k_{pc}A_3 \tag{1.7}$$

$$\frac{dA_3}{dt} = k_{cp}A_2 - k_{pc}A_3 \tag{1.8}$$

where k_a is the rate constant for absorption from the gut into the serum compartment, k_{cp} is the rate constant from the serum out to the peripheral compartment, and k_{pc} is the rate constant back from the peripheral to the serum compartment.

Do differential equations boggle your mind? Just go back to eighth-grade algebra where X was the thing on the left, whatever it was. The only thing different now is that X is replaced by a statement of a rate of change. All the rest is basically the same, so not to worry!

1.9 OUTPUT EQUATIONS: DESCRIBING THE OBSERVATIONS

Having set up our model to describe the overall behavior of the system—with the doses being the *inputs* to the system, and the three compartments being the *states* of the system (amounts of drug in the various compartments at various times)—we now need to describe our observations of the system. These are called the output equations. These *outputs* are often called Y. The most common one describes the observed serum concentrations. From Fig. 1.7 and Eq. (1.7), one can write

$$Y = \frac{A_2}{V} \tag{1.9}$$

in which the amount of drug A in compartment 2 is divided by V, its apparent volume of distribution. This volume can be regarded as a bathtub, into which a calculated or stated amount of drug is diluted by (or distributed into) an apparent volume to correspond to a measured serum concentration Y.

Notice that the *behavior* of the PK system is described by its differential equations. The *inputs* to the system are the doses. The *responses* of the system are the *output* equations, as in Eq. (1.9). The *parameters* of the system are V and k, etc. Such equations are widely used to describe the behavior of many other systems and processes. Radioactive decay and compound interest are only two examples out of many.

1.10 PARAMETERIZING THE MODEL: VOLUME AND CLEARANCE OR VOLUME AND RATE CONSTANT?

One can describe a model of drug behavior in terms of either the apparent distribution volume V and rate constant k_e, or V and clearance (which is $V \times k_e$). Except for some extremely subtle points, either describes drug behavior equally well. Many people (see below) firmly believe that clearance is a "more physiologic" parameter, as we conventionally use the term for creatinine clearance, for example. Clearance gives us a convenient number to relate to a physiologic function, such as the volume of blood filtered per minute by the glomeruli. The concept has become deeply entrenched in much of the thinking in the PK community.

However, there is a problem with the use of clearance clinically, as clearance is the product of V and k. If all you perceive is clearance, you cannot perceive the relative contribution of V and k to clearance. They are comingled and cannot be separated. The basic relationship is

$$\text{Clearance} = kV \tag{1.10}$$

In this relationship, it is equally true that

$$k = \frac{\text{Clearance}}{V} \tag{1.11}$$

and also that

$$V = \frac{\text{Clearance}}{k} \tag{1.12}$$

No parameter is independent. All are closely interrelated. Knowledge of any two permits calculation of the third.

1.11 THE CLEARANCE COMMUNITY IN PK

A group within the PK community strongly feels that clearance and V are independent parameters, and it maintains that k is "dependent" on clearance and V. This viewpoint is well stated in Ref. [3]. It is extremely interesting to read. While its author agrees to the interconnected relationships described here in Eqs. (1.10) through (1.12)—and also that when data is available, it is perfectly easy to use either V and k or V and clearance—he nevertheless maintains that clearance and V are independent. He supports this statement by saying that the physiological processes of elimination and of distribution of a drug within the body are independent of each other, while maintaining that k is dependent upon these two. However, clearance, V, and K are all related by Eqs.(1.10)–(1.12).

From what we can see, the processes of distribution and elimination of a drug may well be physiologically independent. However, there is no clear evidence that V and clearance are mathematically independent. We respectfully suggest that k is a more direct clinical descriptor of elimination than clearance, which is why it is called an elimination rate constant, and that clearance is simply the product of V and k. He (and many others) discusses the effect of a change in one of these three parameters upon the other two. There are descriptions of many things that *may* happen, but not necessarily of what *must* happen. There is much discussion, for example, of what can happen after a change in V as the concentration of drug in that compartment changes. However, much of this seems to be invoked only to keep constant the value of the term on the left side of the equation in Eqs. (1.10) through (1.12). There is no discussion of what happens as the parameters start and *continue changing* over time.

Interestingly, there seems to be essentially no discussion at all of this issue in conventional PK, as there is in the aerospace community, for example, where none of the equations of conventional

PK apply to orbital calculations, as the force of gravitational attraction is changing from moment to moment as a satellite orbits the Earth. The Earth is flatter at the poles, with less gravitational attraction, and bulging at the equator, with more gravitational attraction, and all this must be accounted for during each instant of calculating the orbital track of an object. The quite similar issue of changing parameters from moment to moment in an unstable patient is ignored in all conventional PK equations, which assume that V and k, for example, are at least piecewise constant during any defined period of time, and the effects of a change are considered only before and after a change. There is no discussion of what happens as changes are actually *taking place*.

If one asks simply, what are the minimum parameters both necessary and sufficient to describe the behavior of a PK system under conventional assumptions of constant coefficients, there are only two; V and k. Clearance, the product of V and k, is not needed at all. It is actually an unnecessary parameter. All that is needed are the differential equations, the parameters V and k, the inputs to the system, and its outputs, as described above. No need for clearance. Nevertheless, there continues to be an unending controversy about this issue of clearance and V or k and V. There are also intercompartmental clearances described between compartments and assumed volumes in an unobserved peripheral compartment, for example. If one accepts the assumptions, then the equations work.

It is also interesting to see how often PK equations will be written to describe a process and use Cl/V rather than k. It is as if authors will do almost anything in order not to use k. However, no assumptions such as the assumed volume of an unobserved peripheral compartment are necessary to describe such behavior. It is quite adequate to describe PK behavior in terms of amounts, inputs, outputs, V, the rate constants, and the output equations. Clearance is simply not needed.

On the other hand, there is one situation where it is essential to use clearance. That is when a patient is on a fixed dose in a steady state on that regimen, and the only available data is a single sample. In that case, only a single parameter can be estimated from the data, and that is clearance. *Any* combination of V and k can result in the observed concentration. If V is small, then the peak concentration after a dose is high and the k is large, or the V can be large and the k will be small. Neither V and k nor V and clearance can be estimated in this data-poor setting, only clearance.

In any real-world setting, with two or more data points taken at different times (see Chapter 8), then V and k can both be estimated directly, and there is no need for clearance.

Further, the word "clearance" has the colloquial connotation of elimination. Because of this, it is very often regarded as being synonymous with elimination. For example, a drug is said to be "cleared" from the body. However, to be precise about the meaning of the word "clearance" in the present context, one must look at Eqs. (1.10) through (1.12) for the precise pharmacokinetic definition of the word.

1.12 A CURRENT CLINICAL ISSUE: "AUGMENTED RENAL CLEARANCE" IN THE ICU

Many acutely ill patients receiving aminoglycoside therapy are well known to have abnormally large apparent volumes of distribution. These facts have also been described as increased clearance. However, when one describes drug behavior in terms of overall clearance, the different physiological processes governing fluid changes (often reflected in V) cannot be separated from those governing the rates of movement of drug from one compartment to another, which are reflected in k.

We would respectfully suggest that it appears to be more useful, for clinical purposes, to separate these two clinical processes whenever possible, and therefore to describe drug behavior in general in terms of V and k. Later on, in Chapter 9, we will see that V and k often move in opposite directions in such patients, and that parameterizing a model in terms of clearance may not tell us what we really want to know about our patient, as both V and k are comingled when the model is parameterized as V and clearance. Clearance muddies the waters of clinical understanding, especially of an unstable patient's separate problems of fluid balance and drug behavior, along with dialysis, renal replacement therapy, and extracorporeal membrane oxygenation (ECMO) therapy in these settings, often the ICU, as discussed in Chapter 9.

1.13 PROPERTIES OF SYSTEMS: OBSERVABILITY, IDENTIFIABILITY, AND CONTROLLABILITY

A system is considered *observable* if and only if a unique input leads to a unique output. It is considered *identifiable* if and only if a single unique set of model parameter values can be calculated from data of the inputs and the observed outputs. It is considered *controllable* if and only if a single input (dosage regimen) can be found in order to achieve a clinically desired output. It is by far the best if all three properties are present in a PK system.

The biggest problem is that of identifiability. In even the simple example of oral administration of a drug, where the model has only an oral and a serum compartment and only the parameters k_a, V, and k_e (not even a peripheral compartment as in Fig. 1.7), a unique set of parameter values *cannot* be calculated from a given data set. Instead, for such an oral drug, there are actually two sets of parameter values that can be found. Each set describes the system behavior identically well, to the smallest decimal a computer can handle.

The first set is where the system is set up as described. The second set is where the rate constants are reversed so that k_a is actually k_e and k_e is actually k_a. In that situation, a different apparent volume of distribution V is found. However, the output resulting from these two sets of parameter values is identical. In one case, the k_a is more rapid. In the other, the k_e is faster. This has been called the "flip-flop problem."

In this simple case, the solution is easy. One only has to decide which of the two equally good solutions one prefers to use. If one decides that k_a is faster, one simply writes k_a as $k_e + x$. Then the faster k_a solution is the only one which can be found, and the identifiability problem is solved. If the k_e is more rapid, then one simply writes it as $k_a + x$. In either case, the problem is resolved. This also provides the mathematical foundation for the fact that sustained release preparations of drugs have behavior that is basically similar to that of long-acting drugs.

As the model of drug behavior becomes more complex, the problem of parameter identifiability becomes more difficult to resolve. However, an intravenously administered drug having a single peripheral compartment is uniquely identifiable from observations only of serum concentrations, while one having more than one peripheral compartment is not, unless there are also observations reflecting behavior from some other compartment. Situations of this type have become interesting areas of research for mathematicians.

1.14 NONLINEAR DRUG SYSTEMS

1.14.1 MICHAELIS—MENTEN SYSTEMS

So far, in all the discussion in this chapter, we have assumed that the rate of transfer of drug from one compartment to another is strictly (linearly) proportional to the amount of drug in that compartment.

However, some drugs have behavior that is not linear. Two examples are notable. The first is Michaelis—Menten (MM) behavior. In this case, the rate of transfer reaches a maximum and cannot increase further. It is no longer linearly proportional to the amount in a compartment. This is the case, for example, with the reabsorption rate of filtered glucose by the renal tubule. This reabsorptive process eventually reaches a maximum, and any remaining unabsorbed glucose spills over into the urine. It also describes the effect of a drug as the number of available receptor sites becomes progressively more and more filled by the drug until all are saturated or occupied. This process is described by

$$V = \frac{V_{max} C}{K_m + C} \tag{1.13}$$

where V represents the velocity of a process, V_{max} is the true maximum velocity, C is the measured concentration of the substance, and K_m is the concentration of substance at which the velocity is half maximal. The MM equation can also describe drug effect. In that case, V is usually called E (often as a change in effect from a reference baseline state), V_{max} as E_{max}, and Km as EC50. Phenytoin and Voriconazole are both examples of drugs having MM behavior.

1.14.2 HILL SYSTEMS

In addition, the effects of drugs may also require description by a Hill equation, in which there is real sigmoid behavior. The Hill equation is an extension of the Michaelis—Menten equation, and was developed by A.V. Hill to describe the relationship between the partial pressure of oxygen and the oxygen saturation of hemoglobin. The behavior of many other drug effects can be well described by these nonlinear processes [4].

The basic Hill equation is

$$E = E_0 + \frac{E_{max} C^n}{EC_{50}^n + C^n} \tag{1.14}$$

where E is the effect, E_0 is the baseline effect before application of the drug, C is the concentration of the drug, E_{max} is the true maximum drug effect, EC_{50} is the concentration at which the effect is half maximal, and n is the Hill coefficient that describes the degree of sigmoidicity. When $n = 1$, the relationship reduces to the Michaelis—Menten equation above in Eq. (1.13).

A good example of the Hill equation is shown in Fig. 1.5 of the introduction, with one such equation describing the relationship between drug concentration and the incidence of the effects we like to see (called "therapeutic effects") and another describing those we do not like to see (called "toxic effects"). A very good and readable discussion of this interesting equation, which is applicable to a wide variety of situations and is very understandable in words, is given in Ref. [4].

However, one cannot calculate the behavior of these nonlinear systems directly as one can with the linear processes discussed earlier. These nonlinear equations require more complicated computational methods (integration routines) to describe their behavior over time. Larger linear systems than the ones described here (with more compartments) also require the use of integration routines.

1.15 CONCLUSIONS

Using these basic tools to describe PK and PD behavior, we can understand much better what happens when we place a patient on a certain drug dosage regimen and then observe his clinical behavior. We also now have a tool (the PK/PD model) to "see" into a patient and better understand the behavior of the drug, and a patient's clinical response to a drug dosage regimen. In addition, we now have a useful tool with which to calculate the precisely individualized dosage regimen we choose to give in order to achieve a certain clinically selected specific target serum concentration and clinical therapeutic goal. This goal may be a desired serum or peripheral compartment concentration at a desired time after the dose, or an effect such as a target leucocyte or platelet count in the future, as we learn better how to model and control drug effects. With this information, we should be able to take a patient to a tolerable degree of hematological toxicity, for example, to maximize the antitumor effect of a drug, and yet keep therapy within the bounds of tolerable clinical toxicity for each individual patient.

REFERENCES

[1] Bonate P. Pharmacokinetic—pharmacodynamic modeling and simulation. 2nd ed. New York: Springer; 2011. ISBN−10. 144199484X.
[2] Shargel L, Yu A, Wu-Pong S. Applied pharmaceutics and pharmacokinetics. 6th ed. New York: McGraw − Hill Education/Medical; 2012. ISBN−10. 007160393X.
[3] Mehvar R. Teachers topics. The relationship among pharmacokinetic parameters: effects of altered kinetics on the drug plasma concentration-time profiles. Am J Pharm Educ 2004;68(2), Article 36.
[4] Goutelle S, Maurin M, Rougier F, Barbaut X, Bourguinon L, Ducher M, et al. The Hill equation: a review of its capabilities in pharmacological modelling. Fundam Clin Pharmacol 2008;22:633−48.

DESCRIBING DRUG BEHAVIOR IN GROUPS OF PATIENTS

2

R. Jelliffe

CHAPTER OUTLINE

Now that we have our basic descriptions of pharmacokinetic behavior, let us apply them to see how we can study and describe drug behavior in groups or populations of subjects or patients. This is called population pharmacokinetic and dynamic (PK/PD) modeling. The *models* have the basic structures discussed in Chapter 1, but the specific *methods* used here to study their behavior are those of population PK/PD modeling.

2.1 EARLY APPROACHES TO MODELING

2.1.1 THE NAÏVE POOLING APPROACH

In this approach, all the data from all the subjects are pooled into one set of data, which is then fitted using a method such as weighted nonlinear least squares regression (What is this? See a brief description in Chapter 7). One obtains parameter estimates as if all the subjects were made into one single subject. However, because of this, there is no way to determine the variability between the various subjects in their behavior and all subjects must receive exactly the same square regression.

2.1.2 THE STANDARD TWO-STAGE (S2S) APPROACH

First this approach uses a method such as weighted nonlinear least squares regression to fit the model parameter values but for each individual subject or patient, one at a time. Second, it averages

Individualized Drug Therapy for Patients. DOI: http://dx.doi.org/10.1016/B978-0-12-803348-7.00002-2

everything. It calculates the population mean and standard deviation (SD) for each of the model parameter values. The method requires at least as many data points *from each patient* as there are model parameters to be estimated.

2.1.3 THE ITERATIVE TWO-STAGE BAYESIAN (IT2B) APPROACH

One can begin this approach by using the standard two-stage method as described above, to obtain the initial means and SDs of the model parameters. That completes the first iteration of the IT2B approach. These values are then used as the Bayesian prior (see Chapter 7, Monitoring the Patient: Four Different Bayesian Methods to Make Individual Patient Drug Models) for the next stage. Using this population prior, each subject's data are first examined to obtain the maximum a posteriori probability (MAP) Bayesian parameter estimates for each subject [1]. Then, once again, the means and SDs of the parameter values are obtained, thus completing that second stage again. That result then becomes the Bayesian prior for the next iteration, and so forth. This iterative process is repeated until a convergence criterion is reached. While this has been a popular approach for many years, it is not optimal because the model parameters are *assumed* to have normal or Gaussian distributions, and this is often not the case. Often, a lognormal distribution is assumed instead. What makes these approaches suboptimal is the fact that any assumption at all is made concerning the shape of the model parameter distributions in the population. We will soon see how such constraining assumptions can be dispensed with entirely.

2.2 TRUE POPULATION MODELING APPROACHES

2.2.1 PARAMETRIC MODELS WITH ASSUMED AND CONSTRAINED PARAMETER DISTRIBUTIONS

True population modeling was introduced by Beal and Sheiner [2−4] with the nonlinear mixed effects modeling (NONMEM) approach that was first made available, and is currently still available, in the NONMEM software (Icon, Inc.). This widely used method uses PK/PD models in which the model parameter values (volumes, rate constants, etc.) are assumed to have certain shapes such as the normal or Gaussian distribution over the population, or lognormal shapes, in which the logarithms of the parameters are assumed and constrained to have normal distributions. Others, such as bimodal distributions, are possible. The key thing here is that the shape of the parameter distributions over the population is always assumed and constrained in advance, before the analysis is done, and this shape is specified and defined by a specific equation, whose *parameters* are then estimated. The common equation that describes the normal or Gaussian distribution has the parameters of mean and SD. That is why we estimate means and SDs so often. This approach [2−4] was a big step forward in its time.

This process is often described as nonlinear mixed effect modeling, as the parameter distributions are centered about a mixture of typical (mean) parameter values (the "fixed effects"), with distributions (the SDs) describing the Gaussian dispersion around them (the "random effects"). The overall model is thus called a "mixed effect" model. In this particular type of model, the overall parameter distributions (whatever they actually may be) are broken down into these two components of fixed and random effects. The true parameter distributions in the population are always perceived only within the constraints of the specific assumption that they are normal, lognormal, bimodal, etc.

The structural models (like those described in Chapter 1) are fitted to the data of doses, serum concentrations, and other responses such as effects, which are obtained from each subject or patient. The assumed and therefore specified and constrained parameter distributions (means and SDs) of the model parameter values in the population of patients studied are estimated from the data to obtain the fixed and random effects as defined in the model. They are the *single-valued* parameters of the specific equations that *summarize, specify and constrain* the true parameter distributions, whatever they may be, to their assumed normal or Gaussian shape, such as the parameter means, SDs, and correlations between the various parameters. That is why these are called parametric modeling methods, as they estimate the *parameters* of the *equations* that define and constrain their *assumed* shape. These methods, therefore, use constrained parameter distributions (CPD's). NONMEM also uses an approximate (first-order, conditional expectation, or FOCE) method to estimate the approximate likelihood of the results given the data. Other parametric population modeling methods now compute the likelihood exactly, and are better for it, though still constrained by their parametric assumptions.

There are two general types of CPD population modeling methods: maximum likelihood (ML) and Bayesian. There are both parametric and nonparametric (NP) Bayesian approaches to population modeling. The Bayesian approaches to population PK/PD modeling are very interesting, but are outside the scope of this book at the present time. ML approaches are discussed here.

2.2.2 NONPARAMETRIC (NP) POPULATION MODELS WITH UNCONSTRAINED PARAMETER DISTRIBUTIONS

In contrast to the parametric methods described above that constrain the model parameter distributions to have a predefined assumed and specified shape, NP unconstrained parameter distribution (UPD) methods make no assumptions or specifications at all about the shape of the distributions of the parameter values in the population of patients studied. NP methods do not break up the true distribution into a blend of assumed fixed and random effects as in the parametric models above. Instead, the parameter distributions are entirely unconstrained (UPD).

Further, instead of estimating only *single* summary values to represent the distributions such as the parameter means and SDs, the *entire* parameter distributions are estimated. These NP methods also are within the scope of mixed effect modeling. They simply do it better, without any constraining assumptions about the shape of the parameter distributions.

At this time, it is appropriate to ask what the truly ideal population PK/PD model would be like. In the absolutely ideal case, it would be somehow to directly observe and somehow to know the exact model parameter values present in each subject or patient one has studied. The collection of these exactly known (not estimated) model parameter values for each subject would then constitute the ideal population model. One could never do any better than that.

Note that the model parameter distributions in this ideal and unattainable case are not continuous, but rather are discrete. They are simply the collection of each individual patient's exactly known model parameter values. They will reflect all the many known and as yet undiscovered genetic variations present in populations of patients, such as fast and slow metabolizers, for example. While one can estimate means, medians, SDs, and correlations of these discrete distributions, that process will usually lose information by constraining those distributions into the assumed shapes for which those quantities are estimated, and by using only a single summary value for each parameter rather than the entire distribution in the population. Nothing can substitute for the discrete, exactly observed, ideal model parameter distributions derived from exactly knowing each subject or patient in the population.

NP methods that employ unconstrained population model parameter distributions (UPDs) are the closest approximation to the unattainable ideal described above. In the NP-UPD approach, the estimated population model parameter distributions are discrete, just as in the ideal. The distributions are *supported* at a number of discrete points up to the number of subjects studied, up to one point for each subject.

Each population model *support point* contains an estimate of each discrete model parameter value, plus an estimate of the relative or normalized likelihood of that support point in the overall population. The probabilities of all the support points add up to one. If it is difficult to distinguish between the data of two patients who are quite similar, because of noise in the serum assays or other sources of noise in the clinical environment (such as errors in how doses are prepared, errors in recording when the doses are given, unrecognized changes in parameter values over time, and any incorrect assumptions incorporated into the structural model), then two or more points may coalesce into a single point with an appropriately greater probability. The UPD approach always obtains the results that are most likely given the data, as their distributions are never constrained by any assumptions of shape, and the likelihood of the results given the data is computed exactly, not as an approximation [5−7].

NP-UPD population modeling was introduced into the biomedical community by Mallet [5], building on the work of Caratheodory and Lindsay [6]. Other NP versions were then developed by Schumitzky [7] and were greatly improved by Leary et al. [8]. Their NP adaptive grid (NPAG) software has now been embedded in an environment of the R language by Neely. This software, Pmetrics, is now the leading software for NP-UPD population modeling [9]. A good description of the strengths and weaknesses of this approach is given in [10].

Figs. 2.1−2.3 show the discrete structure of the NP-UPD population parameter distributions in the Pmetrics population model of gentamicin. The total lack of any constraining assumptions about

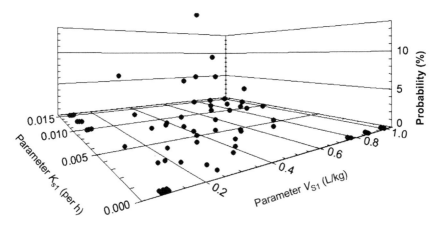

FIGURE 2.1

Three-dimensional plot of the NPAG NP-UPD population model of gentamicin. Left oblique axis: the rate constant K_{S1} for elimination (in h^{-1} per unit of CCr, in mL/min per 1.73 M^2 of body surface area). Right oblique axis: apparent volume of distribution of the central (serum concentration) compartment, in L/kg. Vertical axis: probability. The dots represent the tops of each support point in the population. Nine extra support points of extremely low probability have been added at each corner to extend the range of the population parameter values.

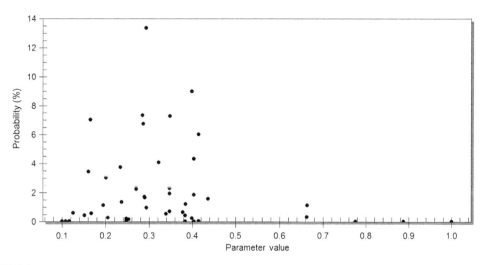

FIGURE 2.2

Plot of the marginal distribution of the parameter V_{S1}, in L/kg, shown in Fig. 2.1. Horizontal axis: V_{S1} in L/kg. Vertical axis: probability. Again, the dots indicate the tops of the support points.

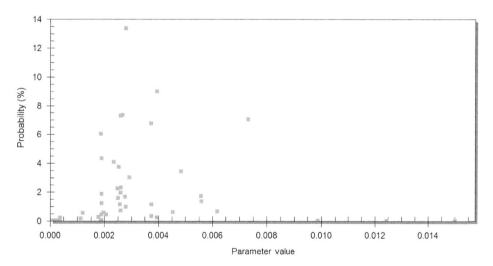

FIGURE 2.3

Plot of the marginal distribution of the parameter K_{S1}. Horizontal axis: K_{S1} (in h^{-1} per unit of CCr, mL/min per 1.73 M^2 of body surface area). Vertical axis: probability. Squares indicate the tops of the support points.

the shape of the model parameter distributions also makes them uniquely well suited to the discovery of unsuspected subpopulations [9].

An example of the ability of the NP-UPD modeling approach to discover unsuspected subpopulations of patients is shown in Fig. 2.4, taken from Ref. [9]. A population was simulated in which

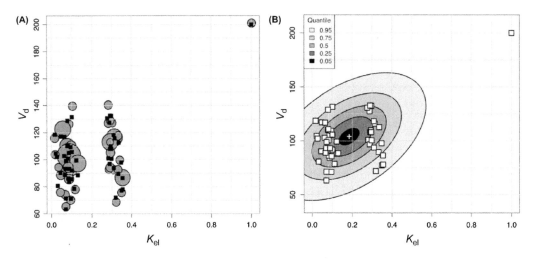

FIGURE 2.4

Analysis of a simulation of two populations plus an outlier. (A) Results of the NPAG analysis. True parameter values of the simulated population are shown as black squares. NPAG-estimated support points are shown as gray circles, the sizes of which are proportional to the probability of each NPAG support point. Both subpopulations, as well as the outlier subject, are detected. (B) Results of the IT2B analysis. The true parameter values of the simulated population are shown as white squares. The bivariate normal parameter distribution estimated by the IT2B parametric method is shown as ellipses of fading darkness corresponding to the percentile of the distribution. The white cross at the center of the ellipse is the mean of each distribution. Neither subpopulation is detected, nor is the outlier subject detected, with IT2B. This performance with IT2B is typical of all parametric methods.

Reproduced with permission from Neely M, van Guilder M, Yamada W, Schumitzky A, and Jelliffe R: Accurate Detection of Outliers and Subpopulations with Pmetrics, a Nonparametric and Parametric Pharmacometric Modeling and Simulation Package for R. Therap. Drug Monit. 34: 467–476, 2012.

the volume of distribution (V_d) was unimodal, with one outlier subject. The elimination rate constant K_e was bimodal, and, again with the outlier subject.

As shown in Fig. 2.4, the NPAG-Pmetrics software closely estimates the true population model parameter distribution of both subpopulations and the outlier subject. In contrast, the parametric approach clearly does not, as it is constrained by the assumptions of normal distributions. Because of this, it fails to detect what is really going on in the population.

In addition, when the data are extremely good, or perhaps when the model is overparameterized, one may even occasionally see the Pmetrics NP-UPD population modeling approach come near the unattainable ideal. Our lab has seen this behavior in two different exploratory results with Pmetrics when used to model the behavior of drugs. While there were minor variations in the probability of the various model support points, they were all extremely close to $1/n$, as in the ideal case, and with one support point for each subject, just as in the ideal case.

In summary, the NP-UPD modeling approach provides more likely results than do parametric methods, as the results are not constrained by any parametric assumptions. This is a very real strength of this approach. The other major clinical strength is discussed in Chapter 3 (Multiple Model (MM) Dosage Design for Clinicians) on maximally precise drug dosing regimens.

REFERENCES

[1] Sheiner L, Beal S, Rosenberg B, Marathe V. Forecasting individual pharmacokinetics. Clin Pharmacol Therap 1979;26:294 305.
[2] Beal S, Sheiner L. NONMEM user's guide I. Users basic guide. San Francisco, CA: Division of Clinical Pharmacology, University of California; 1979.
[3] Sheiner L. The population approach to pharmacokinetic data analysis: rationale and standard data analysis methods. Drug Metab Rev 1984;15:153−71.
[4] Beal S. Population pharmacokinetic data and parameter estimation based on their first two statistical moments. Drug Metab Rev 1984;15:173−93.
[5] Mallet A. A maximum likelihood estimation method for random coefficient regression models. Biometrika 1986;73:645−56.
[6] Lindsay B. The geometry of mixture likelihoods: a general theory. Ann Stat 1983;11:86−94.
[7] Schumitzky A, Nonparametric EM. Algorithms for estimating prior distributions. Appl Math Comput 1991;45:143−57.
[8] Leary R, Jelliffe R, Schumitzky A, Van Guilder M. A unified parametric/nonparametric approach to population PK/PD modeling. Presented at the annual meeting of the Population Approach Group in Europe, Paris, France; June 6−7, 2002.
[9] Neely M, van Guilder M, Yamada W, Schumitzky A, Jelliffe R. Accurate detection of outliers and subpopulations with Pmetrics, a nonparametric and parametric pharmacometric modeling and simulation package for R. Ther Drug Monit 2012;34:467−76.
[10] Bustad A, Terziivanov D, Leary R, Port R, Schumitzky A, Jelliffe R. Parametric and nonparametric population methods: their comparative performance in analysing a clinical data set and two Monte Carlo simulation studies. Clin Pharmacokinet 2006;45:365−83.

DEVELOPING MAXIMALLY PRECISE DOSAGE REGIMENS FOR PATIENTS—MULTIPLE MODEL (MM) DOSAGE DESIGN

3

R. Jelliffe

CHAPTER OUTLINE

Now that we understand the basics of pharmacokinetics and have our nonparametric (NP) population pharmacokinetic and dynamic (PK/PD) models for our drugs, how can we use them best? We can use these NP population models to develop the specific dosage regimen for a patient which hits a desired target most precisely.

3.1 AGAIN, SELECT A SPECIFIC TARGET, NOT A RANGE

An all-too-common practice is to classify serum drug concentrations into subtherapeutic, therapeutic, and toxic ranges or windows. This was discussed in the introduction. It is perfectly possible to develop a drug dosage regimen to maximize the probability that the serum concentrations will be within a selected "window" or range of serum concentrations [1]. The problem is that below whatever breakpoint is set for the lower limit of the range, the benefits are likely to be smaller, with less therapeutic effect, and the risks are likely to be those associated with lack of effect. Within the selected range, there is actually no zone of neutrality, as the beneficial and the potential toxic effects are both increasing throughout this range, and usually at different rates. Above the range, the benefits usually continue to increase, but at a slower rate, and the risks to the patient are more and more associated with toxic effects we do not wish to see.

From the point of view of weighing risks and benefits, and selecting an optimal course of action, the risks of being at or below the "lower limit" of the range are quite different from those

Individualized Drug Therapy for Patients. DOI: http://dx.doi.org/10.1016/B978-0-12-803348-7.00003-4

at the "upper limit." Selecting an optimal risk/benefit ratio for a patient becomes impossible, as there are no specific data with which to optimize this decision. However, the problem, from the patient's point of view, is that a so-called therapeutic range only reflects a general region of serum drug concentrations where most patients, but certainly not all, generally do reasonably well.

Is there a place where the risks and benefits of being slightly above it are not significantly different from being slightly below? Yes, there is. We can choose a *specific* serum concentration target for a patient. If we do not know the patient well, then we might choose a target in the middle of the region where most patients do well, but then attempt to hit that target with maximum precision.

On the other hand, if we already have some information about the relationship between the patient's clinical response to a drug and some data of serum drug concentrations, we can use our conventional clinical judgment to select a new specific target where the patient's response might be expected to be more optimal. Furthermore, since the risk/benefit relationship is hardly different if one is just slightly above or below a specific target goal, we can now employ techniques designed to hit a selected specific target with maximum precision. That is the rationale for the approach we take throughout this book.

3.2 THE SEPARATION PRINCIPLE

This principle states that whenever one separates the process of controlling a system by first, getting *single point summary* estimates of the model parameter distributions, and then, second, using these estimates to control the system (the patient's PK model), the task is inevitably done suboptimally. This is because one can only take action based on estimated central tendencies of parameter distributions which are *assumed* to have a certain shape, and not on the *entire* distributions themselves.

Parametric population models are good examples of separation principle controllers. The reason for this is that there is no way to evaluate the precision of target attainment using such models, as they use only a single summary value for each model parameter. Because of this, there is only one dosage regimen that can be considered, and it must be assumed that it should hit the target exactly. We all know that this never happens.

Fig. 3.1 shows the results of an intravenous infusion regimen of vancomycin derived from the mean parameter values of its population model in the BestDose software. If the patient were to have the exact mean parameter values, then the regimen would hit the target exactly. However, when that regimen, based on the mean parameter values, is given to each of the NP population model support points from which the mean values were derived, we see great variability in the resulting responses. Fig. 3.1 thus illustrates the dangers of dosage regimens based on mean parameter values. It also shows the very real limitations of the separation principle. The goal here was to achieve a target serum concentration of 15 μg/mL at 2, 4, 6, 8, 12, 18, and 24 h into the regimen. A piecewise constant infusion regimen was given to achieve this goal, again based on the mean parameter values in the population model. A very wide spectrum of predicted responses is seen, based on the predicted response from each population model support point.

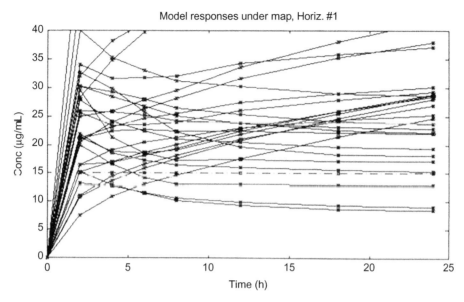

FIGURE 3.1

Continuous piecewise constant IV vancomycin regimen based on population parameter mean values. The dashed horizontal line denotes the target goal of 15 µg/mL, to be achieved at 2, 4, 6, 8, 12, 18, and 24 h into the regimen. Solid lines: predicted responses from each model support point from which the population mean parameter values were derived. Note the great variability in predicted patient responses around the desired target. Five trajectories go off the top of the plot and stay there. Horizontal axis: time into regimen (h). Vertical axis: serum vancomycin concentrations (µg/mL).

Reproduced with permission from Jelliffe R, Bayard D, Milman M, Van Guilder M, and Schumitzky A: Achieving Target Goals most Precisely using Nonparametric Compartmental Models and "Multiple Model" Design of Dosage Regimens. Therap. Drug Monit. 22: 346–353, 2000.

3.3 THE WAY AROUND THE SEPARATION PRINCIPLE: MULTIPLE MODEL DOSAGE DESIGN

The need to achieve maximum precision is optimally satisfied by the multiple support points available in NP population PK/PD models. The collection of the multiple support points in NP models (estimated from the raw data) provides us with a means to overcome the problem posed by the separation principle with its single summary parameter values.

First, we give a candidate dosage regimen to each of the many support points in the NP population model. Each point will generate its own prediction of future serum concentrations resulting from that regimen. Each such point prediction can be weighted by the probability of that support point in the overall population.

Since we have selected a specific target goal at a specific time, we can now examine and compare the ability of various candidate regimens to hit our goal. We can easily calculate the weighted squared error of the failure of each candidate regimen to hit our target. Then we can find the *specific* dosage regimen that minimizes this error. This, then, is the maximally precise regimen,

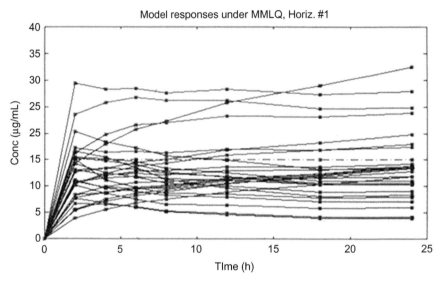

FIGURE 3.2

Results of MM dosage regimen given to the same model support points. The reduction of variability in response about the target is visible. The error in achievement of the target has been minimized. The maximally precise regimen has been developed. No trajectory is outside the plot.

Reproduced with permission from Jelliffe R, Bayard D, Milman M, Van Guilder M, and Schumitzky A: Achieving Target Goals most Precisely using Nonparametric Compartmental Models and "Multiple Model" Design of Dosage Regimens. Therap. Drug Monit. 22: 346–353, 2000.

as it hits our target with the least overall expected weighted squared error. This is multiple model (MM) dosage design [2,3].

An example of MM dosage design is shown in Fig. 3.2. It shows the minimized variability in predicted responses resulting from the MM vancomycin dosage regimen to hit the same targets as in Fig. 3.1 above [2,3]. The predictions are much better centered about the desired target. Remember that while each line on the plot has equal visibility, the probability of each prediction, and therefore its weight, depends on the probability of each support point in the population model.

Notice that the design of the dose itself now becomes an important tool to minimize patient variability in response about a desired goal. This is often more important than having additional covariate information. Furthermore, bear in mind that if you use parametric models, you will never even be aware of this issue of precision because you can never see it, and therefore you will never be able to do it. This is why you never hear of this issue from those who use parametric models such as NONMEM, for example, and other parametric modeling methods to develop drug dosage regimens for patients. Since parametric modeling approaches are used so widely in the pharmaceutical industry, it is not surprising that the drug industry has not shown any awareness of or interest in designing maximally precise drug dosage regimens.

MM dosage design provides, for the first time, dosage regimens for any genetically polymorphic population, known or not yet discovered, which will hit the desired target with minimum expected weighted squared error, based on whatever data is known at the time. In addition, unless the entire NP model parameter distributions are known, one can never know this information and can never know what is truly optimal in a dosage regimen. MM optimal dosage design can never be duplicated with parametric models.

Furthermore, in a randomized controlled clinical trial, MM dosage design significantly outperformed dosage regimens of tacrolimus developed by expert transplant physicians [4].

REFERENCES

[1] Tarlght N, Mentre F, Mallet A, Jouvent R. Nonparametric estimation of population characteristics of the kinetics of lithium from observational and experimental data: individualization of chronic dosing regimen using a new Bayesian approach. Ther Drug Monit 1994;16:258−69.

[2] Jelliffe R, Schumitzky A, Bayard D, Milman M, Van Guilder M, Wang X, et al. Model-based, goal-oriented, individualized drug therapy: linkage of population modeling, new "multiple model" dosage design, Bayesian feedback, and individualized target goals. Clin Pharmacokinet 1998;34:57−77.

[3] Jelliffe R, Bayard D, Milman M, Van Guilder M, Schumitzky A. Achieving target goals most precisely using nonparametric compartmental models and "multiple model" design of dosage regimens. Ther Drug Monit 2000;22:346−53.

[4] Storset E, Asberg A, Skauby M, Neely M, Bergan S, Bremer S, et al. Improved tacrolimus target concentration achievement using computerized dosing in renal transplant recipients − a prospective, randomized study. Transplantation 2015;99:2158−66.

OPTIMIZING LABORATORY ASSAY METHODS FOR INDIVIDUALIZED THERAPY

4

R. Jelliffe

CHAPTER OUTLINE

4.1 INTRODUCTION: WRONG WEIGHTING OF DATA, WRONG PK MODELS, WRONG DOSES

When one measures the concentrations of substances in serum or elsewhere, it is good to do it right. This includes having the proper evaluation of the precision with which a measurement is made. Precision is arguably the most important index of the credibility of a measurement.

Individualized Drug Therapy for Patients. DOI: http://dx.doi.org/10.1016/B978-0-12-803348-7.00004-6

It determines how much meaning or significance we can attach to a measurement such as that of the concentration of a drug in a sample. A precise result should lead someone to pay closer attention to it than to a less precise result.

When we model the behavior of drugs in patients, the procedure used, whatever it might be, should be influenced more by a precise laboratory result than by a less precise one. The fitting procedure should be drawn more closely to a precise measurement than to a less precise one.

Furthermore, an incorrect model of drug behavior based on incorrect evaluations of the credibility of the data will result in incorrect doses of that drug being given to achieve some desired goal such as a target serum drug concentration. The wrong measure of assay precision means the wrong model and the wrong doses given to patients. Because of this, it is important to use the correct measure of assay precision.

4.2 PERCENT COEFFICIENT OF VARIATION IS NOT THE CORRECT MEASURE

It has been standard practice among the clinical laboratory community for decades to describe the precision of an assay as the percent error of the measurement. In its usual procedures of quality control, the laboratory measures several replicates of a sample and calculates the mean and standard deviation (SD) of the measurements, and then goes on to describe the SD as a percent of the mean. This is called the percent coefficient of variation (CV%).

This is an intuitive measure and appears at first glance to make good sense. The problem with this approach, which has also been well documented for the laboratory community for decades, is that as the measurement approaches zero, the CV% increases and finally becomes infinite as the measurement reaches zero. The entire approach using CV% fails [1].

Because of this well-known failure, those in the laboratory community have simply decided that when the CV% reaches a certain value, often 15% or 20%, measurements lower than that value with a higher CV% have reached an unacceptable percent error. The value at which the percent error reaches or exceeds the acceptable percent error has been called the lower limit of quantification (LLOQ), and the laboratory community has simply decided to withhold and censor results below the LLOQ and not to release or report them. Almost no one seems to have questioned this arbitrary practice.

Laboratories, the FDA, and the College of American Pathologists (CAP) have all followed this custom and have censored laboratory results when they are below the so-called LLOQ. This, and the regulatory policies based on this erroneous idea, have significantly impaired the ability of the laboratory to serve the medical community optimally.

4.3 METHODS

4.3.1 CALCULATING THE ASSAY CV%

One obtains replicate samples and measures the concentration of drug present in each. One calculates the mean and SD for each sample, divides each sample SD by the mean sample value, and expresses the result as the percent of the mean (CV%) at each measurement. If CV% is greater than 15% or 20%, that result is usually censored because it is believed to be unacceptably imprecise.

Since CV% increases as the measurement approaches zero, when it exceeds the acceptable CV%, the assay is said to have reached the LLOQ. The result is then deliberately withheld (censored) by the laboratory community and is reported only as being "less than" the LLOQ. The CAP, to evaluate laboratory quality worldwide, sends out samples of known concentration, receives their results back, and publishes them as measures of quality control, including the SD of the overall sample results.

The relationship between CV%, SD, and the assay measurement can be described as

$$CV\% = (\text{Assay SD}/\text{mean assay measurement}) \times 100 \tag{4.1}$$

The key to this relationship is the assay SD, which is obtained by rearranging Eq. (4.1) as shown in Eq. (4.2):

$$\text{Assay SD} = A_1 C \tag{4.2}$$

where A_1 is a number representing the fraction of the assay measurement represented by the CV%, and C is the mean measured concentration. For example, if the CV were 10%, the value of A_1 would be 0.1. In that case, $SD = 0.1C$.

However, Fig. 4.1 and Eqs. (4.1) and (4.2) are not realistic, because the CV% increases as the measured concentration approaches zero and becomes infinite as the measurement reaches zero. Because of the erroneous belief in CV% as a measure of assay precision, intuitive rather than scientific judgments have been made about what constitutes an "acceptable" CV%.

Jusko [2] has discussed the significance of data below the LLOQ. He stated that "low concentrations are meaningful and should not be neglected," and "repeated measurements below the LLOQ can be assigned a lesser weight based on the actual or expected larger CV% of the analytical method." However, he did not offer any specific way to determine these weights.

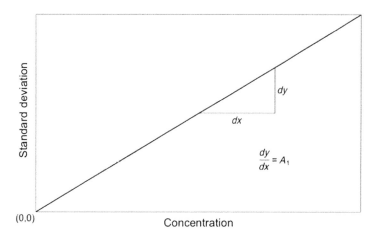

FIGURE 4.1

Diagram of an ideal assay with a constant CV%. The assay SD gets smaller and smaller as the measurement approaches zero, and ideally is zero when the measurement is zero.

Reproduced with permission from Jelliffe R, Schumitzky A, Bayard D, and Neely M: Describing Assay Precision - Reciprocal of Variance is much better than CV%. Therapeutic Drug Monitoring. 06/2015; 37(3):389–94.

The problem is that as the measurement approaches zero, one enters the region of the assay noise present when the true measurement is zero. This is not accounted for in the previous concept of constant CV% as shown in Fig. 4.1 or Eqs. (4.1) and (4.2).

However, it is easy to take this into account. One can simply describe the assay SD when a blank sample is measured in replicate, and call this A_0. Now we have the expression

$$\text{Assay SD} = A_0 + A_1C \tag{4.3}$$

where A_0 is the SD of the blank sample, A_1 is defined as in Eq. (4.2), and C is the mean measured concentration (Fig. 4.2).

This simple addition of a second term describing the SD of a blank sample has a most profound result. One now can accurately describe the assay SD all the way down to and including the blank. There is no longer any need to censor low values. There is, in fact, no LLOQ any more at all. By introducing C_0, one can describe the SD of an assay all the way down to and including zero. We can see that the entire illusory concept of LLOQ has in fact existed solely because of the incorrect impression that CV% is the measure of assay precision!

The assay CV% is usually not constant over the entire range of the assay. It may change with higher measurements. In this case, one can easily add other terms to this relationship. For example, one can use the expression for a third-degree polynomial:

$$\text{Assay SD} = A_0 + A_1C + A_2C^2 + A_3C^3 \tag{4.4}$$

where A_0, A_1, A_2, and A_3 are numbers to be estimated, and C, C^2, and C^3 are the concentration, the concentration squared, and the concentration cubed, respectively. Instead of calculating CV%, we are now calculating the assay SD itself, in the same units as the assay.

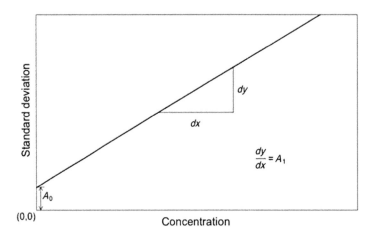

FIGURE 4.2

Diagram of an ideal assay with a constant CV%, but with an extra coefficient describing the assay SD (the measurement noise) when the true measurement is actually zero. The assay SD decreases as the measurement approaches zero, but still remains positive and finite as the blank value is encountered.

Reproduced with permission from Jelliffe R, Schumitzky A, Bayard D, and Neely M: Describing Assay Precision - Reciprocal of Variance is much better than CV%. Therapeutic Drug Monitoring. 06/2015; 37(3):389–94.

If one makes the reasonable assumption that assay noise is normally distributed, it has also been well known for decades that the correct way to describe the width of such a Gaussian bell-shaped curve is by the reciprocal of the variance of that measurement [3]. As before, the key is the assay SD. First, find the assay SD. However, instead of describing it as a percent of the measurement, square it to get the variance (var). The reciprocal of the variance (1/var) is the correct way to describe assay precision [3]. This also has been well known for a long time by the statistical community, but has been, it seems, sadly ignored by the laboratory community.

4.3.2 CALCULATING THE RECIPROCAL OF THE VARIANCE

Interestingly, the usual calculation of an SD also has an error associated with it. The greater the number of samples that are measured in replicate to obtain the estimate of the SD, the smaller is the error in the estimate of the SD. Because of this, one must measure enough replicates to get a reasonable estimate of each sample SD. To do this, we suggest at least five replicates per sample (not just two or three), just as the FDA Guidelines for Industry do [4]. More are always better. The overall relationship between the number of replicates and the error in the estimate of the sample SD [5,6] is described in Eq. (4.5) and shown in Fig. 4.3.

$$\text{ERR of } \sigma \approx \frac{1}{\sqrt{2(n-1)}} \tag{4.5}$$

or, after rearranging, as

$$\frac{\text{ERR}}{\sigma} \approx \frac{1}{\sqrt{2(n-1)}} \tag{4.6}$$

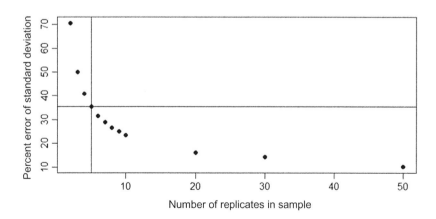

FIGURE 4.3

Plot of the error of the estimate of the true sample SD versus number of sample replicates [5,6]. Probably at least five replicates should be measured, the more the better. Nine replicates, for example, have only half the error of three replicates. The vertical line shows that for five replicates, the ERR is 35.3%.

Reproduced with permission from Jelliffe R, Schumitzky A, Bayard D, and Neely M: Describing Assay Precision - Reciprocal of Variance is much better than CV%. Therapeutic Drug Monitoring. 06/2015; 37(3):389–94.

where ERR is the error of the estimate of the SD (a number from 0 to 1.0), σ is the true value of the SD, n is the number of replicate samples, and $\approx$ means "approximately equal to." The more replicates measured, the more precise the estimate of the SD [5,6]. For triplicate samples, it is somewhat surprising to find that ERR is 0.5 or 50%. For $n = 5$, it is 0.353 or 35.3%. For $n = 9$, it is 0.25 or 25%. It seems prudent to use at least five samples for a reasonable estimate of the SD of each sample. Clearly, the more replicates, the smaller the error in the estimate of the SD.

There must also be a zero-concentration blank sample to determine the SD of the blank, the machine noise of the assay. Additionally, there should be at least a low sample, a medium one, a high one, and a very high one to cover the entire working range of the assay.

The relation between the mean assay concentrations and assay SD can be fitted with a polynomial equation as shown in Eq. (4.4). Many software packages do this, including the makeErrorPoly routine in the USC Pmetrics package for population pharmacokinetic (PK) modeling [7]. This polynomial equation can then be stored in software such as the USC BestDose clinical software [8] to calculate the SD for each single assay sample that goes through the laboratory's assay system, square it to get the variance, and calculate 1/var to provide correct weighting of the assay data for the PK analysis of that drug.

In this way, the optimal PK model, either for an individual patient or for populations of patients receiving a drug, can be made from drug assay data. This also permits optimal individualized drug dosage for each patient [8−10]. Use of such a polynomial to find the assay SD and 1/var provides an easy and practical way to describe and store the correct error pattern of any assay. CV% no longer needs to be used.

4.4 RESULTS: APPLICATION TO REAL ASSAY DATA

4.4.1 EXAMINING AN ASSAY FOR VANCOMYCIN

Fig. 4.4 illustrates this process for vancomycin. The data shown are taken from CAP samples sent to participating clinical laboratories [11]. The figure shows the results of 15 vancomycin quality control samples that were measured by the chemiluminescence assay and reported by 198−202 laboratories (not all laboratories reported on all 15 samples). Sample concentrations ranged from 5.61 to 33.38 µg/mL. Fig. 4.4 shows the relationship between the assay measurements and the SDs of the reported results.

4.4.2 A CAVEAT

Just as with CV%, it is dangerous to extrapolate any polynomial equation beyond the range of its raw data. For example, there is significant doubt from the vancomycin data in Fig. 4.4 about what the assay SD is at the blank and especially at concentrations over 33 µg/mL.

The SD of the vancomycin blank here may be somewhere between about 0.1 and 0.3 µg/mL. This is why one needs specifically to determine the SD of the blank.

Peak vancomycin concentrations are often greater than 33 µg/mL. If we use the first-degree polynomial, a concentration of 60 µg/mL has an estimated SD of 3.547 µg/mL. If we use the second, it is 2.8828 µg/mL. If we use the third, it is only 1.4618 µg/mL. This is due to the downward curvature shown in Fig. 4.4 as the concentrations increase, because of the negative coefficients in

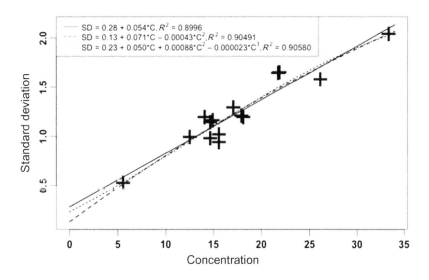

FIGURE 4.4

Relationship between measured serum vancomycin concentrations in CAP quality control samples [11] and the assay SDs. Horizontal axis: measured vancomycin concentrations (µg/mL). Vertical axis: standard deviation (µg/mL).

Reproduced with permission from Jelliffe R, Schumitzky A, Bayard D, and Neely M: Describing Assay Precision - Reciprocal of Variance is much better than CV%. Therapeutic Drug Monitoring. 06/2015; 37(3):389–94.

the second- and third-degree polynomials. All SD estimates above the documented measurement of 33 µg/mL are therefore questionable.

For example, if we estimate the SD for an assumed measurement of 100 µg/mL, a not too uncommon peak value, the first-degree polynomial estimates the SD at 5.723 µg/mL. However, that found with the second degree is only 3.001 µg/mL and the third-degree polynomial results in a total impossibility, as the estimated SD has become negative: -8.787 µg/mL. That simply cannot be. All values of SD must be greater than zero. We now see the dangers. Polynomial estimates, just like CV%, cannot be trusted outside the ranges of their raw data.

4.4.3 ANOTHER EXAMPLE: VORICONAZOLE

At Children's Hospital of Los Angeles, therapeutic drug monitoring (TDM) of voriconazole has employed an Absciex LCMS-MS assay [12,13], a nonparametric population PK model of voriconazole [14], and the USC BestDose clinical software [8]. The assay is a quantitative MRM analytical method by ESI-LC/MS/MS (ABSiex 400 Q-Trap), which was developed utilizing Positive mode to quantitate voriconazole (**m/z 350.1/281.20**) using D3-Voriconazole (**m/z 353.1/284.2**) as an internal standard. The assay is basically linear from 0.0 to 50 µg/mL.

The error pattern of this assay was analyzed using seven samples, each measured in quintuplicate. The samples were a blank, 0.02, 0.5, 5.0, 12.5, 30, and 40 µg/mL. These seven samples gave mean values $\pm$ SDs of 0.00592 $\pm$ 0.000239, 0.177 $\pm$ 0.00118, 0.487 $\pm$ 0.0121, 5.364 $\pm$ 0.8385, 13.94 $\pm$ 0.1342, 29.58 $\pm$ 0.642, and 38.54 $\pm$ 0.381 µg/mL, respectively.

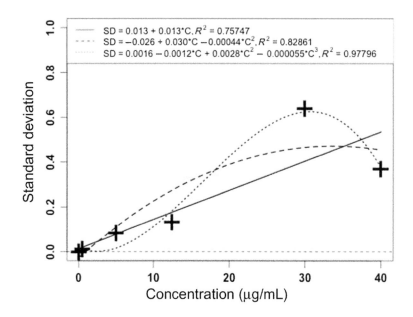

FIGURE 4.5

Plot of voriconazole measured concentrations (horizontal) and assay standard deviation (vertical). The solid line represents the graph of the first-degree polynomial, the dashed line the second-degree polynomial, and the dotted line the third-degree polynomial.

Reproduced with permission from Jelliffe R, Schumitzky A, Bayard D, and Neely M: Describing Assay Precision - Reciprocal of Variance is much better than CV%. Therapeutic Drug Monitoring. 06/2015; 37(3):389–94.

When those data were analyzed with the makeErrorPoly function in Pmetrics [7], the following relationships were found, as shown in Fig. 4.5.

In this figure, the third-degree polynomial fits the data best, as expected, but has a marked downward curve at the high end. This will become dangerous if extrapolated any higher. The second-degree polynomial has a less pronounced downward curve, and may perhaps be useful, as not many measurements are to be expected to be over 40 µg/mL. However, it may well overestimate the assay SD in the more frequent range from 10 to 25 µg/mL. Because of this, and because the data point at 30 µg/mL is the only one departing from the otherwise general tendency to have a linear relationship, we chose to employ the first-degree polynomial in this particular case as providing a reasonable and safe description of the error pattern of this assay. Other assays [15] have higher-order polynomials that fit their particular quality control data well, which in their cases provide better information for those assays than the first-order polynomial shown here.

4.4.4 AN EXAMPLE OF GENTAMICIN

In the Emit gentamicin assay from the Los Angeles County Medical Center, more was done to capture the information over what was taken to be close to the full working range of the assay at that

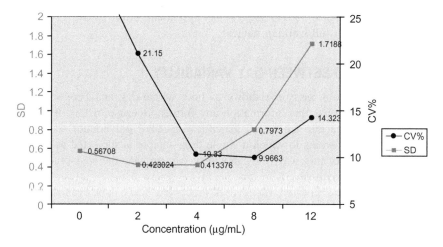

FIGURE 4.6

Relationship between measured gentamicin concentrations and SD, and CV%. Solid squares and left-hand vertical scale: assay SD. Solid circles and right-hand vertical scale: CV%. Note that the relationship between concentrations and CV% is at least as nonlinear as that between concentration and SD.

Reproduced with permission from Jelliffe R, Schumitzky A, Bayard D, and Neely M: Describing Assay Precision - Reciprocal of Variance is much better than CV%. Therapeutic Drug Monitoring. 06/2015; 37(3):389–94.

time. Both the SD and CV% of the assay are shown in Fig. 4.6. The polynomial relationship between the assay and its SD is:

$$SD \ (\mu g/mL) = 0.56708 - 0.10563C + 0.016801C^2 \qquad (4.7)$$

In this figure, the 2.0- and 4.0-μg/mL measurements have almost the same SD, and therefore, both measurements are almost equally precise. However, the higher measurement has a CV of only 10.33%, while the lower one has a CV% essentially twice as large. This quality control data illustrates well both the falsity and the danger of using CV% as a measure of assay precision.

4.5 DISCUSSION: LLOQ IS AN ILLUSION

It is always prudent to carefully examine data covering the entire working range of any assay. The assay SDs should be positive, not negative, and should be realistic. If that is done, it is safe to use the polynomial that fits the data best. Sometimes the full third-degree polynomial is good, especially if its plot is concave upward at the high end. Sometimes one may settle for a second-degree polynomial if it also is either straight or concave upward. Examples of this can be seen in Fig. 4.6 and from CAP data from an earlier report [15]. Furthermore, in that earlier data, the CAP had covered much more of the working ranges of several assays. They often tended to show a gentle upward concavity, which again shows the utility of this method of describing assay errors [15].

The CAP data described above for vancomycin are disappointing in that they only provide an estimate of assay precision over the range of their chosen samples, where measurements are made most often. There is no evidence here to suggest any systematic effort by the CAP to examine the precision of assays over their full working ranges.

4.5.1 WITHIN-DAY AND BETWEEN-DAY VARIABILITY

It has been common to report assay variability as both within-day and between-day variability. However, it is impossible to use this information any further. Because of this, it is probably most useful to incorporate all data into an overall general assay error polynomial, to develop an error model of the many random events to which a single drug sample is subjected as it goes through a laboratory's assay system. In this way, the laboratory can provide the best practical measure of credibility or precision for any assay.

Assay error analysis can be repeated whenever desired. New data can be evaluated with respect to the previous quality control polynomial. If the relationship between sample means and SD has changed, the assay has drifted. One may develop a new polynomial or can re-evaluate the assay itself. On the other hand, if it is similar, the new data can be included with the previous data, developing a still richer and more informative polynomial to use for optimal quality control of that assay.

Those who individualize drug dosage regimens for patients need to fit serum concentration data with the correct quantitative measure of precision so that the optimal pharmacokinetic model can be made for that patient, yielding the drug dosage regimen to hit a clinically selected serum concentration goal for each patient most precisely, using the method of multiple model dosage design [8,9].

Some vancomycin monitoring guidelines have stated that peak concentrations have no clinical significance [16]. We strongly feel that this is not correct. Vancomycin has toxicity as well as therapeutic effect. Its bacterial killing is probably nonconcentration-dependent [17], but this probably is not the case at all for toxicity. Peak concentrations, while having some further effect on killing the organism, clearly represent increased exposure of the patient to a toxic drug. Well-known general strategies for the design of optimal TDM protocols [18] show that even a minimal drug model always has at least two model parameters (volume and either elimination rate constant or clearance) and that a minimum of two samples is therefore required to make an optimal one-compartment, individualized clinical pharmacokinetic model of drug behavior. Vancomycin peak concentrations as well as troughs are needed to properly evaluate possible toxicity and to better estimate the area under the concentration curve. Ignoring these important general principles leads to less informed strategies for individualized dosage regimens of any drug. In addition, vancomycin has at least two-compartment behavior, and such a model is required to obtain realistic estimates of its serum concentration profile over time.

4.5.2 DEFINING THE LOWER LIMIT OF ASSAY DETECTION (LLOD) IS IMPROVED

Because the SD of the blank is rigorously determined, rather than simply setting the smallest possible movement of the detector, one can set a desired criterion of probability (number of blank SDs above the blank, often 2, 3, or 5, for 95% or 99% or greater probability) with which one decides to accept a forensic result as indicating that a substance is present in the sample or not. In this way, the entire procedure can be done with total transparency, without withholding or censoring any data at all, and with clear explanation of the criteria used upon which to base the final decision as to whether a substance is present in a sample or not. Note that when quality control of an assay is done in this way, there is no concentration that can be regarded as "too small to measure." The true measurement will always be recorded, including one that is zero. Furthermore, the sensitivity of various assays can be compared, not through their illusory LLOQ, but rather by rigorous scientific criteria based on the SD of blank samples and the number of SDs above the blank that are felt to be required for a reasonable decision concerning the probable presence or absence of a substance. All this can be done with total transparency and rigorous criteria, without withholding anything. All of this is well documented by experimental data of the superiority and scientific correctness of 1/var as the measure of assay precision, and by decades of such data documenting the clear failure of CV%.

4.6 CONCLUSION

4.6.1 RECIPROCAL OF MEASUREMENT VARIANCE IS THE CORRECT MEASURE OF ASSAY PRECISION

Assay measurement errors consist of additive noise, which is assumed to be independent from one measurement to another and from the model PK parameter values to be estimated. Because of this, if one fits a PK model to assay data, its most correct parameter estimates will be obtained only if each data point is correctly weighted by the reciprocal of its variance as the measure of assay credibility [3]. This is easy to do, with no significant change in cost or effort over CV%. This approach was first described in [19] and was expanded in [15]. The present chapter now provides full, rigorous, mathematical, statistical, and visual support for this improved approach [1,3,5,6].

4.6.2 THE ASSAY ERROR POLYNOMIAL PROVIDES A PRACTICAL WAY TO STORE THE ERROR DATA

After one has obtained the SDs of the assay data from the replicate samples, it is easy and practical to store that error pattern in the form of a polynomial for easy reference in reporting the results of any measurement.

4.6.3 RELATIONSHIP TO OTHER CLINICAL SOURCES OF ERROR IN THE THERAPEUTIC ENVIRONMENT

To describe and determine the additional contribution of the other errors in the clinical environment in which drug therapy takes place, one can calculate an additional noise term in the population PK model of the drug. This other noise term reflects the errors in how drug doses are prepared and given, the errors in recording the times at which the doses are given and blood samples obtained, the errors inherent in any description of drug behavior when a model is used (model misspecification), and any unsuspected and unknown changes in a patient's pharmacokinetic parameter values over time.

Such an error model describes past experience with the drug and provides the Bayesian prior for the clinical process of planning, monitoring, and adjusting drug dosage regimens specifically tailored to the needs of each individual patient [8,9]. In the Pmetrics population modeling package [7], the additional noise present in the clinical environment is called lambda. Using both 1/var and lambda, both laboratory and clinical uncertainties can be independently determined for Bayesian individualization of drug dosage regimens for optimally precise patient care. This permits optimal knowledge about, and understanding of, the separate laboratory and clinical sources of uncertainty in each patient's environment for optimally precise management of drug dosage for that individual patient. See 4.6.5 below.

4.6.4 ONE CAN STOP CENSORING LOW MEASUREMENTS

Using 1/var rather than CV% also eliminates the erroneous perceived need to censor values below some illusory LLOQ. Eliminating LLOQ is a significant benefit to the laboratory. It avoids both wasted samples and a number of ad hoc methods to compensate for such arbitrarily censored data [20,21].

This approach is not limited to drug assays. HIV and HCV PCR results, and many others, can also be reported in this more informed manner. Clinicians now can follow these results all the way down to zero, to document whether or not the illness is optimally treated. If a patient with HIV has a value reported as <50 copies, one patient might have a value of 45, another only 3. This important result has been deliberately withheld to date from those ordering the test, simply because of the erroneous belief in CV% and the illusion of LLOQ. Instead of reporting a result as "less than 50 units/mL," for example, one can report it both ways, for example, as "16 units/mL, below the old LLOQ of 50 units/mL." The SD of that result can always be obtained from the laboratory if the clinician wishes, and, better yet, the TDM personnel have what is needed (and what is correct and optimal!) for correct drug dosage individualization.

The awkward use of CV%, and its documented failure for decades to describe assay precision as the measurement approaches zero, can now be replaced by a more informed and correct measure of assay precision. 1/var is based on sound mathematical and statistical methods and should replace CV%. It provides the correct measure of assay precision. Furthermore, 1/var eliminates the need to censor low data. It eliminates the need for inventing any illusory LLOQ at all. It also improves the ability of any assay to provide more rigorous criteria for forensic detection of the presence or absence of a substance in a sample. FDA regulations dealing with this subject [4] and the quality control policies of the CAP [11], eg, can easily be (and definitely should be) updated in accord with modern statistical and mathematical practice. Dr. Jusko's intuition [2] was on the right track.

4.6.5 OTHER SOURCES OF UNCERTAINTY IN THE CLINICAL ENVIRONMENT

There are also other sources of noise and uncertainty in the clinical environment that surrounds each patient. They consist of the errors in the preparation and administration of the various doses (no dose is ever known exactly), errors in recording when the doses were given and the serum samples were drawn, and the misspecification of the model compared to reality. These can be lumped into another term that we have called lambda, which can be estimated separately from the stated assay error pattern. Thus it is possible to have a not unreasonable estimate of the quality in the clinical environment in which each patient's therapy takes place. Most other modeling approaches do not do this. They consider only a lumped single error pattern and do not consider this important clinical question.

The largest single source of uncertainty in the clinical environment is not knowing when the doses were given [22]. In the usual clinical setting, the nurses go around to the various patients, giving them their 8 am medications, for example.

This is a physical impossibility. No patient—or at the most, only one out of many—gets a dose at exactly 8 am. This discrepancy between when the doses are said to have been given and the time at which they actually were given constitutes the largest single component of the therapeutic imprecision in the clinical environment [22]. In many hospitals, there is either a written or unwritten policy that essentially states that it is acceptable for a nurse to falsely chart a dose as "given when ordered" if it was given within half an hour of when it was ordered. This misguided policy not only makes nurses feel guilty when it is impossible for them to feel otherwise; it defeats and corrupts attempts to individualize dosage regimens for patients.

How can we overcome this problem? It is surprisingly easy. Simply get rid of the check mark that says that the 8 am dose was given. Instead, just look at the clock on the wall and write down in military time (0814, for example) when the dose was actually given. Thus there is not only a record that the dose *was* given at some time, but much more precisely just *when* it was given, to the minute. This overcomes the greatest component of uncertainty interfering with the ability to achieve maximal precision in drug therapy [22]. In addition, one can get cheap digital watches for the nursing staff. All this is so easy! The phlebotomy service can use the same approach to record, also in military time, just when the blood was drawn for the serum concentrations. Some places now have barcodes to record these events. The thing to make sure of is that the barcode is done AT THE TIME of the event and not at any other time.

No one cares if the dose was given as ordered or not. But it is vital to know exactly *when* each dose was given. The same is true for the phlebotomy service. These issues are easily addressed, and are worthwhile and useful for the optimal care of each patient.

ACKNOWLEDGMENTS

The work in this chapter was supported in part by NIH grants GM068968, HD070996, and EB005803, to Drs. Jelliffe and Neely. The authors also wish to acknowledge most gratefully the original suggestion by Thomas Gilman, Pharm. D., Assistant Professor of Pharmacy at the USC School of Pharmacy, when he was with our laboratory in the 1980s, to describe assay error this way. We are sad that Dr. Gilman left the USC School of Pharmacy quite a number of years ago and that there is no further contact information for him.

REFERENCES

[1] Spiegel M. Theory and problems of statistics. Schaum's outline series. New York, NY: Schaum; 1961. p. 73.

[2] Jusko W. Use of pharmacokinetic data below lower limit of quantification values. Pharm Res 2012;29:2628−31.

[3] DeGroot M. Probability and statistics. 2nd ed. Reading MA: Addison-Wesley; 1989. p. 403 and 423.

[4] FDA guidance for industry bioanalytical method validation. <http://www.fda.gov/cder/guidance/4252fnl.pdf>.

[5] Ahn S, Fessler JA. Standard errors of mean, variance, and standard deviation estimators. Technical report. Ann Arbor, MI: The University of Michigan; July 24, 2003.

[6] Seber G, Wild C. Nonlinear regression. New York, NY: Wiley; 1989. p. 536−7.

[7] Neely M. Pmetrics. A software package in R for parametric and nonparametric population modeling and Monte Carlo simulation. Available from: <http://www.lapk.org/>.

[8] Jelliffe R, Bayard D, Schumitzky A, Milman M, Jiang F, Leonov S, et al. A new clinical software package for multiple model (MM) design of drug dosage regimens for planning, monitoring, and adjusting optimally individualized drug therapy for patients. Presented at the 4th international meeting on mathematical modeling. Vienna, Austria: Technical University of Vienna; February 6, 2003.

[9] Jelliffe R, Bayard D, Milman M, Van Guilder M, Schumitzky A. Achieving target goals most precisely using nonparametric compartmental models and "multiple model" design of dosage regimens. Ther Drug Monit 2000;22:346−53.

[10] Bayard D, Jelliffe R, Schumitzky A, Milman M, Van Guilder M. Precision drug dosage regimens using multiple model adaptive control: theory, and application to simulated vancomycin therapy. Selected topics in mathematical physics, professor R. Vasudevan memorial volume. Madras, India: Allied Publishers Ltd; 1995. p. 407−26.

[11] College of American Pathologists (CAP) Survey C-C (2011), p. 132; Survey C-A (2012), p. 128, and Survey C-B (2012), p. 129.

[12] Decosterd L, Rochat B, Pesse B, Mercier T, Tissot F, Widmer N, et al. Multiplex ultra-performance liquid chromatography-tandem mass spectrometry method for simultaneous quantification in human plasma of fluconazole, itraconazole, hydroxyitraconazole, posaconazole, voriconazole, voriconazole-N-oxide, anidulafungin, and caspofungin. Antimicrob Agents Chemother 2010;54(12):5303−15.

[13] Alffenaar J, Wessels A, van Hateran K, Greijjdanus B, Kosterink J, Uges D. Method for therapeutic monitoring of azole antifungal drugs in human serum using LC/MS/MS. J Chromatogr B Analyt Technol Biomed Life Sci 2010;878(1):39−44.

[14] Neely M, Rushing T, Kovacs A, Jelliffe R, Hoffman J. Voriconazole pharmacokinetics and pharmacodynamics in children. Clin Inf Dis 2010;50:27−36.

[15] Jelliffe R, Schumitzky A, Van Guilder M, Liu M, Hu L, Maire P, et al. Individualizing drug dosage regimens: roles of population pharmacokinetic and dynamic models, Bayesian fitting, and adaptive control. Ther Drug Monit 1993;15:380−93.

[16] Rybak M, Lomaestro B, Rotschafer J, Moellering R, Craig W, Billeter M, et al. Therapeutic monitoring of vancomycin in adult patients: a consensus review of the American Society of Health-System Pharmacists, the infectious diseases society of America, and the society of infectious disease pharmacists. Am J Health-Syst Pharm 2009;66:82−98.

[17] Larsson A, Walker K, Raddatz J, Rotschafer J. The concentration-independent effect of monoexponential and biexponential decay in vancomycin concentrations on the killing of *Staphylococcuss aureus* under aerobic and anaerobic conditions. J Antimicrob Chemotherap 1996;38:589−97.

[18] D'Argenio D. Optimal sampling times for pharmacokinetic experiments. J Pharmacokin Biopharmacol 1981;9:739−56.

[19] Jelliffe R. Explicit determination of laboratory assay errors − a useful aid in therapeutic drug monitoring. drug monitoring and toxicology No. DM89-4(DM-56) American society of clinical pathologists check sample continuing education program. Drug Monit Toxicol 1989;10(4).

[20] Bergstrand M, Karlsson M. Handling data below the limit of quantification in mixed effect models. AAPS J 2009;11:371−80.

[21] Beal S. Ways to fit a PK model with some data below the quantification limit. J Pharmacokinet Pharmacodyn 2001;28:481−504.

[22] Jelliffe RW, Schumitzky A, Van Guilder M. Nonpharmacokinetic clinical factors affecting aminoglycoside therapeutic precision. A simulation study. Drug Invest 1992;4:20−9.

EVALUATION OF RENAL FUNCTION 5

R. Jelliffe

CHAPTER OUTLINE

5.1 CLASSICAL ESTIMATION OF CREATININE CLEARANCE (CCr), BASED ON URINARY EXCRETION

Glomerular filtration rate (GFR) has been the most important single index of renal function. Inulin clearance has been the gold standard for determining GFR. However, as creatinine is easily measured and is primarily excreted by glomerular filtration, with only a bit of tubular secretion, it has become the single most useful index of renal function in clinical practice. As GFR decreases, creatinine elimination by renal tubular secretion may remain constant, and so probably represents a greater proportion of creatinine excretion when renal function is significantly impaired.

Individualized Drug Therapy for Patients. DOI: http://dx.doi.org/10.1016/B978-0-12-803348-7.00005-8

Classically, creatinine clearance (C or CCr) has been evaluated by obtaining a 24-h urine specimen, measuring the concentration of urinary creatinine and the urine volume, and obtaining a sample of serum creatinine (SCr) halfway through the urine collection. CCr is then computed as

$$C = UV/P \tag{5.1}$$

or

$$PC = UV \tag{5.2}$$

where U is the measured concentration of urinary creatinine, C is creatinine clearance, V is the 24-h urinary volume, and P is the plasma concentration or SCr. UV thus represents the total 24-h urinary creatinine excretion (usually in mg/day), and P is the serum or plasma creatinine, usually in mg/dL. The idea is to estimate the GFR, which is usually expressed in mL/min or corrected for body surface area as mL/min per 1.73 m^2.

One might ask the following question: is the function of the kidneys simply to make urine or to excrete waste substances? Interestingly, to my knowledge few seem to have asked, for example what the half-time of or the rate constant for creatinine excretion actually is. Nevertheless, CCr remains the most frequently used index of renal function in patients and will probably remain so for the foreseeable future. It is also interesting that in common parlance, the word "clearance" is generally regarded as being synonymous with the word "elimination". However, this is clearly not so, as has been discussed in earlier chapters. Elimination is described by its rate constant K_{el} or by writing that K_{el} = clearance/V. Clearance, in contrast, is K_{el} times V.

5.1.1 ESTIMATION OF CCr WITHOUT A URINE SPECIMEN, BASED ON A SINGLE SCr

There have been two major methods for this estimation, and variants based on them: that of Cockcroft and Gault [1], and that of modification of diet in renal disease (MDRD) [2]. Both of these have been widely employed, and estimates of GFR based on these methods have now been incorporated into routine results supplied with a measurement of SCr by many clinical laboratories.

These methods have been useful for those clinicians who have been content with a general estimate by which to classify a patient's renal function into various ranges or stages of estimated GFR, when the patient is in a stable, steady state.

5.2 PROBLEMS WITH ESTIMATES OF CCr USING ONLY A SINGLE SERUM CREATININE (SCr) SAMPLE

Fig. 5.1 shows the rise over time of SCr following a sudden decrease of CCr, with a sudden decrease in urinary creatinine excretion and the subsequent rise of SCr to a new steady state value. Urinary creatinine excretion also gradually rises as SCr does, until excretion once again equals production and both SCr and urinary excretion become stable again at new equilibrium values. If CCr has not decreased much, the new steady state may be reached within a few days. However, if CCr and urinary excretion are severely decreased, it will require perhaps at least a week before the new steady state is reached.

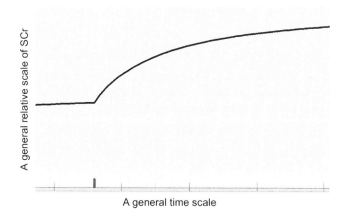

FIGURE 5.1

Time course of the rise in SCr after a decrease in CCr that takes place at the vertical line at the bottom, on the horizontal axis. Horizontal axis: a general time scale. Vertical axis: a general relative scale of SCr concentration. After a change in CCr, SCr begins to change, and several days to at least a week may be required until a new steady state is reached.

Reproduced from Figure 5 in Jelliffe, R., Commentary-Optimal Methodology Is Important for Optimal Pharmacokinetic Studies, Therapeutic Drug Monitoring and Patient Care. Clin Pharmacokin 2015; 54(9):887–892. (doi) 10.1007/s40262-015-0280-4.

If one uses any method based on only a single observation of SCr such as Cockcroft−Gault (CG) or MDRD, when SCr is increasing after a decrease in CCr or decreasing after an increase in CCr, it is most likely that SCr has not reached its new steady state yet. Because of this, the perceived change in CCr is always less than the true change which will not be seen until the SCr reaches its final steady state later on. Furthermore, it is perceived only after renal function has actually changed. With only a single SCr, the estimated change in CCr is too little and is recognized too late.

5.3 ESTIMATING CCr FROM A PAIR OF SCr SAMPLES AT KNOWN TIMES

5.3.1 A DYNAMIC MASS-BALANCE MODEL OF TOTAL BODY CREATININE OVER TIME

A much better estimate of CCr can be achieved by using a pair of SCr samples, C_1 and C_2 at stated times T_1 and T_2, so that the rate of change from the first to the second SCr can be seen. This was first done in [3], and a further version of that approach was done later [4]. In this approach, the basic logic considers the total amount of creatinine in the body at two different times, T_1 and T_2. First, the change in the total amount of creatinine in a patient's body (Delta C) between T_1 and T_2 can be expressed as

$$\text{Delta C} = \text{Production} - \text{Excretion} \tag{5.3}$$

This may be restated as

$$\text{Delta } C = 0.4W(C_2 - C_1) \tag{5.4}$$

and

$$0.4W(C_2 - C_1) = \text{Production} - \text{Excretion} \tag{5.5}$$

where C_1 and C_2 are the SCr's at T_1 and T_2, in mg/dL; W is total body weight, in hundreds of grams; the estimated total volume of distribution of creatinine is felt to be 40% of total body weight; CCr is creatinine clearance, in hundreds of mL/min, and

$$\text{24-}h \text{ urinary creatinine excretion} = C_{\text{avg}} \times \text{CCr} \times 1440 \tag{5.6}$$

Then one can adjust to size for an average body surface area of 1.73 m^2.

5.3.2 CALCULATION OF DAILY CREATININE PRODUCTION (*P*)

5.3.2.1 Age and Creatinine Production

Siersbaek-Nielsen et al. [5] examined the 24-h urinary excretion of creatinine in hospitalized patients who had no clinical evidence of renal disease. The relationship between urinary excretion (*E*) and age (*A*) could be described by

$$E = 29.305 - 0.203\,A \tag{5.7}$$

Furthermore, since all patients were in the steady state, Delta C was zero, and

$$E = P \tag{5.8}$$

In almost every age group studied by Siersbaek-Nielsen et al., the average SCr was 1.1 mg/dL. This information will be useful later.

5.3.2.2 Chronic Uremia and Creatinine Production

Goldman [6] studied patients with chronic uremia of various degrees and found that the greater the degree of chronic uremia, the less urinary creatinine excretion (and therefore production) the patient exhibited. Let PG represent the production found by Goldman. He found the relationship

$$PG = 1344.4 - 43.7C \tag{5.9}$$

One can then bring these two separate data sets and relationships together as follows. First, one can say that, in Goldman's data set, one can use a patient's two SCr values C_1 and C_2 to obtain C_{avg}, and say that

$$PG1 = 1344.4 - 43.7 \times C_{\text{avg}} \tag{5.10}$$

In addition, one can use the average SCr of 1.1 found by Siersbaek-Nielsen as mentioned above, and estimate their figure for production *P* as perceived by Goldman as

$$PG2 = 1344.4 - 43.7 \times 1.1 \tag{5.11}$$

One can then take the ratio *R* of PG1 and PG2, where

$$R = PG1/PG2 \tag{5.12}$$

and use the ratio R to adjust the original estimate of P found by Siersbaek-Nielsen to give a final estimate of production (PF) based on both data sets, as

$$PF = E \times R \tag{5.13}$$

This estimate is for men. For women, 90% of the above value is used, due to their smaller muscle mass. For patients on dialysis, 85% of that final value for men or women is taken, in an attempt to compensate for the further reduction in muscle mass in the sicker and less active dialysis patients. This approach has been implemented in the USC BestDose clinical software [7] and in the MW/Pharm pharmacokinetic software [8] for individualization of drug dosage regimens for patient care. In addition, in the USC BestDose software, the clinician is given an opportunity to enter an estimated muscle mass, as a percent of normal as perceived on gross physical examination, to permit some further refinement of the estimate of production based on perceived muscle mass in muscular, bedridden, or cachectic patients.

5.3.3 CALCULATION OF DAILY CREATININE EXCRETION

Since $C = UV/P$, as in Eq. (5.1), one can rearrange this to

$$PC = UV \tag{5.14}$$

and

$$E = C_{avg} \times CCr \times 1440$$

restated from Eq. (5.6) earlier, where E is in total mg/day, C_{avg} is the average of C_1 and C_2, CCr is in hundreds of mL/min, and 1440 in the number of minutes in a day.

5.4 THE FINAL OVERALL FORMULA

Putting these relationships together, one obtains

$$0.4W(C_2 - C_1)/T = PF - C_{avg} \times CCr \times 1440, \tag{5.15}$$

where W is body weight in hundreds of grams, C_1 and C_2 are in mg/dL, T is the time in days between C_1 and C_2, and C_{avg} is as described above. PF is the final adjusted production rate of creatinine. One can then rearrange this equation and solve for CCr. This value can then be adjusted for the patient's body surface area to give the result in mL/min per 1.73 m^2 of body surface area.

5.5 WHEN DID THE PATIENT'S RENAL FUNCTION CHANGE?

If one uses a method such as CG or MDRD, a change in CCr is perceived only after a change in SCr from a previous value. The underestimated change in CCr is inevitably noted only after the fact. In contrast, when one uses the method described here, CCr is perceived as changing starting from C_1, whenever that was, usually somewhat before the actual change, to C_2. This is because the present method calculates the CCr that makes SCr change from C_1 to C_2 in a patient of the stated age, gender, height, and weight. This may well lead to more responsive tracking and analysis of drug behavior in most unstable patients with high intrapatient variability. While the method may perceive CCr changing somewhat early, at least it is not late and behind the initial event, nor is it inevitably too little.

5.6 UNCERTAINTIES IN THE GOLD STANDARD MEASUREMENT OF CREATININE CLEARANCE

The traditional gold standard measurement of CCr is based on three key measurements: SCr, urinary creatinine concentration, and the 24-h urine volume. Many common laboratory assays have a coefficient of variation of about $\pm 5\%$ for an assay of SCr and about 8% for urinary creatinine. Furthermore, if one is able to collect a 24-h urine specimen with an error of 5%, the errors will propagate approximately as follows. If one squares these errors which are similar to a standard deviation (equivalent to obtaining variances), and adds them, one obtains a total of $25 + 25 + 64 = 114$. Taking the square root of this total, one gets 10.68. Thus the likely coefficient of variation of a classical gold standard determination of CCr is about 11%. Twice this is about 22%. Thus it is likely that the 95% confidence limit about the gold standard determination of CCr is about $\pm 22\%$.

5.7 COMPARISON OF ESTIMATED VERSUS MEASURED CREATININE CLEARANCE

In 15 patients studied in the renal transplant unit at the Los Angeles County−USC Medical Center, 9 men and 6 women, averaging 44.1 years old, and ranging from 21 to 70 years, with an average weight of 135.5 lb, ranging from 105 to 202 lb, who had an average number of 8.5 SCr measurements per patient, ranging from 1 to 25, the present method had an accuracy similar to that found by Jadrny [9].

Furthermore, in 14 patients who had just undergone renal transplantation at the Los Angeles County−USC Medical Center, the standard error of the estimate made with the present method was 14.9 mL/min, with a scatter of about $\pm 25\%$ between estimated and measured values, similar to the 95% confidence limits in the estimate of CCr when obtained by the gold standard (vertical axis) as described earlier. This relationship is shown in Fig. 5.2.

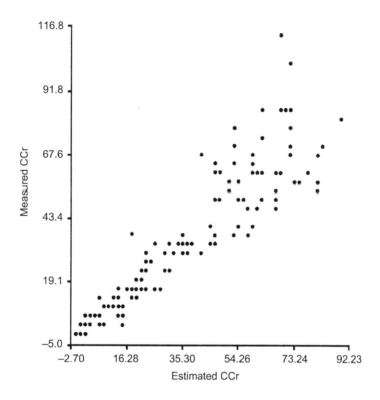

FIGURE 5.2

Comparison of CCr estimated by the method described here (horizontal axis) versus the gold standard—measured CCr using 24-h urine specimens (vertical axis) in 250 observations on 14 patients. The comparison was done starting on the day of surgery, as the transplant took hold and renal function improved thereafter. The scatter shown here is similar to that of the classical gold standard CCr based on a 24-h urine specimen (see text).

Reproduced with permission from Jelliffe R: Estimation of Creatinine Clearance in Patients with Unstable Renal Function,

without a Urine Specimen. Am. J. Nephrology, 22: 320–324, 2002.

5.8 COMPARISON WITH COCKCROFT—GAULT ESTIMATION WHEN SCr IS STABLE

Table 5.1 shows the relationship between the present method (J) and that of Cockroft—Gault (CG) [1] for male and female patients who are 20, 50, and 80 years old. Values are in mL/min per 1.73 m^2 for J and in mL/min for a 72-kg patient for CG.

The table shows that when SCr is stable, the J and CG estimates are quite similar. The advantage of J is seen when SCr is changing, permitting better tracking of drug behavior in unstable patients with changing renal function, as shown in Table 5.2.

Table 5.2 shows the effect of a change in SCr from C_1 to C_2 over 24 h upon the estimate of CCr.

Table 5.1 Comparison of the Present Method (J) With That of Cockroft–Gault (CG)

	Creatinine Clearance Estimate					
	Male (J/CG)			Female (J/CG)		
SCr	20 Years	50 Years	80 Years	20 Years	50 Years	80 Years
0.6	198/200	150/150	102/100	178/170	135/128	92.0/85.0
1.0	117/120	88.7/90.0	60.5/60.0	105/102	79.9/76.5	54.5/51.0
3.0	36.4/40.0	27.6/30.0	18.8/20.0	32.7/34.0	24.8/25.5	16.9/17.0
5.0	20.2/17.1/24.0	15.4/13.0/18.0	10.5/8.9/12.0	18.2/15,4/20.4	13.8/11/7/15.3	9.4/8.0/10.2
10.0	8.2/6.9/12.0	6.2/5.2/9.0	4.2/3.6/6.0	7.3/6.2/10.2	5.8/4.7/7	3.8/3.2/5.1

For SCr from 0.6 through 3.0, values are given as J/CG, while for SCr from 5.0 and 10.0, values are given as J – nondialysis patient/J – dialysis patient/CG.

Table 5.2 Effect of Change in SCr From C_1 to C_2 Over 24 h Upon the Estimate of CCr

C_1 (mg/dL)	C_2 (mg/dL)	Est CCr (mL/min per 1.73 m^2)
0.6	0.6	150
0.6	1.0	102
0.6	3.0	22
0.6	5.0	0.0
1.0	0.6	121
1.0	1.0	89
1.0	3.0	23
1.0	5.0	1.7
3.0	0.6	74
3.0	1.0	62
3.0	3.0	28
3.0	5.0	10
5.0	0.6	74
5.0	1.0	54
5.0	3.0	30
5.0	5.0	15

5.9 SHOULD IDEAL BODY WEIGHT BE USED INSTEAD OF TOTAL BODY WEIGHT?

Since creatinine is produced nonenzymatically from creatine, it might seem logical to use an estimate of nonobese or ideal body weight rather than total body weight in the estimation of creatinine production, especially for obese patients. However, in the author's anecdotal experience with several morbidly obese patients, it has seemed that somewhat better estimates of CCr were obtained using total body weight.

The LAPKB BestDose clinical software [7] provides an option to use either total or ideal body weight, and also, as mentioned earlier, a means for entering an estimate of a patient's apparent muscle mass, based on gross physical examination, as a percent of normal. This accommodates bedridden or cachectic patients on the one hand, or very athletic and muscular patients on the other.

5.10 CHANGING SCr — THE DIRECT CLINICAL LINK BETWEEN THE PATIENT'S CHANGING RENAL FUNCTION AND DRUG BEHAVIOR

To date, much effort has been spent by many on developing the best way to estimate GFR and to link GFR to drug behavior in order to best understand the relationship between renal function and the behavior of drugs. This is especially to be desired for optimal care of acutely ill and highly unstable intensive care unit (ICU) patients. To date, the most precise measurements of GFR are not well suited for the ICU environment.

However, by the process of linking the elimination rate constant of a drug to an estimate of CCr and describing the rate constant as a value (K_{slope}) per unit of estimated CCr, especially when CCr is changing, using the method described in this chapter, one now has a direct link between the behavior of a patient's changing SCr values from time to time through the use of this method of estimating CCr. One can model drug elimination as

$$K_{\text{el}} = K_{\text{slope}} \times \text{CCr} \tag{5.16}$$

It is quite likely, however, that such estimates of CCr for any individual patient may have a systematic bias, based on a systematic bias in the estimation of the volume of distribution of creatinine, or of creatinine production in each patient due to the way in which production has been estimated-total versus ideal body weight, for example. In such cases, if CCr is underestimated, K_{slope} is overestimated, and vice versa.

However, because of this relationship, one now has a direct and self-correcting link between any patient's changing SCr and the overall elimination rate constant, K_{el}, of the drug. This provides a direct empirical link between the patient's changing and unstable renal function and the changing and unstable behavior of the drug. For clinical purposes, this bypasses the need to know GFR precisely, as it links the behavior of the drug directly to the probably biased estimates of CCr, based on the changing values of the patient's SCr, and to its rate of change over time.

Furthermore, when the patient's pharmacokinetic data is analyzed using the interacting multiple model approach described in Chapter 7, one can see not only the direct effect of changing renal function, but also that of dialysis, renal replacement therapy, and extracorporeal membrane oxygenation (ECMO) upon the behavior of the drug. One is in a good position clinically to make optimum use of the patient's data (these patients need much more data and much closer observation than most others) to develop the dosage regimens specifically designed to achieve desired target serum concentrations or effects in the near future, with maximum precision (minimum expected weighted squared error), using multiple model dosage design, as discussed in Chapter 3.

5.11 SUMMARY

Estimation of CCr and of drug behavior from realistically changing rather than assumed stable values of SCr provides a better way to track the behavior of renally excreted drugs in acutely ill and unstable patients, who also may be receiving dialysis, renal replacement therapy, or ECMO. Both SCr and serum drug concentrations can be measured at the beginning and end of such procedures (along with entering a dose of zero at start and end), and also probably at least daily in such patients, along with optimally designed protocols for monitoring serum drug concentrations at the most informative times, as described in Chapter 8. In this way, the behavior of the drug can be tracked most precisely in unstable patients with high intrapatient variability, and maximally precise dosage regimens can be developed to achieve desired target serum drug concentrations for them for the very near future.

REFERENCES

[1] Cockroft D, Gault H. Prediction of creatinine clearance from serum creatinine. Nephron 1976;16:33–41.
[2] Levey AS, Bosch JP, Lewis JB, et al. A more accurate method to estimate glomerular filtration rate from serum creatinine: a new prediction equation. Modification of diet in renal disease study group. Ann Int Med 1999;130(6):461–70.
[3] Jelliffe RW, Jelliffe SM. A computer program for estimation of creatinine clearance from unstable serum creatinine levels, age, sex, and weight. Math Biosci 1972;4:17–24.
[4] Jelliffe R. Estimation of creatinine clearance in patients with unstable renal cunction, without a urine specimen. Am J Nephrol 2002;22:320–4.
[5] Siersbaek-Nielsen K, Moholm Hansen J, Kampmann J, Kristensen J. Estimation of creatinine clearance. Lancet 1971;1:1133.
[6] Goldman R. Creatinine excretion in renal failure. Proc Soc Exp Biol Med 1954;85:446–8.
[7] BestDose The BestDose clinical software is available for evaluation and download at <http://www.lapk.org>.
[8] MWPharm User Manual, Version 3.15, Volume 3, 1995, p. 9.
[9] Jadrny L. Odhad glomerulani filtrace z kreatiniimie. Cas Lek Cesk 1965;104:947–9.

THE CLINICAL SOFTWARE

USING THE BESTDOSE CLINICAL SOFTWARE—EXAMPLES WITH AMINOGLYCOSIDES

6

R. Jelliffe

CHAPTER OUTLINE

6.1 INTRODUCTION—THE BESTDOSE CLINICAL SOFTWARE

The BestDose clinical software for optimal management of individualized drug dosage regimens tor patient care first began back in 1967. It was first known as the USC*PACK software about 1973, and more recently the RightDose and now the BestDose software. It now employs nonparametric (NP) models of the pharmacokinetic behavior of drugs (see Chapter 2) and uses multiple model (MM) design of dosage regimens (see Chapter 3) to hit desired targets with maximum precision (minimum expected weighted squared error). The software employs four different methods of Bayesian analysis (see Chapter 7: Monitoring the Patient: Four Different Bayesian Methods to Make Individual Patient Drug Models) as required to make individual patient PK models in an optimal manner for each patient according to his clinical need and clinical setting.

The present chapter is intended to illustrate the routine use of this software as done for the great majority of clinical situations. The BestDose software is currently available for free evaluation and use from the Web site for our laboratory [1].

Individualized Drug Therapy for Patients. DOI: http://dx.doi.org/10.1016/B978-0-12-803348-7.00006-X

6.2 TWO REPRESENTATIVE DRUGS—AMIKACIN AND GENTAMICIN

Amikacin is a commonly used aminoglycoside antibiotic. Let us consider first how to plan and develop an initial dosage regimen of it for a patient. Then we will consider how to manage a patient who was given gentamicin and has had several past doses and measured serum concentrations, whose renal function has been changing during the time of his dosage history. After that, we will develop an adjusted dosage regimen for him, tailored to the behavior of the drug in him as an individual patient, to hit a desired therapeutic target most precisely. Amikacin and gentamicin are examples of how this software can be used with a number of other drugs. The population model for both drugs was obtained from over 630 patients at seven medical centers in France, some of who were in intensive care units (ICUs) and others who were on various medical services [2].

6.3 PLANNING THE INITIAL REGIMEN

Fig. 6.1 shows the basic screen at the beginning. Across the top, shown better in Fig. 6.2A, are the various tasks and options one can choose such as the "Patient," the "Popmodel," or the population model of the drug you wish to consider using; the "Task," such as fitting the model to the patient's data or simply simulating with the popmodel parameters to see how well the popmodel predicts the

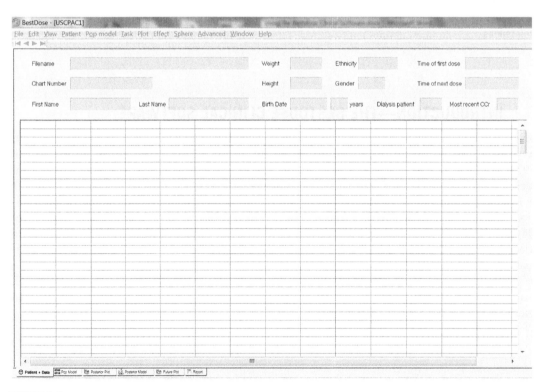

FIGURE 6.1

Basic first screen of BestDose.

patient's data; the "Plot" with its various options; an "Effect" model using a Hill equation to describe the growth of microorganisms and their kill by an antibiotic, which may be useful in some situations (see Chapter 10, Quantitative Modeling of Diffusion into Endocardial Vegetations, the Postantibiotic Effect, and Bacterial Growth and Kill); the "Sphere" option to calculate the drug concentrations at the surface of, or the diffusion into the center of an assumed spherical object such as an endocardial vegetation or a small microorganism; and the "Advanced" options where one selects whether to use the hybrid Bayesian approach or the interacting multiple model (IMM) approach.

Fig. 6.2B shows the bottom of the first screen. Along the bottom are various things relating to the particular patient under consideration: the patient and his relevant data, the data of the popmodel of the selected drug, the posterior plot of the Bayesian posterior model of the behavior of the drug in that patient after fitting it to the data, further details about the patient's Bayesian posterior model, the future plot of the serum concentrations predicted to result from the new dosage regimen given, the report of the analysis of both the past drug behavior, the new dosage regimen, and the predictions of the various areas under curve (AUC) and other numerical results. All of these can be printed out and placed in the patient's chart or pasted into the patient's electronic medical record, if that EMR system permits it.

You can start at the top left and click on "Patient." Select the option "New Patient, Initial Regimen." Fill in the information as in Fig. 6.3.

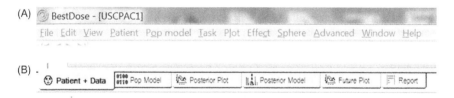

FIGURE 6.2

(A) First screen of BestDose, top of screen. (B) Bottom strip of first screen.

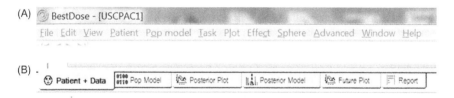

FIGURE 6.3

Entering the patient's data.

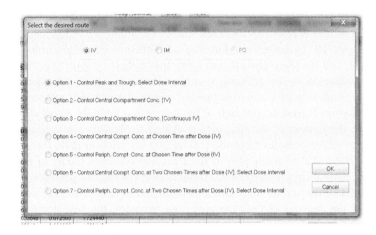

FIGURE 6.4

Menu of options for implementing the dosage regimen.

Here we will consider a 65-year-old male patient, 70 in tall, weighing 70 kg. There is an option at the top right to use the patient's ideal body weight if desired rather than the actual body weight. (Fig. 6.3). You can also select desired units of height and weight.

Then, proceed along the top to "Popmodel," and select the population model of the drug you are using, here amikacin. Then go along the top to "Task" and select "Plan Initial Regimen" for our discussion here.

As shown in Fig. 6.4, note that there are the three possible routes of drug administration and that seven different general dosage options can be chosen. For amikacin, select option 1, "Control Peak and Trough" goal, with later on the dose and dose interval that the software calculates will let you hit your target with the greatest precision. Click "OK."

Next, as shown in Fig. 6.5, BestDose asks about the patient's renal function and estimates a creatinine clearance (CCr) for use for the initial regimen [3]. In the beginning, there is usually only a single serum creatinine (SCr), so enter the SCr as being stable. Enter the patient's present SCr (here 1 mg/dL), and see the estimated CCr of 69.14 mL/min per 1.73 M^2 below. If desired, there is an option to enter the patient's estimated muscle mass (as a percent of normal, evaluated by gross physical examination). This is used mainly to revise the estimate of creatinine production to adjust for cachectic patients with reduced muscle mass and reduced creatinine production. Further, if one clicks that the patient is a dialysis patient, a further 15% reduction in estimated creatinine production is made to better account for production in dialysis patients.

Moreover, one can use this part of the software to compute CCr from any pair of changing SCr values for the stated patient. This is what also happens internally. The software takes the history of the patient's SCr values and computes the CCr between pairs that makes SCr change from the first value and go to the second. The software does this in pairwise fashion throughout the patient's entire history of SCr data. The change in CCr is picked up at the next dose interval. Click "OK." Also, the CCr can be entered directly for each dose interval if desired, as is discussed in Chapter 9, Optimizing Individualized Drug Therapy in the ICU, on ICU patients receiving dialysis, renal replacement therapy, or extracorporeal membrane oxygenation.

As shown in Fig. 6.6, enter the target peak goal, say 45 μg/mL, and the target trough goal, say 3 μg/mL. Use your knowledge or impression of the probable minimum inhibitory concentration

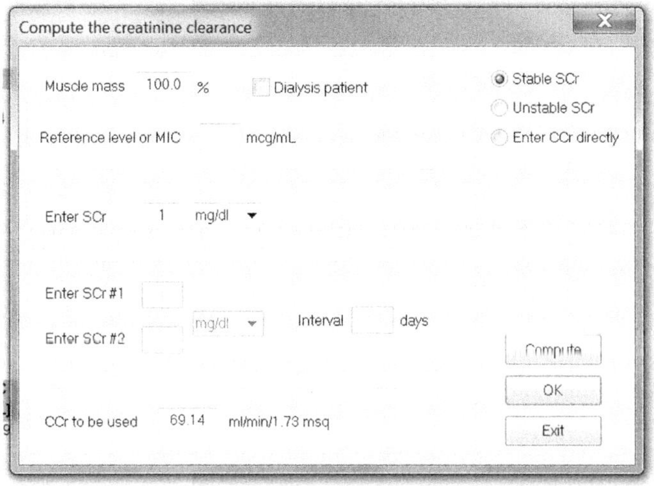

FIGURE 6.5

Entering data of serum creatinine and estimating creatinine clearance.

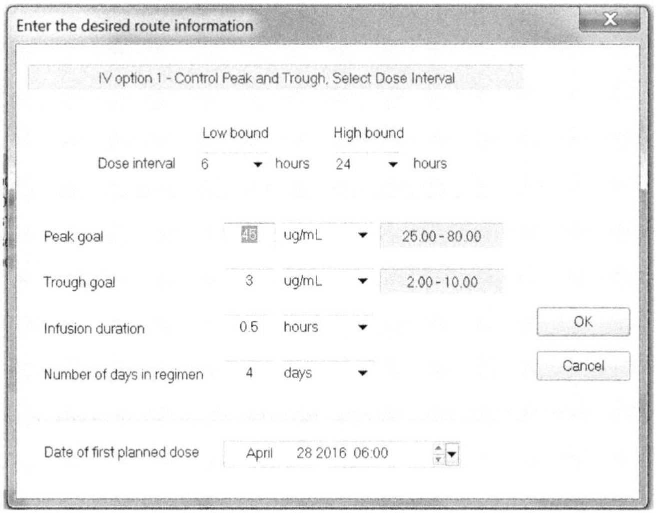

FIGURE 6.6

Entering data to determine the dosage regimen.

(MIC) of the patient's organism in choosing your target. Now enter your desired infusion duration, say 0.5 h, and the number of days for which you wish this initial regimen to be calculated, say 4 days, to see the general format of the regimen.

BestDose uses MM dosage design (see Chapter 3) to develop the regimen for that number of days, calculating and minimizing the weighted squared error with which the various candidate regimens (every 6, 8, 12, 24 h, etc.) hit the desired target goals. It then takes the overall expected weighted squared error for each candidate regimen over the stated number of days, divides it by the number of times the goal is desired to be achieved (4 times daily for every 6 h, once daily for 24 h). It then takes the square root of that to show you this index of the degree of failure of each candidate regimen to hit the desired target, and displays this for you to see. It also suggests the index with the least error. You choose the dose interval you wish to use. Make sure you also approve of or revise the desired lower and upper ranges of the dose interval, at the top right corner. Patients with poor renal function often need to have the upper dose interval extended to 48, 72, or 96 h, for example, in order to achieve the desired trough goal most precisely and not end up with a high trough because you did not extend the dose interval long enough.

BestDose calculates the various candidate regimens and displays their associated error indices on a graph, as shown in Fig. 6.7. You select the dose interval you wish to use. For many

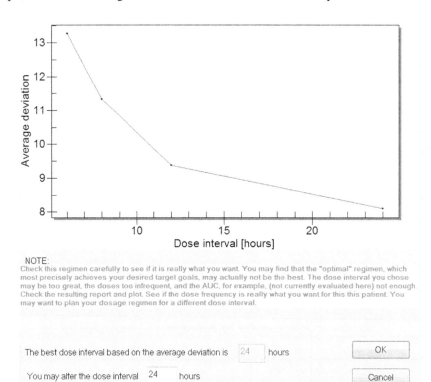

NOTE:
Check this regimen carefully to see if it is really what you want. You may find that the "optimal" regimen, which most precisely achieves your desired target goals, may actually not be the best. The dose interval you chose may be too great, the doses too infrequent, and the AUC, for example, (not currently evaluated here) not enough. Check the resulting report and plot. See if the dose frequency is really what you want for this this patient. You may want to plan your dosage regimen for a different dose interval.

The best dose interval based on the average deviation is 24 hours   OK

You may alter the dose interval 24 hours   Cancel

FIGURE 6.7

Showing the best dose interval. BestDose develops the combination of dose and dose interval to hit the peak and trough targets most precisely.

concentration-dependent drugs such as the aminoglycosides, it is commonly felt that the peak/MIC ratio or the AUC/MIC ratio are the best indices. Do not let that catch you up. The crucial key is the dose interval, or how often the dose is given that hits your desired peak. If the dose interval is too long, the serum concentrations may be below the MIC for too long, and the bugs may start to grow out again (see Chapter 10: Quantitative Modeling of Diffusion into Endocardial Vegetations, the Postantibiotic Effect, and Bacterial Growth and Kill). Once you select your desired dose interval, BestDose displays the ideal dose regimen, the numerical predictions, the predicted AUC, and the running total AUC in both the central (serum) and peripheral (nonserum) compartments. However, if you order this ideal regimen, you may not be in the good graces of the nurses and pharmacists, who must prepare and give the doses.

However, knowing the ideal regimen, you can now go back to the task option at the top, select "Revise Dose Regimen," and replace each ideal dose with your best approximation of it.

Here, for example, the ideal regimen was revised to be 1000 mg every 24 h. Then you can select "Report," which displays the doses and the numerical results predicted from it, as in Figs. 6.8 and 6.9,

Planning Future Therapy							
Route	IV Option 1 - Control Peak and Trough, Select Dose Interval						

Goal 1	45.00 [ug/mL]		Goal 2	3.00 [ug/mL]
Time 1	0.50 [hours]		Time 2	24.00 [hours]

ObjFunc	8.0990	AUC	867.40

Dose #	Date	Time	Dose [mg]	AUC [ug/mL]	Total AUC [ug/mL]	AUC [ug/kg]	Total AUC [ug/kg]
1	04/28/16	06:00	1017.9453	210.3434	210.3434	48.3134	48.3134
2	04/29/16	06:00	997.6988	216.6755	427.0188	85.6189	133.9323
3	04/30/16	06:00	993.2691	219.0994	646.1182	118.5499	252.4823
4	05/01/16	06:00	990.8038	221.2834	867.4017	152.3524	404.8347

Goal #	Time [h]	Goal	WgtAvg	Diff
1	0.50	45.00	44.99	-0.01
2	24.00	3.00	0.93	-2.07
3	24.50	45.00	44.98	-0.02
4	48.00	3.00	1.12	-1.88
5	48.50	45.00	44.97	-0.03
6	72.00	3.00	1.22	-1.78
7	72.50	45.00	44.97	-0.03
8	96.50	3.00	1.25	-1.75

Patient + Data   Pop Model   Posterior Plot   Posterior Model   Future Plot   Report

FIGURE 6.8

Display of ideal initial regimen.

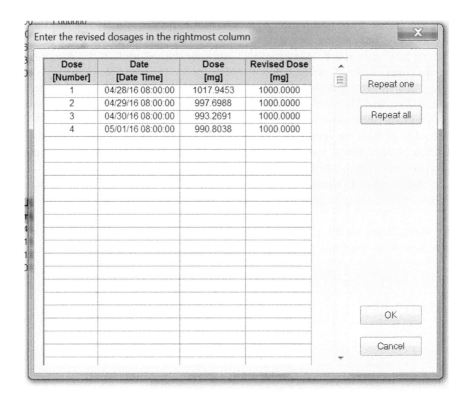

Enter the revised dosages in the rightmost column

Dose [Number]	Date [Date Time]	Dose [mg]	Revised Dose [mg]
1	04/28/16 08:00:00	1017.9453	1000.0000
2	04/29/16 08:00:00	997.6988	1000.0000
3	04/30/16 08:00:00	993.2691	1000.0000
4	05/01/16 08:00:00	990.8038	1000.0000

Repeat one

Repeat all

OK

Cancel

FIGURE 6.9

Display of revised regimen.

and you can also select "Future Plot" to see the plot of it. In Fig. 6.10, instead of showing only the trajectory of the weighted average concentration, we have gone up to the "Plot" option at the top, selected the option to "See Support Points," and clicked to see the 99% most likely support points. Here we can see the real diversity of the predictions due to the diversity among the 637 patients from the seven centers in France from whom this population model was developed [2].

In addition, one can place the cursor anywhere along the plot. When it changes from an arrow to a pointing finger, one can click and see a cross section of all the predictions at that time, as shown in Fig. 6.11, for the very first peak. Not shown here, one also can click, drag the cursor over a selected rectangular field, and release to see a magnified view of the selected field. Type the letter "Z" to remove the magnification.

The great diversity of the predictions also shows the need for TDM here.

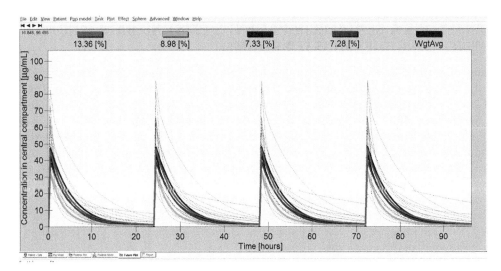

FIGURE 6.10

Future plot of serum concentrations predicted from this regimen, seeing the 99% most likely support points. The most probable prediction, in red, has a probability of 13.36%, as shown at the top left. The weighted average prediction is shown in black.

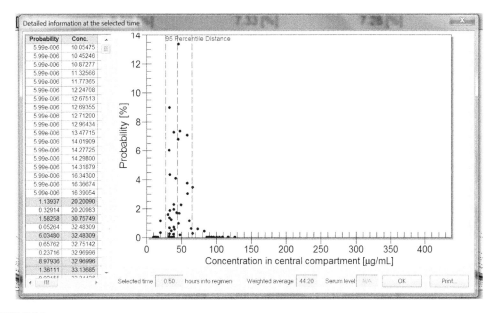

FIGURE 6.11

Profile plot of predicted serum concentrations at the time of the desired first peak of 45 μg/mL. Central dashed vertical line—weighted average prediction—here 45 μg/mL as desired. Vertical dashed lines to its right and left show the 95% ranges of these predictions, from about 27 to 66 μg/mL, similar to 95% confidence limits in an assumed Gaussian or normal distribution. Horizontal axis shows the predicted concentration at the selected time. Vertical axis shows the predicted probability of the predicted concentration.

6.4 ANALYZING A GENTAMICIN PATIENT'S EXISTING DATA, AND DEVELOPING THE ADJUSTED REGIMEN

The patient illustrated here was a 65-year-old man, 70 in tall, weighing 68 kg. He received genta-micin. He was not a dialysis patient. Note the important question in the lower right part of the screen in Fig. 6.12 concerning when you wish to start the first dose in the new future regimen. This serves to end the analysis of the past and to begin the future regimen. BestDose usually has this set to tomorrow as the usual default day. Make sure that you specify the day and time when you want to begin the new regimen. The first dose of the new regimen will be given at that time.

Go to "New Patient, Past History" and click. When the screen comes up, be sure first to click "Cancel" at the bottom left. Then select "New Patient" at the bottom center. Here we have entered that he is age 65, male, and height 70 in, as in Fig. 6.12.

Now, click on "Select Doses" at the top. Choose "gentamicin," as this is what the patient received. The menu to enter the past doses appears. Double click on the row to enter each dose, as shown in this view of two composite screens in Fig. 6.13.

Next, in exactly the same way, go up to the top, and click to enter the serum concentrations, the body weight, and the patient's SCr results, all in the same general format of date, time (0000 to 2359 h), and the value to be entered. Then click "Save to File," give it a name, and save it. Use either

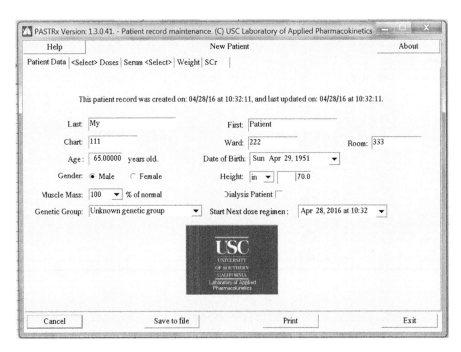

FIGURE 6.12

Entering the patient's data.

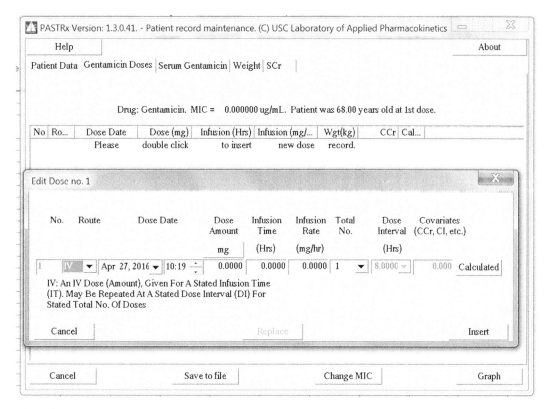

FIGURE 6.13

Ready to enter the patient's doses.

the .mb2 newer format or the older .MB format (see Chapter 9: Optimizing Individualized Drug Therapy in the ICU).

Fig. 6.14 summarizes that data as if it came from a patient whose file had already been saved that way. Under the data of doses, note that the data from the SCr measurements has been used to compute the CCr that makes the SCr change from one value at a stated time to another at another stated time in a patient having the stated age, gender, height, and weight. Here, CCr began at 56.47 mL/min per 1.73 M^2 but changed to 41 as the SCr rose from 1.2 to 1.5, then changed to 27 as SCr rose further from 1.5 to 2.1 mg/dL. The BestDose software uses SCr data pairwise throughout the history of the patient's SCr data to compute the CCr between the pairs.

In addition, the patient's weight can change throughout his history. That is why the weight is entered as are all the other events: day, time, and value. BestDose uses linear interpolation between the weight data to estimate the patient's weight at the start of each dose interval and sets the volume of distribution for each dose interval in that way.

Fig. 6.15 shows the analysis of the data as predicted from the population model alone, before any fitting to the data yet.

Filename	C:\Program Files (x86)\BestDose\patients\GENT2.MB					Weight	68.00 kg		Ethnicity	Not in use		Time of first dose	04/01/80 08:00:00
Chart Number	123					Height	70.00 in		Gender	Male		Time of next dose	04/03/80 16:00:00
First Name	patient		Last Name	alan forrests		Birth Date	04/01/15	65 years		Dialysis patient	NO	Most recent CCr	27.10

Dose	Route	Date	Time	Time	Weight	Descriptor	IV inf. Time	Dose Interv	IV Rate	Amount		
[#]	[IM/IV/PO]	[locale]	[hh:mm:ss]	[Hours]	[kg]	[CCr,Cf]	[Hours]	[Hours]	[mg/Hour]	[mg]		
1	IV	04/01/80	08:00:00	0.00	68.00	56.47	1.000	8.50	80.00	80.00		
2	IV	04/01/80	16:30:00	8.50	68.00	41.34	1.000	9.75	80.00	80.00		
3	IM	04/02/80	02:15:00	18.25	68.00	41.34	0.000	6.00	0.00	100.00		
4	IV	04/02/80	08:15:00	24.25	68.00	41.34	1.000	8.50	100.00	100.00		
5	IV	04/02/80	16:45:00	32.75	68.00	27.10	1.000	15.25	100.00	100.00		
6	IV	04/03/80	08:00:00	48.00	68.00	27.10	1.000	8.00	80.00	80.00		

Level		Date	Time	Time	After dose	After dose				Conc.	
[Number]		[locale]	[hh:mm:ss]	[Hours]	[Number]	[Hours]				[ug/mL]	
1		04/01/80	09:20:00	1.33	1	1.33				3.6000	
2		04/01/80	15:35:00	7.58	1	7.58				1.8000	
3		04/02/80	06:10:00	22.17	3	3.92				5.2000	
4		04/02/80	18:20:00	34.33	5	1.58				9.1000	
5		04/03/80	07:40:00	47.67	5	14.92				4.1000	

SCr		Date	Time	Time	After dose	After dose				Conc.	
[Number]		[locale]	[hh:mm:ss]	[Hours]	[Number]	[Hours]				[mg/dL]	
1		04/01/80	09:20:00	1.33	1	1.33				1.2000	
2		04/02/80	09:00:00	25.00	4	0.75				1.5000	
3		04/03/80	12:00:00	52.00	6	4.00				2.1000	

FIGURE 6.14

Summary of data entered.

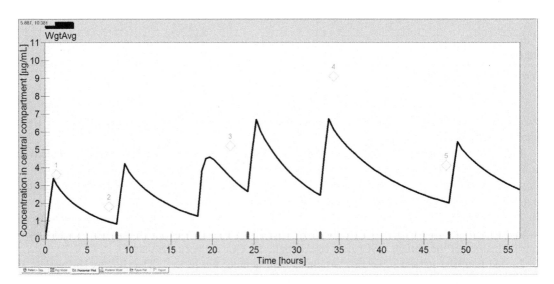

FIGURE 6.15

Analysis of the patient's data from the population model alone before any fitting to the data. Dark line shows the weighted average predicted concentration. Empty diamonds represent the measured but as yet unfitted serum concentrations.

Fig. 6.16 shows the poor prediction of the patient's third serum concentration without fitting to the data yet. The patient clearly is not an average patient, and the predictions are quite variable. The measured concentration of 5.2 μg/mL is far above the weighted average prediction of 3.47 and fairly close to the upper 97.5 percentile value.

Fig. 6.17 shows the same thing as in Fig. 6.15, but now after fitting to the patient's data and obtaining the Bayesian posterior individualized model for this patient. Note the good fit, even in the presence of his changing renal function as his CCr changed from an initial value of 56 to 41 to 27 mL/min per 1.73 M^2 during his history. This also shows the value of estimating CCr based on pairs of changing SCr measurements rather than having to assume that each SCr was a stable value (see Chapter 5: Evaluation of Renal Function).

Fig. 6.18 shows the improved prediction of the same third serum gentamicin concentration that was shown in Fig. 6.16. The percentile distribution is much narrower, showing us graphically just how much our TDM has done for us and how much more precise is our knowledge of the patient at this time.

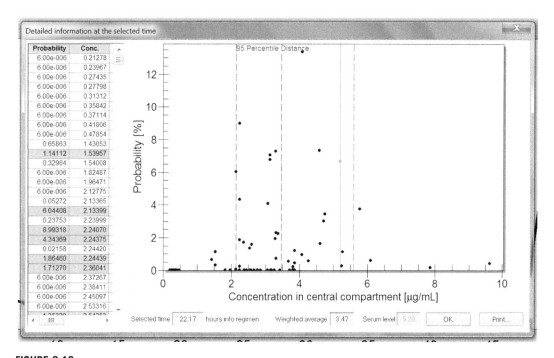

FIGURE 6.16

Prediction of the patient's third serum gentamicin concentration based on the population model alone before any fitting to the data yet. Horizontal axis shows the concentration. Vertical solid line with dot halfway up is the measured concentration of 5.2 μg/mL. Central dashed line is the weighted average prediction of 3.47 μg/mL. Outside dashed lines are the 2.5 and 97.5 percentiles of the distribution. Note the skewness toward the right of the weighted average due to the nonparametric nature of the modeling process, which makes no assumptions at all about the shape of the distributions of the predicted serum concentrations.

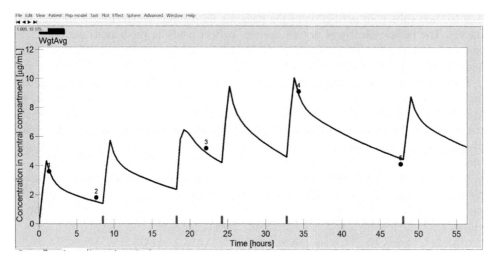

FIGURE 6.17

Plot of patient's weighted average concentration after fitting to his data. Dots represent measured serum concentrations. Note the improved relationship between predicted and measured data after fitting.

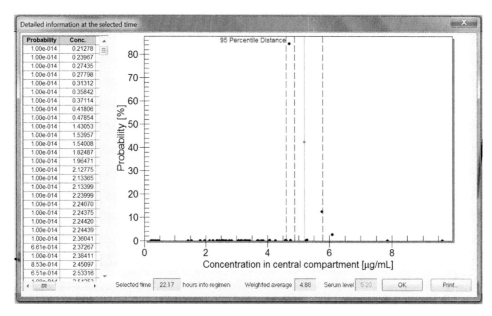

FIGURE 6.18

Profile of predictions of the patient's third serum concentration after fitting to his data. Note the visual evidence of the improved estimation after fitting. This plot shows graphically just what the process of TDM does for our understanding of drug behavior in each individual patient. In addition, note the much greater percent probability with the much fewer predictions, with the maximum probability of 84% now, another of 12%, another of 2.6 %, and all the other predictions with much smaller probability after Bayesian fitting to the data.

6.5 **THE EFFECT MODEL**

We can also examine the possible quantitative effect of the trajectory of the patient's serum concentrations upon the possible kill of the organism. This can be seen with the effect model (see Chapter 10: Quantitative Modeling of Diffusion into Endocardial Vegetations, the Postantibiotic Effect, and Bacterial Growth and Kill), which here describes the relationship between pseudomonas and gentamicin found by Corvaisier et al. [4]. This effect model is another way to evaluate the effectiveness of a regimen in addition to the more usual ones such as peak/MIC or AUC/MIC ratios (Figs. 6.19 and 6.20).

Here in Fig. 6.19 we see that the high trough concentrations, which are often associated with toxicity, are also quite above the assumed MIC of 2 μg/mL here and that bacterial kill continues while the concentrations are above the MIC. This approach lets us step away from the empirical correlations of kill such as peak/MIC or AUC/MIC and begin to examine the possible time course of these bacterial events. This is discussed more fully in Chapter 10, Quantitative Modeling of Diffusion into Endocardial Vegetations, the Postantibiotic Effect, and Bacterial Growth and Kill.

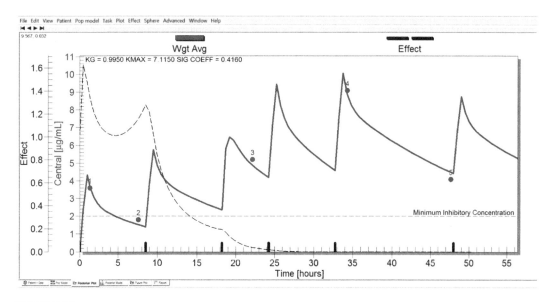

FIGURE 6.19

Possible time course of the kill of pseudomonas by gentamicin. Vertical effect axis shows the possible number of colony forming units, starting with an assumed inoculum of 1.0 (For example think 1 million) relative units of organisms. Thick line shows the weighted average serum concentration over time. Thin dashed line shows the calculated relative number of organisms.

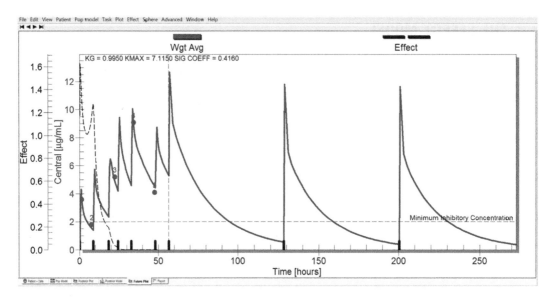

FIGURE 6.20

Plot of predicted future serum gentamicin concentrations and of their possible successful effect here on killing of an organism such as pseudomonas, having an assumed MIC of 2 µg/mL. Other values for MIC can be entered and evaluated as well.

6.6 PLANNING THE NEW ADJUSTED DOSAGE REGIMEN

Here we have gone to "Plan Future Regimen," similar to planning the initial one. We entered as our target goals a peak of 12 µg/mL, a trough of 0.5 µg/mL, a desired infusion time for each dose of 0.5 h, and that we would like to develop the most precise regimen for the next 8 days to see the doses as they approach a steady state. Because the patient's CCr is now down to 27, the ideal regimen is 109, 185, and 185 mg every 72 h. This is revised, just as with the initial regimen before, to 120, 180, and 180 mg every 72 h. Here we get a warning in red that the first dose of 120 mg is more than 10% away from the ideal dose, just to let us know in case we might wish to change it to something else. We click "OK" and see the future plot.

In this case, Fig. 6.20 shows the possible effect [4], again for an assumed MIC of 2 µg/mL. We see that the desired peaks and troughs are closely achieved and that bacterial kill will probably continue, even though we now have achieved more conventional target values for our peak and trough concentrations. The effect scale on the vertical axis of the plot is a relative scale. It starts with an arbitrary value of 1.0 (think 1 million) organisms. We see that even in the presence of reduced renal function, we have been able to develop a dosage regimen for this patient, which achieves our desired target goals with maximum precision (a unique capability of MM dosage design), (see Chapter 3), and that the serum concentration profile over time is likely to continue to be effective clinically, as no further growth is predicted to return.

6.7 SUMMARY

This chapter has shown how to use the BestDose clinical software to develop an initial dosage regimen for a patient, and how to enter and store data of a new patient who has had data of past doses, serum concentrations, and other relevant information, and save the file. We have seen how to analyze this data, make a useful reconstruction of past events, and how to develop a new, adjusted dosage regimen to take that individual patient into the future of his therapy in an optimally precise manner.

REFERENCES

[1] The BestDose clinical software is available for free download and evaluation at <www.lapk.org>.
[2] Jelliffe R, Laffont A, Barbaut X, Girard P, Chapelle G, Pobel C, et al. Pharmacokinetics of amikacin in a large population using the NPEM algorithm. Clin Pharmacol Ther 1994;160 PII-30.
[3] Jelliffe R. Estimation of creatinine clearance in patients with unstable renal function, without a urine specimen. Am J Nephrol 2002;22:320−4.
[4] Corvaisier S, Maire PH, Bouvier d'Yvoire MY, Barbaut X, Bleyzac N, Jelliffe RW. Comparisons between antimicrobial pharmacodynamic indices and bacterial killing as described by using the Zhi model. Antimicrob Agents Chemother 1998;42(7):1731−7.

MONITORING THE PATIENT: FOUR DIFFERENT BAYESIAN METHODS TO MAKE INDIVIDUAL PATIENT DRUG MODELS

R. Jolliffe, A. Schumitzky, D. Bayard and M. Neely

CHAPTER OUTLINE

7.1 INTRODUCTION

Consider the following scenario. You have just seen an advertisement for a product that has caught your interest. You are considering whether or not to buy it. The ad was in a newspaper you like. Your interest in the product is moderate. This constitutes the current state of your information and your interest in the product.

Now consider two differing subsequent experiences. In the first, you now see a TV commercial for that product. It is on a late night channel that commonly carries commercials for a number of questionable products. How has that experience affected your view of that product?

Now consider another possible experience. This time, instead of the TV commercial, someone whom you know well and for whose opinion you have great regard discusses the same product with enthusiasm. How has this experience affected your view of the product?

Individualized Drug Therapy for Patients. DOI: http://dx.doi.org/10.1016/B978-0-12-803348-7.00007-1

In each case, we have (1) an initial impression about the quality of the product. Then we have (2) some new information, and (3) a revised opinion of the product based on each set of information.

The Reverend Thomas Bayes was a Presbyterian minister in Anglican England, living not very far from London. He died in 1760. He was also a mathematician, and he developed a method for expressing the previous scenarios in quantitative form. The three steps in the scenario above are now called:

1. The Bayesian Prior: the estimate of the probability of a certain event prior to obtaining some new information about it — the Bayesian *prior probability.*
2. The *new data.*
3. The revised, or *posterior probability* of that event, after (posterior to) both the initial impression (the prior) and the new data.

Bayes' theorem, as it is now called, is used in an amazing variety of areas, from medicine to finance to the military, as it describes in quantitative terms how we learn from experience. For our purposes, we use it here to make models of the behavior of drugs in individual patients, by

1. Making population pharmacokinetic and dynamic models of drug behavior in patients. These are the Bayesian priors. Each population model needs a measure of its credibility — see Chapter 2.
2. Monitoring the behavior of the drug in an individual patient by drawing blood and measuring the concentration of drug in serum or whole blood, or perhaps dried blood spots in the future, or an effect. Each measurement should have a measure of its credibility — see Chapter 4.
3. One then uses Bayes' theorem to make the individual model, the Bayesian posterior model, to best understand the behavior of the drug in an individual patient who appears to belong to the population of patients who have made up the Bayesian prior.

The Bayesian posterior model is then used to analyze the past and to develop an adjusted dosage regimen of the drug to hit a future target serum concentration or effect at a desired time for that individual patient, with the greatest possible precision — see Chapter 3.

7.2 BUT FIRST, WEIGHTED NONLINEAR LEAST SQUARES REGRESSION

However, let us first start with weighted nonlinear least squares (WNLLS) regression. This is not a Bayesian method, but can be thought of as a stepping stone to a commonly used Bayesian method (see below). WNLLS finds the single-valued model parameter estimates that fit data of an individual patient "best." This procedure finds the single-point model parameter values that minimize the sum of all the weighted squared differences between the estimated values of the data and the data itself. There is no mention or consideration of anything like a population prior.

WNLLS starts with an initial estimate of the model parameter values. It simulates the behavior of the system, using the dosage regimen given to the patient, to predict what the measured serum concentrations might be at the times they were drawn, using the current model parameter values under consideration. It finds the difference between each estimated and its corresponding measured concentration, squares that difference divides it by the variance of each measurement, and adds up all these weighted squared differences to obtain the total sum of the weighted squared differences.

Having done that, the method considers other parameter values that might fit the data better, using, for example, the Nelder-Mead simplex method [1], and eventually finds the parameter values that minimize this total difference. The basic expression that is minimized is the sum of all (Conc. observed—conc. predicted)^2/Var conc predicted. This can be written as

$$Sum\left[\frac{(C_{obs}-C_{pred})^2}{Var\ Conc\ Pred}\right] \tag{7.1}$$

Note that each concentration is weighted by the reciprocal of its variance (Var). Chapter 4 Optimizing Laboratory Assay Methods for Individualized Therapy, deals with the issue of the variance of laboratory assay measurements as the proper measure of the credibility of each measurement, and the estimation of noise and uncertainty in the clinical environment in which each patient's therapy takes place.

This concludes our discussion of WNLLS. Note again that there is no mention of any prior experience with a population model of the drug, only the data for a single patient, and a model whose single-point parameter values are estimated.

7.3 USING BAYES' THEOREM IN ANALYZING DATA, USING PARAMETRIC PK MODELS

This is called maximum a posteriori probability (MAP) Bayesian analysis. It computes the single-point mean model parameter values that are most likely (which have maximum probability) given the population prior and the new data. It has been shown that MAP Bayesian analysis permits better prediction of the future than WNLLS, as it takes into account past experience with similar patients. Remember that parametric PK models assume that the population distribution of each PK model parameter is a normal Gaussian (or lognormal) distribution, which is described by single-valued numbers that summarize the *assumed* shape of the distribution, such as a mean and standard deviation (SD), and remember also that the square of the SD is the variance.

7.3.1 MAP BAYESIAN ANALYSIS

Here a new term is added to the objective function to be minimized: the prior information from past experience with similar patients, in the form of the population model serving as the Bayesian prior. So we now have two terms to minimize in the overall expression. They are:

The sum of all ((Conc. observed − conc. predicted)^2/Var conc predicted). It is exactly like WNLLS, but now there is also another term as shown below:

The sum of all ((Population parameter value − Bayesian posterior parameter estimate)^2/Var population parameter value). All this can be written as in 7.2.

$$Sum\left[\frac{(C_{obs}-C_{est})^2}{Var\ Conc\ est}\right] + Sum\left[\frac{(Pop\ param-Pt\ param\ est)^2}{Var\ Pop\ param\ est}\right] \tag{7.2}$$

Here the fitting procedure minimizes the squared difference between the measured assay concentration and its estimate (weighted by the reciprocal of its variance) while *at the same time* minimizing the squared difference between each population parameter value (each also weighted by the reciprocal of its variance) and each MAP Bayesian posterior parameter estimate for that patient. Thus we have considered both types of data and their credibility, and have arrived at the best overall fit to both types of data, to get the MAP Bayesian posterior model (Pt param est) for each individual patient.

Note that the important job of weighting each type of data, both in the assay data and in the population model parameters, is done by the variance term in the denominator for each type of data. There is the variance of each data point from the patient, which ideally will include both that of the assay plus that in the clinical environment in which the patient's therapy took place. There is also the variance of the model parameter values, which also ideally is the total of both assay and clinical uncertainty in the study from which the population model was made. A precise assay will pull the fit toward the patient's data. A very uniform population model, on the other hand, will keep the fit pulled back toward the population model parameter values. This tug-of-war between the two types of data (the relative credibility of each) determines where the fit will go. It never goes all the way to the assay data as it is held back by the population prior parameter values. This "holding back" of the fit by the population model prior is called "shrinkage" by the PK community.

7.4 BAYESIAN ANALYSIS FOR NONPARAMETRIC (NP) MODELS

Here, for NP models, instead of considering only a single-valued summary point for each parameter that is used to describe the central tendency of the assumed distribution, *each* discrete support point in the population model is considered separately and the *entire* parameter distribution is analyzed. No assumptions at all are made, or need to be made, concerning the shape of the distribution.

The process starts by considering each population model support point in turn. Each support point has its estimated probability in the population. Then the new data from the patient is considered, and the Bayesian posterior probability of that particular support point is calculated.

A support point having model parameter values that predict (fit or describe) the patient's data well becomes much more probable given that data. A support point having parameter values that predict (fit or describe) the data poorly becomes much less probable. In this way, the entire collection of support points has all of its probabilities revised, using Bayes' theorem, based on the data from that individual patient. More details are given in the appendix at the end of this chapter.

Fig. 7.1 shows a three-dimensional (3D) plot of the central volume of distribution (VS1) and the elimination rate constant (KS1) for the population model of gentamicin in the Laboratory of Applied Pharmacokinetics and Bioinformatics (LAPKB) BestDose software. Many points having significant probability are seen in this population model, reflecting the diversity of the patients from which it was made.

Based on this population model, Fig. 7.2 shows the diverse predictions of the third of an individual patient's five serum gentamicin concentrations made using the population model

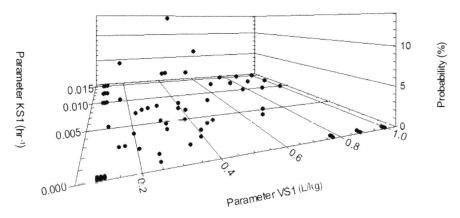

FIGURE 7.1

3D plot of the two-compartment (six-parameter) nonparametric gentamicin population model showing the central (serum) compartment apparent volume of distribution (VS1, L/kg, horizontal axis), the elimination rate constant slope per unit of creatinine clearance (KS1 in hr^{-1}, axis receding from front to back), and the probability of the various support points (vertical). The other four model parameters (Ka, Kint, Kcp, and Kpc) are not shown here. Data from 637 patients in 7 different centers in France has been compressed into 40 support points of significant probability, ranging up to 13.4%. Clusters of nine additional support points of extremely low probability have been added at each corner of the plot to extend the working range of the population model.

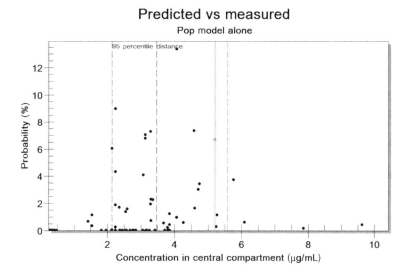

FIGURE 7.2

Plot of the third of the patient's five measured serum concentrations made using only the population model alone, without any fitting. The measured concentration—the dot halfway up the plot, with the solid vertical line through it—is 5.2 μg/mL. Weighted average prediction = 3.47 μg/mL, the dashed central vertical line. Other dots are other predicted concentrations and their probabilities. Note that the 95 percentile distance of the predictions is skewed and ranges widely, from about 2.15 up to about 5.6 μg/mL.

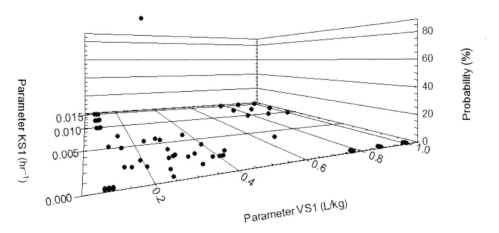

FIGURE 7.3

Plot of an individual patient's nonparametric Bayesian posterior gentamicin model central (serum) compartment apparent volume of distribution (VS1, L/kg, horizontal axis), elimination rate constant slope per unit of creatinine clearance (KS1 in hr^{-1} per unit of creatinine clearance, axis receding from front to back), and probability of support points (vertical). The Bayesian posterior probability has been computed for each model parameter support point given the patient's data. The point with maximum probability is now 84%. Another point (poorly seen) has 12% probability. Still another has 2.6%. These points are the survivors after the Bayesian analysis. They constitute the Bayesian posterior distribution for this individual patient.

alone, before any fitting to the patient's data. Again, note that the most probable support point only has about 13.4% probability, and remember that the probabilities of all the support points total 100%. This figure shows the poor prediction of the individual patient's measured concentration taken at that time, due to the diversity of the PK behavior of gentamicin in the patients making up the population and to the fact that this patient was not an "average" patient.

Fig. 7.3 shows the revised NP Bayesian posterior model after fitting it to data of the five measured serum concentrations obtained from the gentamicin patient described in Chapter 6. Note that there are many fewer support points of significant probability, only those that did a good job of predicting the patient's serum concentration data. The highest point now has 84% probability, the next highest 12%, and the third highest 2.6%. Actually, only the very highest point is well seen in this figure, but all their predictions of the third of the patient's five measured serum concentrations (shown first in Fig. 7.2 before fitting to the data) are also shown in Fig. 7.4.

Fig. 7.4 shows the individual predictions of the same third serum concentration as in Fig. 7.2. Note the greatly increased precision (much narrower 95% distance, now only from about 4.6 to 5.8 μg/mL) with which that measured concentration is now predicted after fitting to the patient's data. This plot shows us graphically what therapeutic drug monitoring (TDM) and proper software can do quantitatively to increase our knowledge of drug behavior in an individual patient.

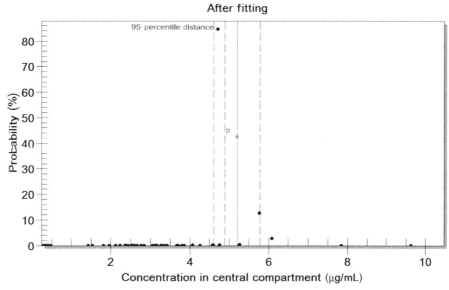

Predicted vs measured

After fitting

FIGURE 7.4

Plot of the third of the patient's five measured serum concentrations made after fitting the population model to the patient's data. The measured concentration—the dot halfway up the plot, with the solid vertical line through it—is 5.2 μg/mL. Weighted average prediction is 4.84 μg/mL, the central dashed vertical line. Other dots: predicted concentrations and their probabilities. Note that the 95 percentile distance of the predictions (the outer two dashed vertical lines) is much narrower now, only from about 4.6 up to about 5.8 μg/mL. This plot shows quantitatively just how much therapeutic drug monitoring can increase our knowledge of drug behavior in individual patients, and thus in the precision with which the adjusted dosage regimen, now based on this individual patient's Bayesian posterior model, can hit the target concentration with the maximally precise dose, using MM dosage design.

7.5 **HYBRID BAYESIAN ANALYSIS**

A limitation of nonparametric PK models is that the model parameters can only exist within a certain stated range. However, some unusual patients will have parameters in an area where there are very few support points, and the knowledge of their parameters may be rendered less precise because of that. In addition, some very unusual patients may have parameters totally outside the stated range. We wished to develop a method to deal with these problems.

The Hybrid Bayesian approach [2] is an ad hoc method that combines the strengths of both the MAP Bayesian and the nonparametric Bayesian methods. It begins with a MAP estimate. Then a grid of extra support points is placed to cover the region of the MAP estimate more widely. Since we now know that this is the area in which the patient's data is going to take the estimate, we know in advance that this region will have considerable probability. We therefore arbitrarily chose to give this grid a default probability of 50% and to combine this grid with the original population model, which is also given 50% default probability, to make an augmented population model. The grid currently can have a total of 16 to 100 points, including the MAP estimate, and it currently has a 5–20% change in value between the support points. One can select any grid and can have any percent change between grid points. Then an NP Bayesian analysis is done as described previously, but on this larger augmented model.

The hybrid analysis provides more support points in the region of the patient's MAP estimate where the patient's parameters may be located when the patient is within the ranges of the population model parameter values, with resulting more precise estimates of the patient's parameter distributions and of the patient's measured serum concentrations. On the other hand, when the patient is quite unusual, even having model parameter values far outside the ranges of the population model, one can still obtain good ad hoc fits to the patient's data by adjusting the weights of the MAP prior downward and revising the relative probabilities of the population model and the grid.

The overall process of the Hybrid Bayesian procedure is shown in Fig. 7.5. The process of computing the MAP estimate is guided by the quantities *imap, mpar, saf,* and *prange,* which are specified by the user.

If *imap* = 1, then only the volume VS1 and elimination rate constant KS1 are optimized in the MAP estimation process, and the remaining model parameters are kept at their population median values. If *imap* = 2, then all parameters of the PK model are optimized, for a total of

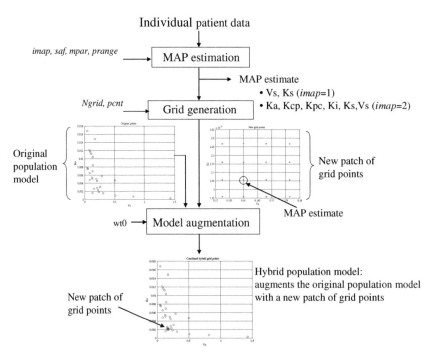

FIGURE 7.5

Process for developing the Hybrid Bayesian augmented population model.

6 parameters in the case of a general three-compartment linear PK model. The Bayesian prior for the MAP estimate is defined by the median parameter values of the population model, *mpar*, and the associated covariance P.

The quantity *saf* is the *sigma-augmentation-factor* with a default value of 1, which is chosen by the user to either increase (*saf* > 1) in order to downweight, or decrease (*saf* < 1) in order to upweight, the contribution of the population prior in the determination of the MAP estimate. For example, it is often useful to downweight the prior by assigning an a *saf* 10 to 25 times greater than that of the original population model SD to overcome the effect of shrinkage and to let the fit go far outside the stated ranges of the population parameters to fit an unusual individual patient if needed.

The quantity *prange* gives hard upper and lower bounds on each of the optimized parameters to suitably constrain the MAP search process. For example, lower bounds on all PK parameters are typically zero since they are not allowed to become negative, and upper bounds can be specified based on practical experience.

As shown in the figure, the MAP estimate is then input to the box marked "Grid Generation," which is guided by the user-specified quantities *Ngrid* and *pcnt*. Grid Generation generates an N × N grid in the region of the parameter space surrounding the MAP estimate, so that the MAP estimate is one of the interior grid points. Here the value of *N* is specified by *Ngrid*, with a default value of 4, but it can be 6, 8, or 10. The default 4 × 4 grid is shown in the right central part of Fig. 7.5, where the MAP estimate corresponds to the 10th grid point out of 16 (counting from left-to-right, top-to-bottom). The quantity *pcnt* specifies the spacing between grid points as fixed percentage offsets as a percent of the MAP estimate values. A default value of 5% is used for *pcnt*, but it can also be 10% or 20% if desired.

The lower box in the figure marked "Model Augmentation" combines the original population model with the new patch of grid points to create the final augmented Hybrid model Bayesian prior. Here, the user specifies the quantity *wt0*, which weights the original population model points relative to the new patch of MAP grid points according to the formula: Hybrid Model = $wt0 \times$ (original population model points) + $(1 - wt0) \times$ (MAP grid points). This form of the weights ensures that the total probability sums to unity. A default value for *wt0* is set to 0.5, or 50%. A value of more than 50% indicates that the original population model is to be trusted more than the MAP patch in treating the individual patient, while a value of less than 50% indicates that the population model is to be downweighted and that the MAP patch is to be trusted more. At times it may be useful to assign a probability of only 5% to the original population model, with 95% to the MAP estimate and patch, for example.

These features provide great flexibility to the hybrid procedure, which can let it use a population model for a drug that has been developed from adults, and yet, with downweighting, to do a good job of fitting data from a child receiving the drug and to permit development of a dosage regimen using maximally precise multiple model dosage design for that child. Later, as more and more children are cared for this way, their data can then be used to make a population model for children in its own right. Having done that, the entire procedure can then be moved down to use the population model for the children as the prior for Hybrid Bayesian estimation in newborns. Thus the hybrid procedure has the great strength of permitting its use as a *tool to bridge Bayesian data analysis from one population to another*. In addition, it provides a good tool to model the effect of significant drug interactions in individual patients, such as that between digoxin and quinidine, as shown in the following example.

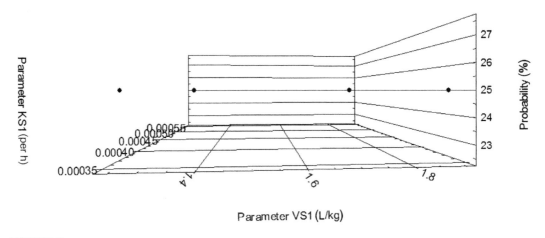

FIGURE 7.6

Population model of digoxin in adult patients. Each dot represents the top of 16 support points, resulting in a total of 64 support points [3] whose means and SDs closely approximate the results obtained by Reuning et al. [4]. Note that each collection of 16 support points has a probability of 25%, for a total of 100%, in this population model of digoxin.

Fig. 7.6 shows the population model for digoxin in adult patients [3]. This plot is unusual, as this model was made not from analyzing data of patients, but rather by taking the results of a study previously done by Reuning et al. [4], who obtained means and SDs for the various parameter values. Then, we used software developed specifically for this application [5] to locate, in this case, four dots in the plot, each dot representing the highest of 16 (for a total of 64) support points, which are specifically described in [3]. The total parameter weighted means and SDs closely approximate the original ones obtained by Reuning et al. [4]. This procedure permits development of digoxin dosage regimens using maximally precise multiple model dosage design.

The Hybrid Bayesian procedure was also used to analyze data of an unusual patient who was on both digoxin and quinidine. She had very high serum digoxin concentrations for the dose she was receiving. Her Hybrid Bayesian posterior model is shown in a 3D plot in Fig. 7.7. The great majority of the plot is occupied by her MAP Bayesian estimate and the 64-point grid patch on the left, of which the MAP Bayesian estimate is the highest point in this plot (usually but not always so, when analyzing different patients). The total probability of the grid patch here is 95%. The original population model is off to the right of the plot. Each of the four dots (each of which has 16 support points, for a total of 64 support points for the 4 dots) in the original population model now has a probability of only 1.25%, as a total probability of 5% was allotted to the original population model, and 95% to the MAP estimate and its adjacent grid points.

Interestingly, while the patient's VS1 was much decreased to between about 0.5 and 0.8 L/kg (perhaps about 1/3 of the original population VS1), further analysis of this patient's model revealed not just that her clearance was about 1/3 or 1/4 of usual, as is often described in the literature when a one-compartment model has been used in the past, but also that the uptake of digoxin into her peripheral nonserum compartment had been significantly inhibited. This corresponds to the fact

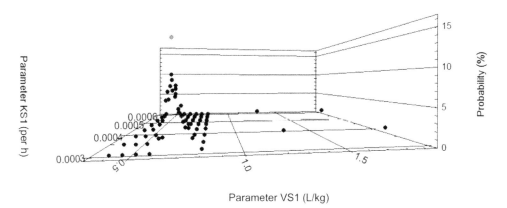

FIGURE 7.7

Hybrid Bayesian posterior display of VS1 and KS1. Note that all six model parameters, however, were fitted to the patient's data. Also note how, with downweighting of the original population model, the procedure can reach far beyond its stated parameter ranges and capture the Bayesian posterior of this patient who has a highly significant interaction between digoxin and quinidine. The four dots on the right represent the ranges of the original population parameters shown in Fig. 7.6.

that quinidine is known to compete with digoxin for binding sites on the Na−K ATPase on cell membranes. Her digoxin had been kept back in her central serum compartment due to such inhibition. When the total amounts of digoxin in both central and peripheral compartments were added up, the total calculated amount of digoxin in her body (both the central and peripheral compartments) was not very different from that found one week later, after quinidine was withdrawn, when her serum digoxin concentrations had fallen significantly, but digoxin uptake into her peripheral nonserum compartment had also increased significantly at the same time to a more normal value for that dose. This patient's data strongly suggest that the digoxin−quinidine interaction causes a redistribution of digoxin from the peripheral back to the central compartment, on the same dose of digoxin. The Hybrid Bayesian procedure permits such analyses to be done for very unusual patients.

Thus when data is obtained from a patient such as a child, but no population model of that drug yet exists for the child, or from a patient having a significant drug−drug interaction, the Hybrid Bayesian procedure, ad hoc though it is, can provide a highly useful means to analyze data of a patient who is clearly outside the range of an available population model to serve as a Bayesian prior. The Hybrid permits useful analysis and understanding of an unusual patient's data with better care, in the form of maximally precise dosage regimens, using multiple model dosage design.

7.6 THE INTERACTING MULTIPLE MODEL (IMM) BAYESIAN APPROACH TO UNSTABLE ICU PATIENTS

A significant limitation has been present with all current fitting procedures discussed so far. It is that all the model parameters are assumed to be fixed and unchanging throughout the entire period of data analysis. This presents a severe problem when caring for acutely ill and highly unstable patients in ICU settings. Indeed, it is clear that while the problem of high *interindividual* variability can be minimized by the use of nonparametric population models, MM dosage design, and TDM with NP Bayesian analysis and MM dosage design of the new adjusted regimen, the other problem of patients having high *intraindividual* (inter-occasional) variability has remained intractable until now. Indeed, some have even suggested that TDM may not be useful in patients with high intraindividual variability. This problem has now been significantly reduced by the use of the interacting multiple model (IMM) Bayesian approach. IMM was introduced into the pharmacokinetic literature by Bayard and Jelliffe [6], based on a method originally developed for tracking abruptly changing targets [7,8]. It permits the patient's model parameters to change with time. Specifically, the patient's parameters are allowed to change by jumping from one support point of the population model to another at random time instants. In undergoing such a jump, the patient's state (amounts in various compartments, serum concentrations, etc.) propagates continuously. A support point is also allowed to jump to itself, which is equivalent to having no jump at all. The current BestDose software implementation allows these jump opportunities to be whenever a new dose is given or a new serum concentration data point is obtained from TDM. In explaining the measured serum concentrations, IMM considers multiple scenarios in which the state of the patient may jump from one support point to another, and then gives highest probabilities to the most likely jump scenarios. It has been shown to track the changing behavior of gentamicin and vancomycin better than other methods in acutely unstable postcardiac surgical patients [9]. Patients with high intra-individual variability now can have their drug behavior tracked with much greater precision than before, so that dosage regimens for them can be much better and more precisely planned for them for the very near future. More will be said about this in Chapter 9, Optimizing Individualized Drug Therapy in the ICU.

7.7 USING THE AUGMENTED POPULATION MODEL FROM THE HYBRID AS THE BAYESIAN PRIOR FOR SUBSEQUENT IMM ANALYSIS

A current limitation of the IMM procedure is the finite number of population model support points to which the patient's data can jump as the new data becomes available. However, the hybrid procedure with a large number of added points in the grid around the MAP estimate, as shown in Fig. 7.7, provides many new support points which can cover a wide range of values to which the patient's data can jump as the patient's new data becomes available and the IMM algorithm suggests that it would be more likely to do so. Preliminary efforts strongly suggest that adding these extra support points, made with a Hybrid Bayesian augmented population model, may well improve and deepen our understanding of the evolution of the patient's model parameters over time. Further work in this direction is in progress.

7.8 CONCLUSION

We now have four ways to perform Bayesian analysis of the relationship between a population model prior and new data coming from an individual patient, to model that patient's drug behavior in a manner best suited to each patient's clinical needs. We now have the tools to move forward and calculate the most precise adjusted dosage regimen based on our observations of that patient. A subsequent chapter will consider the most informative and cost-effective strategies to obtain serum concentrations and other measurements for observing our patients optimally and learning about them as rapidly and as cost-effectively (fewest samples, optimally chosen) as possible.

REFERENCES

[1]   Nelder JA, Mead R. A simplex method for function minimization. Comp J 1965;7:308−13.
[2]   Jelliffe R, Bayard D, Leary R, Schumitzky A, Van Guilder M, Botnen A, et al. A Hybrid Bayesian method to obtain Bayesian posterior parameter distributions in nonparametric pharmacokinetic models for individual patients. Laboratory of Applied Pharmacokinetics Technical Report 2011-1.
[3]   Jelliffe R, Milman M, Schumitzky A, Bayard D, Van Guilder M. A two-compartment population pharmacokinetic-pharmacodynamic model of digoxin in adults, with implications for dosage. Ther Drug Monit 2014 (epub ahead of print).
[4]   Reuning R, Sams R, Notari R. Role of pharmacokinetics in drug dosage adjustment 1. Pharmacologic effects, kinetics, and apparent volume of distribution of digoxin. J Clin Pharmacol 1973;13:127−41.
[5]   Milman M, Jiang F, Jelliffe R. Creating discrete joint densities from continuous ones: the moment-matching, maximum entropy approach. Comput Biol Med 2001;31:197−214.
[6]   Bayard D, Jelliffe R. A Bayesian approach to tracking patients having changing pharmacokinetic parameters. J Pharmacokinet Pharmacodyn 2004;31(1):75−107.
[7]   Blom HAP. An efficient filter for abruptly changing systems. Proceedings of the 23rd conference on decision and control. Las Vegas, NV; December 1984.
[8]   Blom HAP, Bar-Shalom Y. The interacting multiple model algorithm for systems with Markovian switching coefficients. IEEE Trans Automat Contr 1988;33:780.
[9]   Macdonald I, Staatz C, Jelliffe R, Thomson A. Evaluation and comparison of simple multiple model, richer data multiple model, and sequential interacting multiple model (IMM) Bayesian analyses of gentamicin and vancomycin data collected from patients undergoing cardiothoracic surgery. Ther Drug Monit 2008;30:67−74.

APPENDIX: MORE DETAIL ON NONPARAMETRIC BAYESIAN ANALYSIS

The NP model is a collection of n support points; call them $Q_1, \ldots, Q_n$ each with their corresponding probabilities $w_1, \ldots, w_n$. For example, in Fig. 7.1, each $Q_i =$ (ie, the model parameter values $VS1_i$ and $KS1_i$) and their probabilities that $(VS1, KS1) = (VS1_i, KS1_i)$ is w_i.

However, a PK model can have more than two parameters. For example, in the two-compartment model, with first-order absorption, $Q = (Ka, Kint, KS, Kcp, Kpc, Vol)$. An NP population model with n support points is defined by the collection of support points $\{Q_i\}$ and their corresponding probabilities $\{w_i\}$, for $i = 1, \ldots, n$. Each individual Q_i represents the collection of parameter values of the collection Q, and all the w_i's sum to unity.

The Bayesian posterior probability of a support point is calculated as follows. Continuing the general notation given previously, let A be the event that $Q = Q_i$, and let B be the event that the patient's data Y is observed. So a particular support point is considered and put together with the patient's data. The NP population model gives the prior probabilities: $P(A) = P(Q = Q\_i) = w\_i$, for $i = 1, \ldots, n$.

The posterior probability is given by Bayes' theorem:

$$P(A|B) = P(B|A)P(A)/P(B) \tag{7.3}$$

Here, the term $P(A|B)$ is the posterior probability that $Q = Q\_i$ given the data Y. This is what we want to know.

The term $P(B|A)$ is the probability that the data Y comes from the model when $Q = Q\_i$. This is called the *Likelihood* of the event $Q = Q\_i$ and is directly calculated from the PK model.

The term $P(B)$ is the probability that the data Y comes from *any* of the discrete parameter values $\{Q\_j, j = 1, \ldots, n\}$. This is just the sum of $P(Y|Q = Q\_j) * P(Q = Q\_j)$ over all support points $\{Q\_j\}$. This can be written as

$$\text{Sum}\{P(Y|Q = Q_j) * w_j, j = 1, \ldots, n\} \tag{7.4}$$

since $P(Q = Q\_j) = w\_j$. The final formula for the posterior probabilities can then be written as:

$$P(Q = Q_i|Y) = \left[P(Y|Q = Q_i|Y) * w_i \right] / \left[\text{Sum}\{P(Y|Q = Q_j) * w_j, j = 1, \ldots, n\} \right] \tag{7.5}$$

MONITORING EACH PATIENT OPTIMALLY: WHEN TO OBTAIN THE BEST SAMPLES FOR THERAPEUTIC DRUG MONITORING

8

R. Jelliffe, D. Bayard and M. Neely

CHAPTER OUTLINE

8.1 INTRODUCTION

When we consider the subject of individualizing drug dosage regimens for patients, we do so because drugs that require such individualization have narrow therapeutic ranges, and it is important to manage such therapy with maximum precision. Once again, never choose a range. Always choose a specific target goal. However, be sure to choose that target individually for each patient according to that patient's specific perceived needs. Then hit the target with maximum precision with the dosage regimen.

Therapeutic drug monitoring (TDM) has often been done to check the achievement of desired serum drug concentrations. This has usually been done by sampling drug concentrations in the steady state at the end of a dose interval (the trough), just before a next dose is to be given. Relatively little attention has been paid to doing TDM at other times. This can be greatly improved upon, as we will see further on.

Individualized Drug Therapy for Patients. DOI: http://dx.doi.org/10.1016/B978-0-12-803348-7.00008-3

Samples taken at the trough have also been popular because errors in recording when doses were given and blood samples drawn have the least effect upon the actual measurement when it is taken at that time.

However, such a policy, which has somehow become "routine TDM" policy for years, without any rigorous scientific justification that we can find, actually selects the sample containing the *least* information about the pharmacokinetic behavior of the drug. There are an infinite number of trajectories over which a serum drug concentration can proceed from that present when the dose is given to that present at the trough. None of this information is captured when only trough samples are obtained. Think what just another sample, obtained at just about any other time, can do to improve things here. With a pair of samples, the number of possible trajectories is greatly reduced.

In addition, it is physically impossible to give any drug dose exactly when ordered. Only the most unusual patient ever gets a dose at exactly 8 am, for example. Furthermore, there is no record of when the dose was actually given, usually only a check mark saying that the dose was given, but never when. Simulation studies have shown, using realistic clinical scenarios, that lack of precise knowledge of when doses were given is the single biggest obstacle and source of imprecision in the management of individualized drug therapy [1], and that careful recording of these events by properly trained personnel can and does make significant improvements in therapeutic precision [2].

It is easy to do much better. The only thing necessary is to look at the wall clock or a digital watch, and instead of putting a check mark, simply to record to the minute, in military time, when the dose was actually given: for example, at 0817. No one cares if the dose was given when ordered or not. But it is vitally important to know *when* the dose was *actually* given. These current hospital policies need updating.

The same goes for the phlebotomy service. The phlebotomy personnel also can easily look at the clock or their watch and record, military time, when the sample was drawn.

8.2 OPTIMIZING THERAPEUTIC DRUG MONITORING (TDM) PROTOCOLS AND POLICIES

The important thing is to learn, as rapidly as possible, and with the fewest samples (to be most cost-effective), how the drug is behaving in each individual patient, so we can dose the patient best (most precisely). We usually have in mind a desired target goal of a certain serum concentration at a desired time, or perhaps a desired area under the curve (AUC) over a stated dose interval. We use our population model of the drug to develop the initial dosage regimen. Then we monitor the patient later on, to check what we have done.

This sounds natural enough, but it is actually quite a suboptimal approach. What we really want to do is to start as before, with the initial dosage regimen, to hit our target most precisely. But we also want to combine this with a thoughtful and formal plan to learn as quickly as possible how the drug is behaving in the patient. We do not want to leave the patient at risk of our not knowing this until perhaps too late. So we want to optimize the process of learning about a patient as rapidly as possible, while treating him/her at the same time, in order to achieve our target goal with maximal precision over the whole course of treatment, from what is often an urgent beginning, when it is most important to achieve a target goal as rapidly as possible, and then to keep it there afterward.

There are two basic approaches to this. The first is called D-optimal design and its variants: ED, EID, and E-log-D optimal [3]. These use parametric PK models and are designed to learn the patient's model parameter values most precisely. The other is the new multiple model optimal (MMopt) design, which is especially well suited for nonparametric models [4,5]. Furthermore, in addition to learning the model parameters optimally, MMopt can also help us to optimize specific practical clinical tasks of dosing to achieve a target serum concentration at a desired time or of achieving a desired AUC with maximal precision. Such a practical and task-oriented optimal design is an entirely new approach [5]. Let us examine these in turn.

8.3 D-OPTIMAL DESIGN AND ITS VARIANTS

D-optimal design was presented to the PK community by D'Argenio [3], who showed, by comparing it with a conventional clinical strategy for monitoring lidocaine infusion regimens, that significant increases in the precision of parameter value estimation can be obtained. This strategy, however, requires that the model parameter values should ideally be known in advance in order to compute the optimal times at which to observe them. However, the other strategies based on D-optimal design such as ED, EID, and E log D optimal (see further discussion on this topic later in this chapter) have managed to avoid this "catch-22." These designs are all called D-optimal because they optimize the *determinant* (remember high school algebra?) of a matrix of covariances describing the uncertainties between the various model parameters. Remember that the standard deviation (SD) squared is the variance of a parameter. But what about the shared uncertainties between two parameters? They are described by the covariance between them, which is the correlation coefficient between the two parameters, times the SD of one parameter times the SD of the other.

D-optimal design finds the times that minimize these covariances, to find the times that minimize the overall uncertainties among the various parameters. In doing this, D-optimal design thus finds the times at which the serum concentrations are maximally sensitive to small changes in the model parameter values.

ED-optimal design finds times which maximize an expected value of this determinant. EID-optimal design minimizes the expected value of the determinant of the inverse covariance matrix. E log D, which is also called API, maximizes the expected value of the logarithm of the determinant of the covariance matrix.

All such D-optimal-based strategies require that the number of observations (serum concentrations, for example) be at least as great as the number of model parameters to be estimated. For a simple one-compartment model of a drug, having the two parameters of apparent volume of distribution (V) and elimination rate constant (K_{el}), two samples are required. For the common model having an absorptive, a central serum concentration compartment, and a peripheral nonserum compartment, six samples are ideally required, one for each of the six model parameters. In addition, for some dosage formats such as a fixed-rate infusion or an initial loading infusion followed by a maintenance infusion, the final optimal time is achieved only after a final steady state has been reached. This may well be too long to wait for the urgent clinical needs of some patients. However, D-optimal strategies can be designed for any desired period of study.

8.4 D-OPTIMAL TIMES ALSO DEPEND UPON THE DOSAGE FORMAT

8.4.1 INTERMITTENT INTRAVENOUS (IV) INFUSION

D-optimal design and its variants find the time(s) at which a small change in a model parameter value causes the greatest change in the serum concentration. Fig. 8.1 shows that in the format of intermittent intravenous (IV) administration such as for an aminoglycoside, if the volume V were to change by a certain percent, the resulting profile of all the serum concentrations would change appropriately, and that (other things being equal, such as the assay SD being constant over the assay range) the time at which the greatest change in the serum concentrations occurs is at the peak, at the end of the infusion. Getting a sample at any other time will tell us less about V. This is quite different from the common suboptimal strategy of obtaining a so-called "peak" a half-hour after the end of an aminoglycoside infusion, for example. That obsolete strategy was discussed in the Introduction, as an example of an optical illusion. Also, avoid getting the sample from the IV line. Get it from another site, but at the end of the IV infusion, after all the drug is in.

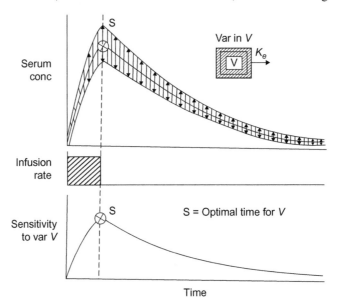

FIGURE 8.1

To best estimate the apparent volume of distribution (V) of a one-compartment pharmacokinetic model of a drug, the time when the peak is reached, at the end of an intravenous infusion, is most informative. Sampling at any other time gives less information about V, as the change in serum concentration (with a constant assay SD) is less than at the peak. *Conc*, concentration; *Var V*, variation in *V*.

Reproduced with permission from Jelliffe R: Commentary - Optimal Methodology is Important for Optimal Pharmacokinetic Studies, Therapeutic Drug Monitoring, and Patient Care. Clinical Pharmacokinetics. 2015. 54: (9) 887–892.

Now, starting from the peak, elimination takes place. Fig. 8.2 shows this phase. Here a change in the K_{el} causes a change in the excretion rate. If you have a hand calculator that can do exponentials, take some value of K_{el} and run it over several values of time and find e^{-kt}. Now take a slightly different

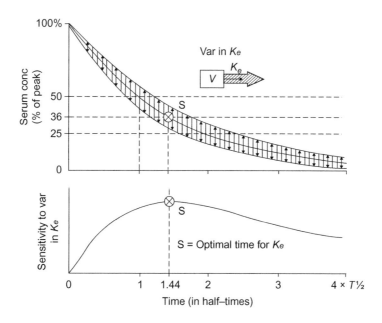

FIGURE 8.2

Getting a sample when the serum concentration has fallen to about 1/3 of the peak value gives the most information about the elimination of the drug. *Conc*, concentration; K_e, elimination rate constant; $T\frac{1}{2}$, half-time; *Var*, variation.

Reproduced with permission from Jelliffe R: Commentary - Optimal Methodology is Important for Optimal Pharmacokinetic Studies, Therapeutic Drug Monitoring, and Patient Care. Clinical Pharmacokinetics. 2015. 54: (9) 887–892.

K_{el} and do the same. You will see that the greatest difference between the two values of e^{-kt} is when its value is 0.36, or 36% of the original peak. Fig. 8.2 also shows that while it is best at that point, there is a general good region there where sensitivity of the serum concentrations to a change in K_{el} is great, but that a trough taken at a later time than 36% is actually less informative about what we really want to know, which is how the drug is behaving and being excreted in that patient. Of course, if the trough comes before the 36% point is reached, then the trough is the best time.

8.4.2 CONTINUOUS IV INFUSION

If the drug is given as a continuous infusion at a fixed rate, then the process to optimize the observations is essentially based on the mirror image of Fig. 8.2. Fig. 8.3 shows that the first optimal point is reached when the concentration has reached 64% of its final steady state value (all but 36% equilibrated), and the second point is reached only after a final steady state has been achieved.

8.4.3 A LOADING FOLLOWED BY A MAINTENANCE INFUSION

If the drug is given as a loading infusion followed by a maintenance infusion that is designed to maintain the concentration achieved at the end of the loading infusion, then the first D-optimal time is at the end of the loading infusion (similar to the peak in Fig. 8.1), and then at the final steady state, similar to S2 in Fig. 8.3. These times are shown in Fig. 8.4.

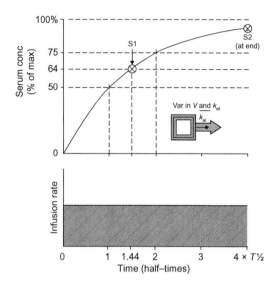

FIGURE 8.3

The two D-optimal times to get samples during a fixed-rate infusion without any loading infusion are sample 1 at S1, when the drug has reached 64% of its final steady state value (has all but 36% equilibrated), and sample 2 at S2, at or after the final steady state has been reached. *Conc*, concentration; K_{el}, elimination rate constant; $T\frac{1}{2}$, half-time; *Var*, variation.

Reproduced with permission from Jelliffe R: Commentary - Optimal Methodology is Important for Optimal Pharmacokinetic Studies, Therapeutic Drug Monitoring, and Patient Care. Clinical Pharmacokinetics. 2015. 54: (9) 887–892.

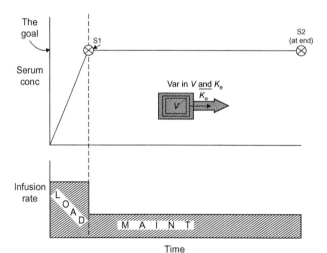

FIGURE 8.4

The D-optimal times for monitoring a dosage regimen given as an intravenous loading infusion followed by a maintenance infusion are S1, at the end of the loading infusion, and S2, at or after a steady state is reached. *Var*, variation.

Reproduced with permission from Jelliffe R: Commentary - Optimal Methodology is Important for Optimal Pharmacokinetic Studies, Therapeutic Drug Monitoring, and Patient Care. Clinical Pharmacokinetics. 2015. 54: (9) 887–892.

Note that the D-optimal times for parameter estimation may well not be optimal for the patient. The patient's clinical situation may not permit waiting for a final steady state, for example. In such cases, it is far better to redefine the period of study to that which is appropriate for the clinical urgency, and to optimize the sampling strategy to be within the patient's often much shorter time constraints. Furthermore, almost any TDM protocol is better than getting only a trough sample at a steady state!

8.5 MULTIPLE MODEL OPTIMAL (MMopt) DESIGN

All the given D-optimal designs and their variants are based on the use of parametric models that assume normal or lognormal distributions for their parameters, and all are designed only to help us learn a patient's model parameters.

In contrast to these approaches, MMopt design [4] is best suited for NP models, in which the parameter distributions are not constrained to have any particular shape. They simply are what they are, given the data.

Fig. 8.5 is another representation of a hypothetical NP population model with parameters V and K_{el} on the two horizontal axes, and the probabilities on the vertical axis. Only a few support points are shown here for clarity.

Let a dose be given to the reference support point, and the others as well. Assume for this discussion that this corresponds to the leftmost support point in Fig. 8.5. Let an experiment be implemented in which measurements are taken on the response of that support group and the others as well at several

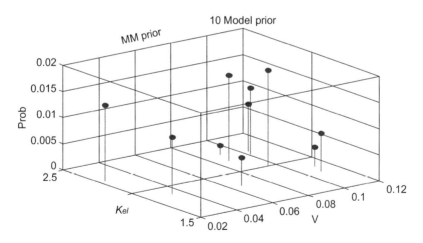

FIGURE 8.5

An nonparametric population model with its support points. Ideally, if a dose is given to the leftmost point, the response of that point should be unique and clearly distinguishable from those of all the others. Its MAP Bayesian posterior should be more probable than that of any other, because of its unique set of parameter values. Horizontal axes, V and K_{el}; Vertical axis, probability.

specified sample times, after which the MAP Bayesian posterior is computed. Intuitively, if the sample times were chosen well, one would expect that the probability of the leftmost point in the Bayesian posterior would be greatly increased relative to its prior probability. It could then be said that the experiment was "informative" in the sense of discriminating the reference support point from the rest of the support points. In fact, if were very informative, the reference support point probability would rise above the rest and be the highest. This is the basic idea behind MMopt. Specifically, MMopt chooses sample times that maximize the probability that the highest probability point in the Bayesian posterior (the MAP estimate) corresponds to the true subject under consideration. The probability that the MAP estimate is wrong (the probability that the MAP estimate does not correspond to the reference support point) is called the Bayes risk. Clearly it is desired to minimize the Bayes risk. For practical reasons, MMopt minimizes an overbound on the Bayes risk that provides an approximate answer, but has the advantage of saving an extremely great amount of computation.

What about the effect of assay error and other clinical sources of noise on the measurements? For simplicity, consider that the population model is composed of only two support points, and let a measurement be taken at a single sampling time. This situation is shown in Fig. 8.6.

The response separation r(t) in Fig. 8.6 is simply the distance between the two responses at the sample time t. Turning the diagram "sideways" yields the arrangement shown in Fig. 8.7. Here the spacing between the two peaks corresponds to the response separation, and the fatness of each Gaussian depicts the amount of measurement noise on each measurement. With this illustration, the gray area corresponds exactly to the probability of making a classification error, ie, the Bayes risk. From statistics, this is a hypothesis testing problem, where the gray area corresponds to the

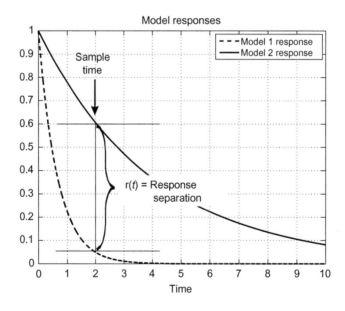

FIGURE 8.6

Responses associated with a model having only two support points. The response separation r(t) between the two model responses is depicted at a specific sample time.

probability of an error associated with making the two classical types of wrong decisions (eg, false negatives and false positives). To minimize the Bayes risk, it is desired to pull the two Gaussian pulses as far apart as possible. The increased separation shrinks the gray area by minimizing the overlap of the Gaussian tails. Physically, this corresponds to choosing a sampling time when the two support point responses are most separated.

Hence, for a two support point model, MMopt minimizes Bayes risk (classification error), by choosing a sampling time that maximizes response separation. This sampling time is generally different from what would be obtained using the D-optimal design considered earlier. The difference is due to the fact that MMopt addresses the true NP nature of the model, something not considered by D-optimal design.

When there are more than two support points, the experiment design problem becomes more complicated. Here, in the practical situation where there are population models having many support points, MMopt minimizes the Bayes risk overbound through a process that best separates the "ensemble" of responses by comparing them two at a time, for all combinations of support points.

Table 8.1 compares the performance of MMopt with that of the three main variants of D-optimal design that are not caught by the catch-22 of having to know the parameter values in advance in order to compute the optimal times at which to observe the system. Furthermore, using MMopt, one does not need to have as many samples as there are parameters in the model, as is required for D-optimal design and the variants ED, EID, and E log D (API in the table). It is shown in Table 8.2 for a two-parameter model, but one can have one, two, or three samples for MMopt, if

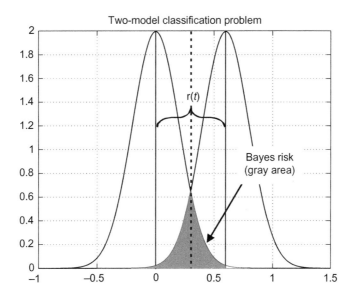

FIGURE 8.7

Bayes risk is depicted as the gray area between curves, corresponding to the sum of false negative and false positive error probabilities. Bayes risk decreases as response separation r(*t*) increases, which "pulls apart" the two Gaussian distributions and shrinks the gray area between them.

Table 8.1 Comparison of the Capabilities of the Three Major Variants of D-Optimal Design With MMopt

Comparison Table				
	ED	**EID**	**API**	**MMopt**
Invariant under regular *linear* reparametrization[a]	Yes	Yes	Yes	Yes
Invariant under regular *nonlinear* reparametrization[a]	No	No	Yes	Yes
Allows taking fewer than p samples, $p = $ # of parameters	No	No	No	Yes
Can handle heterogeneous model structures	No	No	No	Yes
Gives known optimal solution to two model example[a]	No	No	No	Yes
Captures main elements of minimizing Bayes risk	No	No	No	Yes

[a]*Proved in Bayard et al., PODE 2013 [4].*

Table 8.2 Comparison of Performance of MMopt With ED Optimal Design for One, Two, and Three Sample Scenarios

Design Metric	Samples (h)			Bayes Risk (prob)	99% Conf (prob)
	1-Sample Design				
Bopt*	4.25			0.5474	± 0.0015
MMopt	4.25			0.5474	± 0.0015
	2-Sample Design				
MMopt	1	9.5		0.2947	± 0.0014
EDopt	1	24		0.3272	± 0.0014
	3-Sample Design				
MMopt	1	1	10.5	0.2325	± 0.0013
EDopt	1	1	24	0.2617	± 0.0013

*MMopt matches the true Bayesian risk (evaluated by Bopt) in a one-sample design (the only one that is computationally feasible), and is better than EDopt for the two- and three-sample designs.

desired. The more samples, the less risk of misclassification. In addition, Table 8.2 shows that the Bayes risk of misclassification is always less with MMopt than with the other methods, such as EDopt, shown here.

8.6 NEW SPECIFIC CLINICAL TASKS THAT CAN ALSO BE OPTIMIZED WITH WEIGHTED MMopt (wMMopt)

It also turns out that MM optimal design can be used to optimize other things besides model parameter estimation. One can attach a special weight or penalty associated with the misclassification.

Table 8.3 Ability of MMopt and wMMopt_C_1 to Achieve a Desired AUC Compared to the True Bayesian Optimal Design Bopt_C_1

Design Metric	Samples (h)			RMS Error (AUC Units)	99% Conf (AUC Units)
	1-Sample Design				
Bopt_C_1	12.5			3.6194	± 0.0273
wMMopt_C_1	14			3.7729	± 0.0166
MMopt	4.25			16.7924	± 0.1145
	2-Sample Design				
wMMopt C_1	1	13		2.1102	⊥ 0.0125
MMopt	1	9.5		2.2575	± 0.0232
EDopt	1	24		2.6159	± 0.0174
	3-Sample Design				
wMMopt_C_1	1	10.25	10.25	1.6967	± 0.0078
MMopt	1	1	10.5	1.9991	± 0.0192
EDopt	1	1	24	2.4194	± 0.0174

MMopt, MMopt for parameter identification only. wMMopt C_1, MMopt for optimal AUC control; EDopt, ED optimal design. Optimal times are different when it is desired to optimize AUC control, and the RMS error is smaller, with good 99% confidence limits.

This penalty can be the failure to hit a desired target serum concentration at a desired time or to achieve a desired AUC, for example. In this way, weighted MMopt (wMMopt) design can be specifically tailored to the achievement of such desired practical clinical tasks [5]. This brings a unique, new, clinically oriented, and practical capability to optimal design. It can be used not only for parameter estimation, but also to optimize specific tasks that are really important for the patient clinically, such as finding the optimal times to monitor the patient to ensure maximally precise achievement of target serum concentrations or AUCs. This new capability is shown in Table 8.3.

8.7 CONCLUSION

We have now seen how the standard D-optimal design and its variants perform in defined clinical situations, and their comparison with the new and improved MM and weighted (wMM) optimal design.

It is also likely that MM optimal designs will be different for each individual patient. The reason for this is that the design looks not at the general structure of the model, but instead is concerned only with tracking trajectories generated by various support points, which can actually be generated by different structural models. One can easily imagine that different combinations of body weight and renal function will generate trajectories that will cross each other (making classification more difficult) at different times, and that the times at which they will be most separated (making classification easier) will also be different for each patient. Thus, it is highly likely that as this new method becomes used in clinical therapy, each patient will have his own unique set of optimal times to get samples for TDM. Both MMopt and wMMopt are now being implemented in the new BestDose clinical software for modeling and controlling large and nonlinear models of multiple interacting drug systems.

REFERENCES

[1] Jelliffe RW. Control of serum tobramycin levels: contributions of the pharmacy, ward care, serum assay, phlebotomy service, and a smart infusion pump. 22nd Annual meeting of the American Association for Medical Instrumentation. Los Angeles, CA; May 16−20, 1987.

[2] Charpiat B, Breant V, Dumarest C, Maire P, Jelliffe RW. Prediction of future serum concentrations with Bayesian fitted pharmacokinetic models: results with data collected by nurses versus trained pharmacy residents. Ther Drug Monit 1994;16:166−73.

[3] D'Argenio D. Optimal sampling times for pharmacokinetic experiments. J Pharmacokin Biopharmacol 1981;9:739−56.

[4] Bayard D, Jelliffe R, and Neely M. Bayes Risk as an Alternative to Fisher Information in Determining Experimental Designs for Nonparametric Models. Presented at the Population Optimum Design of Experiments Conference, Lilly Laboratories, Erl Wood Manor, Windlesham, Surrey, UK. June 15, 2013. Slides and abstracts at http://www.maths.qmul.ac.uk/∼bb/PODE/PODE2013.html.

[5] Jelliffe R, Bayard D, Neely M. MMopt − an optimal TDM protocol strategy based on Bayes risk and weighted Bayes risk. An oral presentation at the 14th congress of the International Association for Therapeutic Drug Monitoring and Clinical Toxicology, Rotterdam, The Netherlands, October, 14, 2015.

OPTIMIZING INDIVIDUALIZED DRUG THERAPY IN THE ICU

9

R. Jelliffe

CHAPTER OUTLINE

9.1 INTRODUCTION

In the intensive care unit (ICU), we care for very unstable patients. Their clinical status changes rapidly from day to day and hour to hour. They may be in shock. They may be either overhydrated or underhydrated, and their renal function may be changing rapidly. All of these things happen in the most unpredictable ways.

9.2 RENAL FUNCTION

The usual ways of evaluating renal function by using single samples of serum creatinine (SCr) such as the Cockroft-Gault and Modification of Diet in Renal Disease methods are not useful in the ICU. They are useful only when the patient is stable. When renal function is unstable, those methods are inevitably late in recognizing the change and also inevitably underestimate the magnitude of the change. What is needed, especially in the ICU, is a method that considers the rate of change of SCr and calculates the creatinine clearance (CCr) that makes the SCr go from one

Individualized Drug Therapy for Patients. DOI: http://dx.doi.org/10.1016/B978-0-12-803348-7.00009-5

value at one time to another at a later time in a patient of stated age, gender, height, and weight. These issues are discussed more fully in Chapter 5, Evaluation of Renal Function.

9.3 APPARENT VOLUME OF DISTRIBUTION, DRUG ELIMINATION, AND CLEARANCE

Words often carry ambiguous and unintended meanings. Clearance is such a word. When we say that a drug is cleared from the body, the meaning is taken by almost everyone to be synonymous with saying that the drug is eliminated from the body. However, let us examine this more closely.

Elimination of a drug refers to its specific rate of elimination in amount of drug per unit time, — the rate constant for elimination (K_{el}) or the half-time of elimination ($T1/2$), the time when half the drug is eliminated. Both $T1/2$ and K_{el} give direct information about the rate of elimination of a drug.

Clearance (Cl), on the other hand, is quite different. It is the elimination rate constant K_{el} multiplied by the apparent volume (V) into which the drug appears to be distributed. It is, therefore, not the same as elimination at all. Instead, it is a volume of fluid that is cleared at a certain rate. The following expressions describe what is happening.

$T1/2 = 0.69315/K_{el}$	(1)	The units are time to move half the amount.
$K_{el} = Cl/V$	(2)	The units are 1/time = vol times 1/time divided by vol.
$V = Cl/K_{el}$	(3)	The units are vol = vol times 1/time divided by 1/time.
$Cl = V^*K_{el}$	(4)	The units are vol/time = vol times 1/time

We can see that V has direct units of volume, K_{el} has direct units of 1/time, and $T1/2$ has units of time. When V and K_{el} are multiplied together to give clearance, the direct information about the amount of drug actually moved from one compartment to another during a specific time period becomes obscured. One only perceives the volume of fluid cleared per time and not the specific amount of drug actually moved in a given time.

Many people in the pharmacokinetic community, but not in the wider mathematical community, feel quite strongly that Cl is somehow an "independent" parameter, and that V and K are somehow dependent and are derived from Cl. Many feel that Cl is the "most physiologic" parameter. An interesting exposition of this point of view is given in [1].

It is clear, however, that one has a choice in parameterizing any PK model. One can choose to do it either as V and Cl or as V and K_{el}. The real question is what is most useful clinically. V and K_{el} both convey direct information about the behavior of the drug. Cl, however, comingles the separate contributions of V and K and is much less useful clinically.

One can describe the behavior of a PK/PD system by differential equations describing amounts of material in various compartments, with rate constants describing the rates of exchange between compartments. The doses are the inputs to the system. The outputs of the system, when they are concentrations, are the amount of substance in a compartment divided by an apparent volume of the compartment into which they are distributed. Clearance is actually an unnecessary parameter here for clinical purposes. V and K_{el} are what give us direct specific clinical information about the behavior of the patient's PK system. Clearance simply combines them, obscuring the values of each, and adds no new information. You have to divide it by V (obtaining K_{el}) to get direct information about the rate of drug movement.

Measurement or estimation of CCr has become the main method of evaluating renal function. It is an attempt, using clinically available data, to estimate glomerular filtration rate (GFR), which is regarded as the main index of renal function. It is probably because CCr and GFR are so widely used that we have become accustomed to think of the word clearance as somehow being synonymous with elimination of waste products.

This is not so. One might ask if we have kidneys simply to make urine or rather to excrete various waste substances. GFR measures only the ability of the kidney to filter plasma and make urine. It gives no direct information about the quantitative ability of the kidney to excrete any of the many substances that are eliminated. I would actually be much more interested, for example, in information about the half-time of creatinine in a patient or the elimination rate constant of any other substance of interest. The actual ability of the kidney to eliminate a specific substance is a subject almost never discussed, to my knowledge, but that ability is actually a more specific and informative true measure of renal function than GFR.

9.4 INCREASED AND CHANGING V AND "AUGMENTED RENAL CLEARANCE" IN ICU PATIENTS

ICU patients quite often have a large V, which often gets smaller as they recover. Drs. Marcus Haug and Peter Slugg at the Cleveland Clinic used earlier versions of our clinical software [2] in the 1980s. As they would fit clusters of serum gentamicin concentrations doing TDM on their patients, they noticed that the patient's large V would get smaller as patients would recover from their illnesses. They called this "Vd collapse" and used it as a marker and index of the patient's recovery from his illness [3]. It is now widely known that V is often increased in acutely ill ICU patients [4,5]. More recently, this has been described as "augmented renal clearance" in ICU patients [6,7]. However, it is not clear whether V or K_{el}, or some combination of both, is actually what is increased due to the comingling of V and K_{el} that takes place when the term clearance is used. The volumes of intracellular, extracellular, and vascular fluid compartments are what can change rapidly and unpredictably in patients in the ICU due to possible changes in capillary permeability, fluid therapy, and cardiac output. However, "augmented renal clearance" has become commonly used to describe drug behavior in ICU patients, but it is clearly evident from the text in [7], for example, that clearance is regarded as being synonymous with elimination. The elevated CCr found in these patients is assumed to suggest that renal function is what is enhanced, along with the enhanced clearance of many drugs seen in these ICU patients. What is needed to clarify the situation is direct information about V and K_{el}.

The V in PK models is an apparent volume inferred mathematically by fitting models to data. One makes physiologic interpretations of these parameters with caution. V is stated sometimes to be reduced, possibly due to hypovolemia in some patients, and increased in many others, possibly due to changes in capillary permeability or to overhydration. An interesting discussion is given in [7].

9.5 TRACKING DRUG BEHAVIOR OPTIMALLY IN UNSTABLE PATIENTS

All procedures to fit a model to patient data until recently have assumed that the model parameters are fixed and unchanging throughout the entire period of the data analysis. This imposes a severe limitation on our ability to understand the behavior of drugs in unstable ICU patients as we do TDM and analyze their data.

Stimulated by this problem, our laboratory, guided by Dr. David Bayard, developed a new and unique procedure to analyze data in unstable patients [8]. It is based on the Interacting Multiple Model (IMM) method employed in the shipping and aerospace communities to track objects such as ships, to best avoid collisions, and aircraft, either for air traffic separation and control, or for air defense, to best track aircraft taking evasive action [9−11]. The IMM method has been documented to track the behavior of gentamicin and vancomycin better than other methods [12].

9.6 AN ILLUSTRATIVE CHRONIC DIALYSIS PATIENT WITH SEPSIS

A number of years ago, a 73-year-old patient on chronic hemodialysis pulled out his Foley catheter and was admitted to our Los Angeles County−USC Medical Center ICU with a *Proteus* sepsis. The ICU had just recently implemented 24-h pharmacist coverage. He was treated with conventional doses of gentamicin for the time, and conventional TDM for that time was done, using the method of linear regression upon the logarithms of the serum concentrations. The serum concentrations were less than would be expected from the usual volume of distribution found in general medical patients. The pharmacists duly noted in the chart that his *V* was larger than usual. They wanted to present the physicians with the evidence, but they did not wish to be so bold as to suggest that his dosage probably should be increased. The physicians were glad to have the pharmacists aboard, but because of their lack of pharmacokinetic training did not know what an apparent volume of distribution was, and apparently did not ask. Gentamicin was ordered by the physicians but given by the pharmacists, usually after an episode of hemodialysis.

The patient improved and was able to leave the ICU for a general medical floor. However, there was no similar pharmacist coverage there. He received no gentamicin for about a week until a new group of residents came on service, found the problem, began gentamicin again, and our laboratory was eventually asked to see the patient and analyze his data.

The doses he had received and the specific method of data entry to include the episodes of dialysis—or extracorporeal membrane oxygenation (ECMO) or renal replacement therapy of any type—are shown in Fig. 9.1. The contribution of the apparatus can be seen and included in the patient's history by giving the patient a dose of zero of whatever drug is being considered (here gentamicin) at the start of the procedure. It was estimated, using only my gross clinical impression, that the dialysis apparatus might contribute an extra apparent CCr of 50 mL/min/1.73 M^2 in addition to his baseline CCr.

Then, at the end of each procedure, the same thing was done. A dose of zero was again given, and his CCr was set back to his baseline. Note that in such cases one must calculate the patient's baseline CCr beforehand using the routine to do this in the BestDose software, and then to enter all the patient's CCr values directly rather than having them calculated by the software in the usual

[#]	[IM/IV/PO]	[locale]	[hh:mm:ss]	[Hours]	[kg]	[CCr,CI]	[Hours]	[Hours]	[mg/Hour]	[mg]
1	IV	08/01/85	00 00 00	0 00	70 30	3 00	0 500	19 33	200 00	100 00
2	IV	08/01/85	19 20 00	19 33	70 30	53 00	0 100	3 00	0 00	0 00
3	IV	08/01/85	22 20 00	22 33	70 30	3 00	0 100	1 00	0 00	0 00
4	IV	08/01/85	23 20 00	23 33	70 30	3 00	0 500	72 00	100 00	50 00
5	IV	08/04/85	23 20 00	95 33	70 30	3 00	0 500	14 77	220 00	110 00
6	IV	08/05/85	14 06 00	110 10	70 30	53 00	0 100	3 00	0 00	0 00
7	IV	08/05/85	17 06 00	113 10	70 30	3 00	0 100	5 50	0 00	0 00
8	IV	08/05/85	22 36 00	118 60	70 30	3 00	0 500	35 50	160 00	80 00
9	IV	08/07/85	10 06 00	154 10	70 30	53 00	0 100	3 00	0 00	0 00
10	IV	08/07/85	13 06 00	157 10	70 30	3 00	0 100	5 00	0 00	0 00
11	IV	08/07/85	18 06 00	162 10	70 30	3 00	0 500	38 00	200 00	100 00
12	IV	08/09/85	08 06 00	200 10	70 30	3 00	0 500	52 90	200 00	100 00
13	IV	08/11/85	13 00 00	253 00	70 30	53 00	0 100	3 00	0 00	0 00
14	IV	08/11/85	16 00 00	256 00	70 30	3 00	0 100	66 00	0 00	0 00
15	IV	08/14/85	10 00 00	322 00	70 30	53 00	0 100	4 00	0 00	0 00
16	IV	08/14/85	14 00 00	326 00	70 30	3 00	0 100	56 60	0 00	0 00
17	IV	08/16/85	22 36 00	382 60	70 30	3 00	0 500	39 40	200 00	100 00
18	IV	08/18/85	14 00 00	422 00	70 30	53 00	0 100	1 50	0 00	0 00
19	IV	08/18/85	15 30 00	423 50	70 30	3 00	0 100	31 50	0 00	0 00
20	IV	08/19/85	23 00 00	455 00	70 30	3 00	0 500	41 00	200 00	100 00
21	IV	08/21/85	16 00 00	496 00	70 30	53 00	0 100	3 00	0 00	0 00
22	IV	08/21/85	19 00 00	499 00	70 30	3 00	0 100	1 50	0 00	0 00
23	IV	08/21/85	20 30 00	500 50	70 30	3 00	0 500	20 50	200 00	100 00
24	IV	08/22/85	17 00 00	521 00	70 30	4 00	1 000	17 00	95 00	95 00

FIGURE 9.1

History of gentamicin doses and episodes of dialysis. Note that at the start of the first dialysis (dose 2) the patient was given a dose of zero (far right column), and his estimated baseline creatinine clearance of 3 mL/min/1.73 M^2 was increased by 50 units to 53 (Descriptor, CCr,CI—fifth column from right). At the end of dialysis (dose 3), he received another dose of zero, and his estimated creatinine clearance was set back to his baseline of 3 mL/min/1.73 M^2. This was repeated at dose numbers 6−7, 9−10, 13−14, 15−16, 18−19, and 21−22. This procedure permits inclusion of a patient's episodes of dialysis, ECMO, or renal replacement therapy into the pharmacokinetic history of his drug therapy and into the quantitative evaluation of his evolving clinical situation.

way. In doing this, it also may be useful (safer from errors in file writing and reading) to save the patient's data file not in the usual format of .mb2 but in the older format, which one can select when saving the file, of .MB.

When the model of gentamicin was fitted to the patient's data entered in this way, the results are shown in Fig. 9.2. The episodes of dialysis are seen as sharp, almost vertical notches in the weighted average profile of his serum concentrations. So can the lack of gentamicin be seen after leaving the ICU until the new team found the problem, restarted gentamicin again, and asked us to analyze the patient's data. Unfortunately, control of the infection had been lost by then, and despite the restarted gentamicin therapy, the patient died at the right side of the plot.

This patient's case illustrates the fact that not only do messages in the chart need to be very clearly stated, but also that physicians, especially ICU physicians, badly need training in the application of pharmacokinetic concepts and methods. These approaches most definitely need to be taught to medical students as meaningful clinical tools.

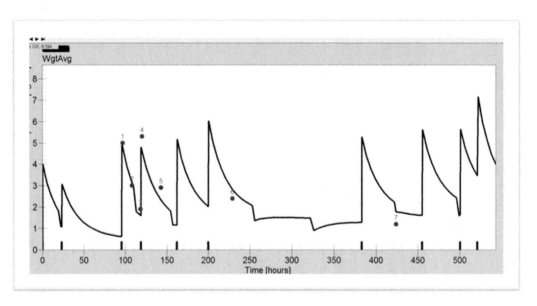

FIGURE 9.2

Screen plot of weighted average serum gentamicin concentrations during the patient's hospital course.
Black line: weighted average serum gentamicin concentrations. Dots: measured serum gentamicin concentrations.
Vertical notches show episodes of dialysis, with some rebound increase in serum concentrations due to movement
from the peripheral compartment back into the central (serum) compartment after dialysis.

This patient's case is shown here to illustrate how procedures such as dialysis, renal replacement
therapy, and ECMO can easily be accommodated into the patient's record and taken into account in
the optimal management of drug dosage in these clinical situations.

9.7 IMM ANALYSIS OF THE PATIENT'S DATA

Let us now look at the same patient's data using the IMM approach. This is shown in Fig. 9.3.

Notice how the fit is improved using the IMM approach. As each new dose is given or each
new data point is encountered, the fit goes to the new data, the model parameter distributions are
updated, and the model proceeds onward until information from another new data point is found.

Fig. 9.4 shows the changing V and K_{slope} (K_{el} per unit of CCr) as the patient proceeded through
his history. With what we now know about optimal sampling, coupled with thoughtful measurements of the drug and also SCr at the beginning and end of each dialysis or other procedure, we
can come to a much improved understanding of a patient's highly variable situation throughout his
course of therapy. However, it takes good data to do this. The reason for getting both an SCr as
well as a drug measurement at the beginning and end of dialysis, etc., is that we can calculate the
apparent CCr conferred by the apparatus, so we can take this information into account as needed in
the management of future cases when drug concentration data may not be available. Then we can

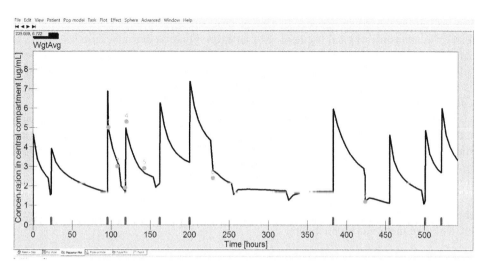

FIGURE 9.3

IMM improved fit to the patient's data.

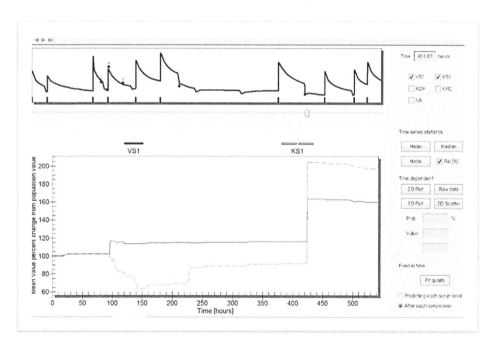

FIGURE 9.4

Plot of the patient's relative (percent) changes in V (here VS1) and K_e (here KS1) during his hospital course. The big change at about 420 h comes after a long period without any information and then a serum concentration drawn just after dialysis. Again, note that V and K_e change independently, sometimes together and sometimes not. This reflects the clinical situation throughout his hospital course, as perceived by each data point as it becomes available.

have information that a certain apparatus, with specific settings for each patient, confers a certain apparent CCr (such as my clinical impression of an extra 50 units) during its use.

Once again, we can do much better in getting good data now. We can use our newer optimal monitoring strategies to best track the patient's drug behavior with the fewest samples. We can also get samples at start and end of each dialysis procedure. We should get an SCr probably every day at least and use the method of estimating CCr described in Chapter 5.

Unstable ICU patients need much more data than has usually been obtained. One reason for this may be that it has commonly been felt that TDM is often not useful in patients with high intrapatient variability, which is what these patients most certainly have. The IMM clinical software for - tracking unstable patients with high intrapatient variability (also known as interoccasional variability) now liberates us from this limitation and provides us with a means to permit much improved care. Now we can get and use, much more intelligently than before, the more frequent and richer TDM data required for these patients and the IMM clinical software designed especially for them, and give them much better care.

9.8 ANOTHER PATIENT, HIGHLY UNSTABLE, WITH HIGH INTRAINDIVIDUAL VARIABILITY

In 1991, courtesy of Dr. Evan Begg, we analyzed data of a 54-year-old woman who presented with a pyelonephritis. She was treated at first with tobramycin 80 mg every 8 h. Her first trough was 0.4 µg/mL, and the following peak was only 4.6 µg/mL. She did well initially, but after a week, she surprisingly developed quite severe septic shock. She was followed closely, more serum concentrations for TDM were obtained, and her dosage was increased. Her SCr also increased from 0.6 at first, to 3.7 mg/dL. On her increased dosage, her tobramycin peaks rose to 5.9 and then to 10.1 µg/mL. She eventually recovered and was discharged home.

When her tobramycin model was fitted to her data in our usual way, the NP fit was extremely poor, as shown in Fig. 9.5. This shows the current problem of trying to do good TDM for unstable patients with high intraindividual and interoccasional variability. The problem is that the patient's model parameters were changing very greatly during the patient's hospital course, and until now, there has been no way to accommodate and account for these highly variable changes during the process of TDM.

Fig. 9.6 shows the much improved fit using the IMM approach, now implemented in the BestDose clinical software [13].

Fig. 9.7 shows the really important results: the changing V and K_{slope} over time revealed by the IMM sequential Bayesian analysis. Note that V and K_{slope} change independently of each other, sometimes going in the same and sometimes in opposite directions. While some changes may appear volatile, perhaps due to errors in recording the times of dosage and sampling, other changes appear quite significant and provide a better fit to, and estimate of, the patient's state over time, as seen in Fig. 9.6.

Figs. 9.6 and 9.7 show the unique ability of the IMM approach to unstable patients with high intrapatient and interoccasional variability, with Fig. 9.7 displaying the changes in V and K as separate issues, with each requiring its own special management approaches.

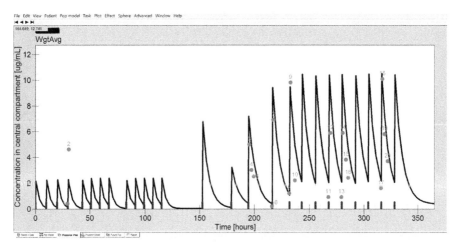

FIGURE 9.5

Patient's model fitted to her data of doses given and concentrations measured. Note the extremely poor fit achieved. Thick line: trajectory of weighted average estimated concentrations after fitting to the data. Dots: measured tobramycin concentrations.

Reproduced with permission from Jelliffe R, Schumitzky A, Bayard D, Van Guilder M, Leary R, Botnen A, Gandhi A, Maire P, Barbaut X, Bleyzac N, Bondareva I, and Neely M: Pharmacokinetic Methods for Analysis, Interpretation, and Management of tdm Data, and for Individualizing Drug Dosage Regimens Optimally, in "Handbook of Analytical Separations", Volume 5, "Drug Monitoring and Clinical Chemistry", ed. by Hempel G, Elsevier, pp. 129– 168, 2004.

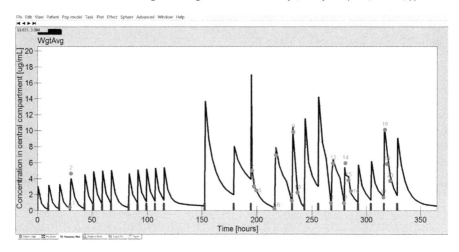

FIGURE 9.6

Fitting the patient's model to the data, using the IMM sequential Bayesian method. Note the great improvement in the fit due to being able to estimate the patient's changing model parameters as each new dose or serum concentration data point becomes available. Labels as in Fig. 9.5.

Reproduced with permission from Jelliffe R, Schumitzky A, Bayard D, Van Guilder M, Leary R, Botnen A, Gandhi A, Maire P, Barbaut X, Bleyzac N, Bondareva I, and Neely M: Pharmacokinetic Methods for Analysis, Interpretation, and Management of tdm Data, and for Individualizing Drug Dosage Regimens Optimally, in "Handbook of Analytical Separations", Volume 5, "Drug Monitoring and Clinical Chemistry", ed. by Hempel G, Elsevier, pp. 129– 168, 2004.

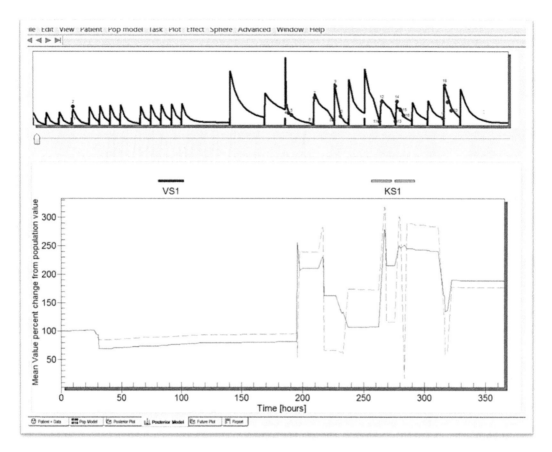

FIGURE 9.7

The top part recapitulates the fit shown in Fig. 9.6. The bottom part shows the percent changes in the patient's estimated mean V (here VS1) and K_{slope} (here KS1) throughout her hospital course, as analyzed with the IMM sequential Bayesian approach employed in the current BestDose clinical software. Note the changes in V and K_{slope} after each new data point becomes available. Some changes appear volatile and may be due to errors in recording times of dosing and drawing of serum samples, but there are also clear changes that are not discoverable by other methods of analysis. In this way, changes in the elimination of tobramycin can be better separated from changes in V, and both can be seen as distinct and separate therapeutic issues. Such changes cannot be perceived by any other current clinical PK software, which assumes that all parameter values are constant through the data analysis.

9.9 TWO NEW MOVES TO FURTHER IMPROVE THE IMM APPROACH

One limitation of the current IMM approach is the number of support points available in the population model and their specific locations. We are currently working to use the hybrid Bayesian approach first, adding a grid of up to 100 extra points widely scattered over the parameter space of its augmented population model, to provide many more available support points for the IMM procedure to jump to when such a jump is more likely given the data. As we have worked on this feature, it has seemed that the more support points available for the IMM software to jump to, the more plausible is the behavior of the drug during its times of high intrapatient variability.

In addition, it may well be useful to enter all values of the patient's CCr simply as 1 mL/min/ 1.73 M^2. When this is done, what one will see is not the K_{slope} per unit of CCr but rather the actual elimination rate constant itself. When the proper data are available of serum drug concentrations at start and end of each procedure, in addition to those around the various doses, then all results will be the actual K_{el}'s themselves, unrelated to the patient's CCr. Then there will be good raw results of the contribution of each apparatus and also of the drug behavior itself at various times.

9.10 SUMMARY

The cases shown here only describe patients receiving aminoglycoside therapy, and from fairly long ago. However, the clinical situations they illustrate are entirely general ones, and the approaches shown here are totally relevant today for any patient in any ICU, receiving any drug, along with dialysis, renal replacement therapy, or ECMO.

Unstable patients clearly require more data to manage them properly than do stable patients who are not so ill. It is likely that such patients will need an SCr at least daily to best track their changing CCr, coupled with optimally chosen times for sampling drug concentrations, as described in Chapter 8. In this way we can learn more rapidly and precisely just how the drug is behaving in the patient over time and have a better idea of his renal function and fluid balance status and needs as well. Further, it is most useful to enter a dose of zero at start and end of any dialysis or similar procedure and also to draw a SCr and a drug concentration at both the start and the end of it.

To summarize again, the following procedures should help us to best perceive the separate issues of fluid balance and drug elimination to improve the care of highly unstable ICU patients with high intrapatient and interoccasional variability in their model parameters:

1. Parameterizing the model as V and K_{el} rather than V and clearance.
2. Entering doses of zero and getting simultaneous samples of drug concentration and SCr at start and end of dialysis, renal replacement therapy, or ECMO, as described.
3. Using optimal TDM strategies, as discussed in Chapter 8, Monitoring Each Patient Optimally: When to Obtain the Best Samples for Therapeutic Drug Monitoring.
4. Using nonparametric rather than parametric PK/PD models of drug behavior, as discussed in Chapter 2, Describing Drug Behavior in Groups of Patients.
5. Using nonparametric Bayesian methods to make individual models, as discussed in Chapter 7: Monitoring the Patient - Making Individual Models.
6. Using MM dosage design to achieve maximal precision of dosage, as discussed in Chapter 3, Multiple Model (MM) Dosage Design for Clinicians.
7. Using the IMM approach as needed for very unstable patients, as discussed in Chapter 7, Monitoring the Patient - Making Individual Models.
8. Evaluating CCr using pairs of changing SCr data throughout the patient's course, as discussed in Chapter 5, Evaluation of Renal Function.

REFERENCES

[1] Mehvar R. Teachers topics. The relationship among pharmacokinetic parameters: effects of altered kinetics on the drug plasma concentration-time profiles. Am J Pharm Educ 2004;68(2):36.

[2] Jelliffe RW, D'Argenio DZ, Schumitzky A, Hu L, and Liu M. The USC PC-PACK programs for planning, monitoring, and adjusting drug dosage regimens. Presented at the American Association of Medical Instrumentation, Washington, DC, 1988; May 14–18.

[3] Haug M. Pharm D, personal communication.

[4] Niemiec P, Allo M, Miller C. Effect of altered volume of distribution on aminoglycoside levels in patients in surgical intensive care. Arch Surg 1987;122:207–12.

[5] Haug III MT, Slugg PH. Antibiotic pharmacokinetics. In: Sivak E, Higgins T, Seiver A, editors. The high risk patient: management of the critically ill. Media, PA: Williams & Wilkins; 1995. p. 1338–64.

[6] Udy A, Roberts J, Shorr A, Boots R, Lipman J. Augmented renal clearance in septic and traumatized patients with normal plasma creatinine concentrations: identifying at-risk patients. Crit Care 2013;17: R35. <http://ccforum.com/content/17/1/R35>.

[7] Udy A, Roberts J, Boots R, Paterson D, Lipman J. Augmented renal clearance. Clin Pharmacokinet 2010;49:1–16.

[8] Bayard D, Jelliffe R. A Bayesian approach to tracking patients having changing pharmacokinetic parameters. J Pharmacokinet Pharmacodyn 2004;31(1):75–107.

[9] Blom H. An efficient filter for abruptly changing systems. Proceedings of the 23rd Conference on Decision and Control, Las Vegas NV, December 1984, p. 656–8.

[10] Blom H, Bar-Shalom Y. The interacting multiple model algorithm for systems with Markovian switching coefficients. IEEE Trans Autom Control 1988;33:780–3.

[11] Mazor E, Averbuch A, Bar-Shalom Y, Dayan J. Interacting multiple model methods in target tracking: a survey. IEEE Trans Aerosp Electron Syst 1998;34:103–23.

[12] Macdonald I, Staatz C, Jelliffe R, Thomson A. Evaluation and comparison of simple multiple model, richer data multiple model, and sequential interacting multiple model (IMM) Bayesian analyses of gentamicin and vancomycin data collected from patients undergoing cardiothoracic surgery. Ther Drug Monit 2008;30:67–74.

[13] The BestDose software is available free for evaluation at <www.lapk.org>.

QUANTITATIVE MODELING OF DIFFUSION INTO ENDOCARDIAL VEGETATIONS, THE POSTANTIBIOTIC EFFECT, AND BACTERIAL GROWTH AND KILL

10

R. Jelliffe

CHAPTER OUTLINE

10.1 INTRODUCTION

In this chapter, we will consider the connection of nonlinear pharmacodynamic models to the basic linear pharmacokinetic model and show some applications in clinical software describing possible drug diffusion into endocardial vegetations, the simulation of a postantibiotic effect (PAE), and the modeling of bacterial growth in the absence of a drug and its kill by an antibiotic.

10.2 DIFFUSION INTO ENDOCARDIAL VEGETATIONS

A problem in managing patients with bacterial endocarditis is that it is extremely difficult to estimate whether or not the drug is able to kill the organisms all the way into the center of a vegetation. To help with this, a diffusion model was made, as shown in Fig. 10.1.

Individualized Drug Therapy for Patients. DOI: http://dx.doi.org/10.1016/B978-0-12-803348-7.00010-1

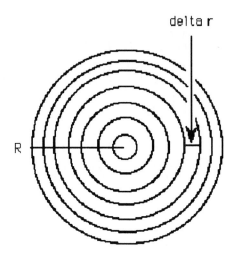

FIGURE 10.1

Diagram of concentric layers in a spherical model of a possible endocardial vegetation. A spherical shape was assumed, having concentric layers. Diffusion takes place from layer to layer, delta r. The sphere is assumed to be homogenous with diffusion taking place in all directions, with a constant coefficient of diffusion. Diffusion is also assumed to be dependent on the concentration of drug in which the object is located (serum concentration) and its profile over time. Vegetation size and shape can be assessed by transesophageal echocardiography.

Reproduced with permission from Jelliffe R, Schumitzky A, Leary R, Botnen A, Gandhi A, Maire P, Barbaut X, Bleyzac N, and Bondareva I: Optimizing Individualized Dosage Regimens of Potentially Toxic Drugs, in Pharmacokinetic Applications in Drug Development, ed by Rajesh Krishna, Ph.D., Kluwer Academic/Plenum Publishers, pp 477–528, 2003.

Eq. (10.1) here was used to model the diffusion:

$$\frac{\partial C}{\partial t} = \frac{1}{r^2} \times \frac{\partial}{\partial r}\left[D \times r^2 \times \frac{\partial C}{\partial r}\right] \tag{10.1}$$

where C represents the concentration in the sphere at time t, at a distance r from the center of the sphere. D represents the coefficient of diffusion in the sphere, and $\times$ indicates multiplication.

When D is assumed constant, the equation becomes

$$\frac{\partial C}{\partial t} = D \times \left[\frac{\partial^2 C}{\partial r^2} + \frac{2}{r} \times \frac{\partial C}{\partial r}\right] \tag{10.2}$$

The vegetation is assumed to be immersed in the surrounding blood, and the serum drug concentration is assumed to attain an equilibrium value with the very outer layer of the sphere. The medium has the changes in concentration over time that constitute the profile of the serum drug concentration. This changing serum concentration is the input to the spherical model [1].

The diffusion coefficient found by Bayer et al. for aminoglycosides in experimental endocarditis [2,3] was used. The model has become part of the BestDose clinical software for individualizing drug dosage regimens [4]. The model can also, by appropriate choice of sphere diameter and diffusion coefficient, simulate a microorganism and a post-antibiotic effect (PAE) of a desired duration.

10.2.1 SIMULATED VEGETATIONS OF VARIOUS DIAMETERS

Let us consider a 65-year-old man, 70 in tall, weighing 70 kg with a serum creatinine of 1 mg/dL. Suppose he has an endocardial vegetation seen by echocardiography on his aortic valve. We wish to evaluate the ability of an amikacin regimen designed to achieve serum peaks of 45 µg/mL and troughs of approximately 5 µg/mL to penetrate the vegetation and reach effective concentrations when the vegetation has a diameter of 0.5, 1, or 2 cm. Let us use the findings of Bayer et al. [2,3] to compute the time course of possible amikacin concentrations in the center of these three different vegetations. Then let us examine their possible ability to kill an organism having an estimated minimum inhibitory concentration (MIC), of 8 µg/mL.

Using the current BestDose [4] software for amikacin, our patient's creatinine clearance is about 69 mL/min/1.73 M^2 [5]. The ideal dose interval to achieve that peak and trough exactly, adjusted for the patient's renal function and employing an IV infusion of 0.5 h, is 10.231 h. Let us select a more practical dose interval of 12 h. The revised dosage regimen is 850 mg for the first dose and then 750 mg every 12 h thereafter.

On this regimen, predicted serum concentrations are 43 µg/mL peak and 3.2 µg/mL trough. The peak is 5.38 times the stated MIC. Serum concentrations are predicted to be at least the MIC for 66% of each dose interval. The area under the curve (AUC) to MIC ratio for the first 24 h is 48.8. The plot of these predicted serum concentrations is shown in Fig. 10.2.

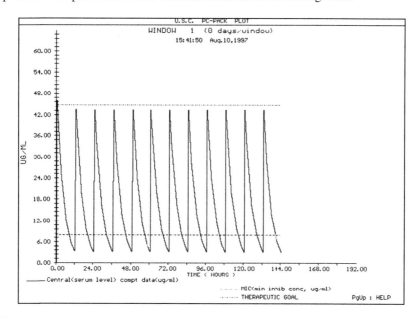

FIGURE 10.2

Predicted time course (for the first 6 days) of serum amikacin concentrations for the patient described. Upper horizontal dotted line shows the initial stated target peak serum concentration of 45 µg/mL. Lower horizontal dashed line shows the estimated organism MIC of 8 µg/mL.

Reproduced with permission from Jelliffe R, Schumitzky A, Leary R, Botnen A, Gandhi A, Maire P, Barbaut X, Bleyzac N, and Bondareva I: Optimizing Individualized Dosage Regimens of Potentially Toxic Drugs, in Pharmacokinetic Applications in Drug Development, ed by Rajesh Krishna, Ph.D., Kluwer Academic/Plenum Publishers, pp 477–528, 2003.

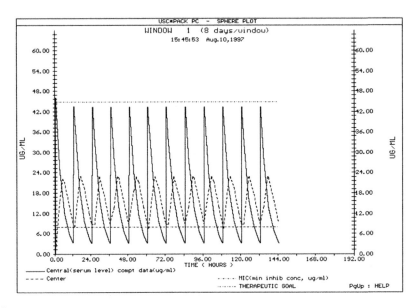

FIGURE 10.3

Predicted time course (the first 6 days) of amikacin concentrations (dashed line) in the center of a simulated endocardial vegetation of 0.5 cm. Solid line shows the predicted serum concentrations, and other lines and symbols are as in Fig. 10.2. The predicted endocardial concentrations rise promptly and are consistently at least the assumed MIC of 8 μg/mL.

Reproduced with permission from Jelliffe R, Schumitzky A, Leary R, Botnen A, Gandhi A, Maire P, Barbaut X, Bleyzac N, and Bondareva I: Optimizing Individualized Dosage Regimens of Potentially Toxic Drugs, in Pharmacokinetic Applications in Drug Development, ed by Rajesh Krishna, Ph.D., Kluwer Academic/Plenum Publishers, pp 477–528, 2003.

Now let us see if this serum concentration profile produces adequate penetration of the vegetation in each of the three sizes and whether or not the regimen might kill effectively there, in addition to the central (serum level) compartment.

Fig. 10.3 shows the predicted concentrations in the center of the simulated vegetation having a diameter of 0.5 cm. The concentrations rise rapidly above the MIC and stay above it, suggesting that this regimen might kill organisms having an MIC of about 8 μg/mL fairly promptly in the center of this particular vegetation. The concentrations in the center of the sphere lag behind the serum concentrations by about 3 h to 4 h.

On the other hand, if the diameter of the vegetation were 1 cm, the drug should take about 12 h to diffuse to the center and reach the MIC. The rise and fall of drug concentrations would be much more damped, as shown in Fig. 10.4.

If the diameter of the vegetation were 2 cm, diffusion to the center should take four times as long as for the 1-cm vegetation and fully 16 times as long as for the 0.5-cm vegetation. The time course of the computed concentrations in the center would be as shown in Fig. 10.5. For every doubling of the diameter of the sphere, four times as much time (the square of the ratio of the diameters) will be required to reach an equal concentration in the center of the sphere. It would take over 52 h to reach the MIC in the center of the 2-cm vegetation, and significant growth of organisms might well take place before that.

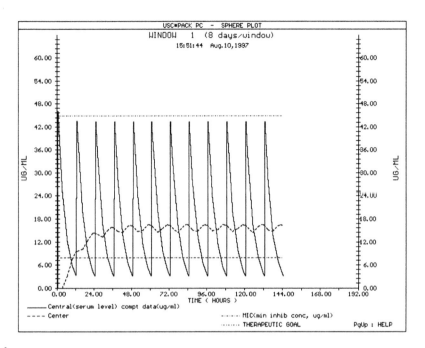

FIGURE 10.4

Predicted time course (the first 6 days) of amikacin concentrations (dashed line) in the center of a simulated endocardial vegetation of 1 cm. Solid line shows the predicted serum concentrations. Other lines and symbols are as in Fig. 10.3. The predicted endocardial concentrations rise more slowly and have smaller oscillations from peak to trough. However, once the estimated MIC is reached, they are consistently above the MIC of 8 μg/mL.

Reproduced with permission from Jelliffe R, Schumitzky A, Leary R, Botnen A, Gandhi A, Maire P, Barbaut X, Bleyzac N, and Bondareva I: Optimizing Individualized Dosage Regimens of Potentially Toxic Drugs, in Pharmacokinetic Applications in Drug Development, ed by Rajesh Krishna, Ph.D., Kluwer Academic/Plenum Publishers, pp 477-528, 2003.

10.3 SIMULATING A SMALL MICROORGANISM

Fig. 10.6 shows computed drug concentrations in the center of a small sphere, simulating a microorganism having a diameter of 0.1 micron, three simulated layers of diffusion, and a diffusion coefficient of 1.5×10^{-14}. This particular simulated sphere has the special property that in its center the concentrations of drug fall below the MIC about 6 h after the serum levels do, simulating (without making any suggestions or conclusions about mechanism of action) a PAE of about 6 h. The organisms will not begin to grow again for about 6 h after the serum concentrations fall below the MIC.

The effects of these computed concentrations in the center of these spheres are discussed in the section on modeling bacterial growth and kill. We see here that the process of diffusion into and out of spherical porous objects such as endocardial vegetations and small microorganisms can be described with these models.

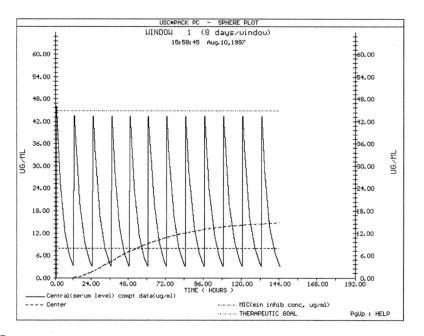

FIGURE 10.5

Predicted time course (the first 6 days) of amikacin concentrations (dashed line) in the center of a simulated endocardial vegetation of 2 cm. Solid line shows the predicted serum concentrations, and other lines and symbols are as in Fig. 10.3. The predicted endocardial concentrations appear to have a lag time, then rise much more slowly and are much more damped, with essentially no oscillations from peak to trough. Once the estimated MIC is reached, the concentrations are consistently above 8 μg/mL, but two full days are required before even the MIC is reached.

Reproduced with permission from Jelliffe R, Schumitzky A, Leary R, Botnen A, Gandhi A, Maire P, Barbaut X, Bleyzac N, and Bondareva I: Optimizing Individualized Dosage Regimens of Potentially Toxic Drugs, in Pharmacokinetic Applications in Drug Development, ed by Rajesh Krishna, Ph.D., Kluwer Academic/Plenum Publishers, pp 477–528, 2003.

10.4 MODELING BACTERIAL GROWTH AND KILL

10.4.1 GENERAL CONSIDERATIONS

Let us consider an organism in its logarithmic, most virulent phase of exponential growth in the absence of any antibiotic. It will have a doubling time equivalent to a half-time but for growth rather than kill (see Chapter 1) and a rate constant for this growth. The killing effect of the antibiotic can be modeled as a Michaelis–Menten or Hill model. Such a model generates a rate constant for this kill. The rate of growth or kill of an organism depends upon the difference between these two rate constants. The killing effect will be determined by the E_{max}, representing the maximum possible rate constant (shortest possible half-time) for kill. It will also depend upon the EC50 (the concentration at which the effect is half maximal) and the time course of the serum concentrations achieved on the dosage regimen the patient is given. Both the growth

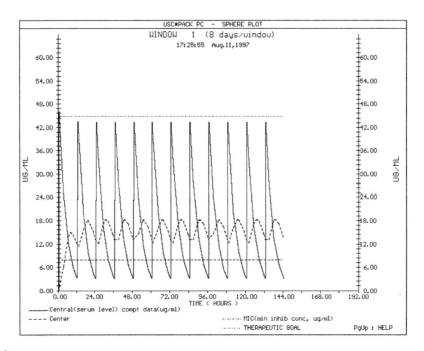

FIGURE 10.6

Plot of computed amikacin concentrations (the first 6 days) in the center of a simulated microorganism. Diffusion coefficients in the very small sphere diffusion model have been adjusted so that concentrations in the center of the organism lag behind the serum concentrations and, if they fall below the MIC, would do so approximately 6 h after the serum concentrations do, thus simulating a postantibiotic effect of about 6 h.

Reproduced with permission from Jelliffe R, Schumitzky A, Leary R, Botnen A, Gandhi A, Maire P, Barbaut X, Bleyzac N, and Bondareva I: Optimizing Individualized Dosage Regimens of Potentially Toxic Drugs, in Pharmacokinetic Applications in Drug Development, ed by Rajesh Krishna, Ph.D., Kluwer Academic/Plenum Publishers, pp 477–528, 2003.

rate constant and the E_{max} can be found from available data in the literature for various organisms. The general growth versus kill equation is

$$\frac{dB}{dt} = (K_g - K_k) \times B \tag{10.3}$$

and

$$K_k = \frac{E_{max} \times C_t^n}{EC_{50}^n + C_t^n} \tag{10.4}$$

where B is the number of bugs, set to 1 relative unit (think 1 million organisms) at the start of therapy. K_g is the rate constant for growth, K_k is the rate constant for killing, E_{max} is the maximum possible rate of killing, EC_{50} is the concentration at which the rate of killing is half maximal, n is the Hill or sigmoidicity coefficient, and C_t is the concentration of drug at the site of the effect (serum, peripheral compartment, effect compartment, or in the center of a spherical model of diffusion) at any time t.

The EC_{50} can be found from the MIC of the organism, or from a clinical impression of what it might be. This relationship was developed by Zhi et al. [6], and independently by Schumitzky [7]. The MIC is modeled as the concentration at which the rate constant for kill is equal to but opposite in direction to the rate constant for growth. The MIC is the concentration that offsets growth. At the MIC, there is neither growth nor decrease in the number of organisms. At the MIC:

$$\frac{dB}{dt} = 0, \text{ and } K_k = -K_g \tag{10.5}$$

and

$$\text{MIC} = \left(\frac{K_g \times EC_{50}^n}{E_{max} - K_g} \right)^{1/n} \tag{10.6}$$

In this way, the EC_{50} can be found from the MIC and vice versa.

The input to this effect model can be from the central or from the peripheral compartment concentrations of a pharmacokinetic model, or from the center (or any other layer) of one of the spherical models of diffusion. The sphere may represent an endocardial vegetation or a small microorganism. For an organism, one can also adjust the sphere diameter and diffusion coefficient so that the concentrations in the center of the small sphere lag behind the serum concentrations and cross below the MIC about 6 h after the serum concentrations do, to simulate a PAE of 6 h. The effect relationship here was modeled by Bouvier D'Ivoire and Maire [8], from data obtained from Craig and Ebert [9], for the relationship between pseudomonas and an aminoglycoside.

In the previous section, we considered a 65-year-old man, 70 in tall, weighing 70 kg, having a serum creatinine of 1 mg/dL. We also assumed that he had a vegetation on his aortic valve, seen by echocardiography, that might be either 0.5, 1, or 2 cm in diameter. We wanted to evaluate the ability of an amikacin regimen designed to achieve serum peaks of 45 and troughs of about 5 µg/mL to reach effective concentrations within the vegetation in these three cases. We applied the findings of Bayer et al. [2,3] to predict the time course of amikacin concentrations in the center of the three vegetations.

The patient's dosage regimen consisted of an initial dose of 850 mg of amikacin followed by 750 mg every 12 h thereafter. On that regimen, predicted serum concentrations were 43 µg/mL for the peak and 3.2 for the trough. The MIC of the organism was assumed to be 8 µg/mL.

The computed concentration of amikacin in the various vegetations was shown in the previous section. Fig. 10.7 is a plot not only of the predicted time course (the first 6 days) of serum amikacin concentrations for the patient described here but also of its ability to kill microorganisms using the model made by Bouvier D'Ivoire and Maire [8], based on the data of Craig and Ebert [9]. In Fig. 10.7, there is no assumption of any PAE. The serum concentration profile is presented as the input to the effect model, which is assumed to be bathed in the serum.

The model always assumes an initial inoculum of one relative unit - 1 million organisms for example. The serum concentration profile resulting from that regimen appears to diffuse into the organism and to kill it well in this particular situation. As the serum concentrations fall below the MIC with the first dose, however, the organisms begin to grow again. However, the second dose kills them again, with slight regrowth later on in that dose interval. The third dose reduces the number of organisms essentially to zero. This effect model suggests that such a serum concentration profile should kill an organism having an MIC of 8 µg/mL, even though

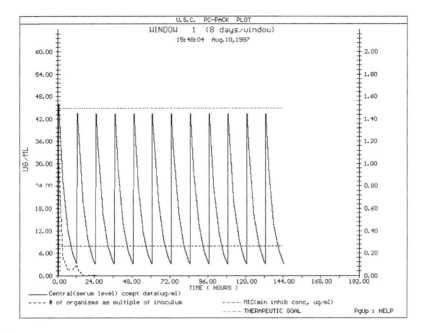

FIGURE 10.7

Predicted killing effect of the regimen. Input from the central (serum) compartment profile of serum concentrations. The regimen is likely to kill well for a bloodstream infection (sepsis). Solid line and left-hand scale show serum concentrations. Dashed line and right-hand scale show the relative numbers of organisms, with 1.0 relative unit present at the start of therapy. Upper horizontal dotted and dashed line show the original peak serum goal of therapy. Lower horizontal dashed line indicates the patient's MIC of 8 μg/mL.

Reproduced with permission from Jelliffe R, Schumitzky A, Leary R, Botnen A, Gandhi A, Maire P, Barbaut X, Bleyzac N, and Bondareva I: Optimizing Individualized Dosage Regimens of Potentially Toxic Drugs, in Pharmacokinetic Applications in Drug Development, ed by Rajesh Krishna, Ph.D., Kluwer Academic/Plenum Publishers, pp 477–528, 2003.

the serum concentrations are below the MIC about one-third of the time, as the high peaks are effective in the killing.

Fig. 10.8 shows the predictions in the center of the simulated endocardial vegetation having a diameter of 0.5 cm. Here the organisms grow almost four-fold, to almost four relative units, before the concentrations in the center of the vegetation reach the MIC and start to kill. The organisms are reduced essentially to zero by 24 h, suggesting that such a regimen might kill well in the center of this 0.5-cm diameter vegetation.

Fig. 10.9 is a similar plot, but of the simulated vegetation having a diameter of 1 cm. Now one sees a significant lag time of 3–4 h before any visible concentrations are reached in the center of the vegetation. The MIC is not reached until about 10 h. During that time, the organisms have grown from 1 to about 150 relative units. However, once the MIC is reached, killing begins, although not quite as fast as with the smaller vegetation, due to the slower rate of rise of drug concentration in the center of the larger vegetation. However, killing appears to be essentially

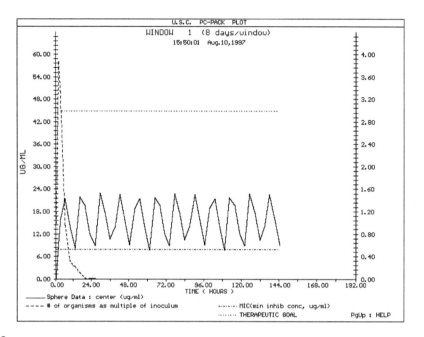

FIGURE 10.8

Calculated killing effect in the center of the 0.5 cm diameter vegetation. Good and fairly prompt killing is seen. Solid line and left-hand scale indicate drug concentrations in the center of the vegetation. Dashed line and right-hand scale indicate the relative numbers of organisms, with 1.0 relative unit present at the start of therapy. Upper horizontal dotted and dashed line show the original peak serum goal of therapy. Lower horizontal dashed line shows the patient's organism's assumed MIC of 8 μg/mL.

Reproduced with permission from Jelliffe R, Schumitzky A, Leary R, Botnen A, Gandhi A, Maire P, Barbaut X, Bleyzac N, and
Bondareva I: Optimizing Individualized Dosage Regimens of Potentially Toxic Drugs, in Pharmacokinetic Applications in Drug
Development, ed by Rajesh Krishna, Ph.D., Kluwer Academic/Plenum Publishers, pp 477–528, 2003.

complete after approximately 40 h. This suggests that the above regimen, of an undefined duration might also be adequate to kill in the center of a 1 cm of vegetation but with less confidence of success than with the smaller vegetation of 0.5 cm diameter.

As shown in Fig. 10.10, things are much worse for the 2 cm vegetation. Diffusion into the center is much (four times) slower. There is a lag of about 12 h before visible concentrations are first seen, and about 52 h are required before they reach the MIC. During this time, the number of organisms has increased from 1 relative unit to over 1 million units. However, after about 5 days, due to the continued presence of drug concentrations in the center of the vegetation approaching 12−15 μg/mL, killing appears to take place, and after about 6 days, the number of organisms approaches zero. Such a dosage regimen might be inadequate in the center of a 2-cm simulated vegetation and might require much more aggressive therapy, surgery, or both.

Fig. 10.11 shows the calculated concentrations in the center of the small simulated microorganism used in the previous section to model the time course of a 6-h PAE. There is a lag of

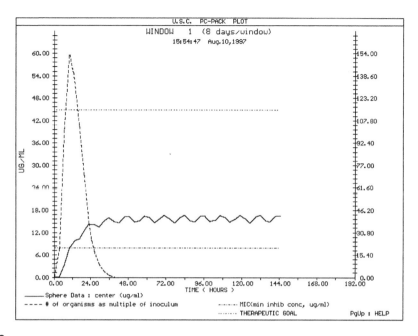

FIGURE 10.9

Killing effect computed for the center of a simulated vegetation of 1 cm diameter. The effect is delayed as it takes longer for diffusion to reach the center. Solid line and left-hand scale indicate drug concentrations in the center of the vegetation. Dashed line and right-hand scale indicate the relative numbers of organisms, with 1.0 relative unit present at the start of therapy. Upper horizontal dotted and dashed line show the original peak serum goal of therapy. Lower horizontal dashed line shows the patient's organism's MIC of 8 μg/mL.

Reproduced with permission from Jelliffe R, Schumitzky A, Leary R, Botnen A, Gandhi A, Maire P, Barbaut X, Bleyzac N, and Bondareva I: Optimizing Individualized Dosage Regimens of Potentially Toxic Drugs, in Pharmacokinetic Applications in Drug Development, ed by Rajesh Krishna, Ph.D., Kluwer Academic/Plenum Publishers, pp 477–528, 2003.

about 6 h between the fall of the serum concentrations and that of the concentrations in the center of this hypothetical microorganism. If the dosage interval were to be greater so the concentrations in the center of the microorganism might fall below the MIC, they would do so approximately 6 h after the serum concentrations fall below the MIC, thus simulating a PAE of approximately 6 h.

One might ask what the contribution (if any) of such a PAE to overall therapy might be. As shown in Fig. 10.12, the outcome is similar to that shown in Fig. 10.7. Killing is delayed until concentrations above the MIC are reached. In both cases, killing is then rapid and prompt. One can see that due to the diffusion model there may be a delay of approximately 6 h before the concentrations in the hypothetical microorganism reach the MIC. During that time, the number of organisms has grown from 1 to about 5.4 relative units. However, after that time, the concentrations are always above the MIC. Significant killing begins and continues, with the organisms being reduced essentially to zero by about 36 h.

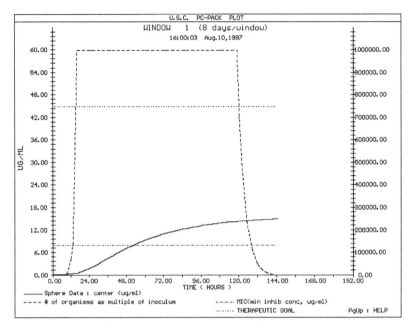

FIGURE 10.10

Calculated killing effect in the center of a 2-cm simulated vegetation. Diffusion to the center is much delayed, while bacterial growth continues. Killing is also very delayed. Solid line and left-hand scale indicate drug concentrations in the center of the vegetation. Dashed line and right-hand scale indicate the relative numbers of organisms, with 1.0 relative unit present at the start of therapy. Upper horizontal dotted and dashed line show the original peak serum goal of therapy. Lower horizontal dashed line shows the patient's assumed MIC of 8 μg/mL.

Reproduced with permission from Jelliffe R, Schumitzky A, Leary R, Botnen A, Gandhi A, Maire P, Barbaut X, Bleyzac N, and Bondareva I: Optimizing Individualized Dosage Regimens of Potentially Toxic Drugs, in Pharmacokinetic Applications in Drug Development, ed by Rajesh Krishna, Ph.D., Kluwer Academic/Plenum Publishers, pp 477–528, 2003.

10.5 AN ILLUSTRATIVE CASE

These diffusion and effect models became of significant clinical interest when they were used to analyze retrospectively data obtained much earlier, back in 1991, from the highly unstable patient from Christchurch, New Zealand, seen through the courtesy of Dr. Evan Begg. She had a pyelonephritis and received tobramycin, 80 mg approximately every 8 h to 12 h. She was having a satisfactory clinical response to therapy when, on about the sixth day, she suddenly and unexpectedly went into septic shock. She then received much more aggressive tobramycin and eventually recovered. The MIC of her organism was 2 μg/mL. The analysis of bacterial growth and kill described below was not done until several years later, after the models of diffusion and growth and kill had been developed. However, the interacting multiple model (IMM) procedure had not yet been developed.

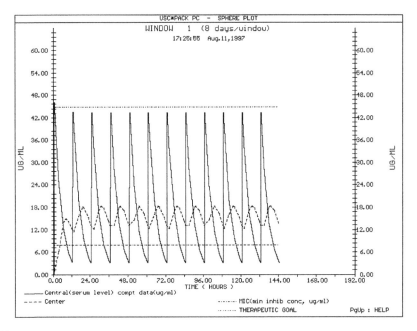

FIGURE 10.11

Computed amikacin concentrations in the center of a hypothetical microorganism in which concentrations fall below the MIC about 6 h after the serum concentrations do, thus simulating (regardless of mechanism) a postantibiotic effect (PAE) of about 6 h. Solid line and left-hand scale indicate serum drug concentrations. Dashed line and right-hand scale show computed concentrations in the center of the microorganism simulating the PAE. Upper horizontal dotted and dashed line indicate the original peak serum goal of therapy. Lower horizontal dashed line shows the patient's MIC of 8 µg/mL.

Reproduced with permission from Jelliffe R, Schumitzky A, Leary R, Botnen A, Gandhi A, Maire P, Barbaut X, Bleyzac N, and Bondareva I: Optimizing Individualized Dosage Regimens of Potentially Toxic Drugs, in Pharmacokinetic Applications in Drug Development, ed by Rajesh Krishna, Ph.D., Kluwer Academic/Plenum Publishers, pp 477–528, 2003.

Fig. 10.13 shows the computed concentrations of drug in the center of the 0.1 µ sphere, simulating an organism with a PAE of 6 h. In the first phase of the analysis, she appeared to be a general medical patient (not an intensive care unit patient) having a satisfactory clinical response to her tobramycin therapy. However, at the end of this time (from 120 h to 148 h into therapy) she unexpectedly relapsed on about day 6 of therapy, went into septic shock, and became an ICU patient.

Note the damped response in the center of the small sphere to the sharp peaks and troughs of the serum concentrations. As data accumulate in the future, this diffusion model may permit improved modeling of these events during a patient's clinical care compared to current indices such as peak/MIC and AUC/MIC.

The patient's peak serum tobramycin concentrations initially were low. Her measured serum peak was 4.6 µg/mL, and her trough was 0.4 µg/mL. Fig. 10.14 describes the growth and kill of the

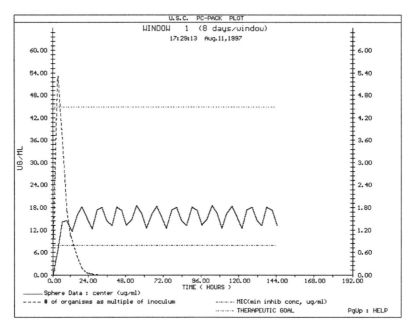

FIGURE 10.12

Killing effect predicted for the simulated postantibiotic effect (PAE) of 6 h, using the computed concentrations in the center of the simulated microorganism as input to the effect model. Solid line and left-hand scale indicate drug concentrations in the center of the microorganism simulating the PAE. Dashed line and right-hand scale indicate relative numbers of organisms, with 1.0 relative unit present at the start of therapy. Upper horizontal dotted and dashed line indicate original peak serum goal of therapy. Lower horizontal dashed line shows the patient's MIC of 8 µg/mL.

Reproduced with permission from Jelliffe R, Schumitzky A, Leary R, Botnen A, Gandhi A, Maire P, Barbaut X, Bleyzac N, and Bondareva I: Optimizing Individualized Dosage Regimens of Potentially Toxic Drugs, in Pharmacokinetic Applications in Drug Development, ed by Rajesh Krishna, Ph.D., Kluwer Academic/Plenum Publishers, pp 477–528, 2003.

organisms in response to events in her serum concentration compartment, while Fig. 10.15 shows the same events as viewed with the sphere model simulating the presumed 6-h PAE.

Note in both figures that few organisms are present at the start of therapy. Growth becomes visible in Fig. 10.14 after the gap between doses in the center of the plot and then becomes exponential during day six of therapy after the last dose on that plot. This plot ends just before the next dose, which was given during her second period, that of septic shock.

Fig. 10.15 extends this examination to show the contribution of the PAE, where the concentrations in the center of the small sphere are evaluated with respect to their ability to kill the organisms. Note that the regimen again appeared to be effective at first, but the organisms again grew out exponentially when the concentrations fell below the MIC for a significant time. However, this growth took place later than in Fig. 10.14, which shows the calculated events without any PAE. The contribution of the PAE here is seen to be modest but perhaps useful by delaying

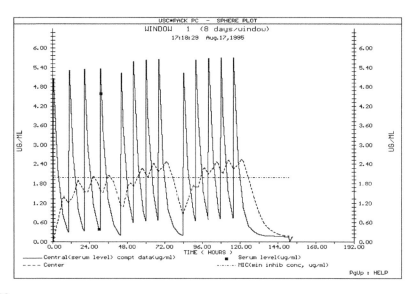

FIGURE 10.13

Patient receiving tobramycin. Measured serum concentrations (small rectangles) and the Bayesian fitted model for the first part of her therapy before she became clinically septic. Small solid rectangles show measured serum concentrations. Solid line and left-hand scale indicate fitted serum drug concentrations. Dashed line and right-hand scale indicate concentrations in the small organism simulating the 6 h postantibiotic effect. Horizontal dashed line indicates the patient's MIC of 2 μg/mL.

Reproduced with permission from Jelliffe R, Schumitzky A, Leary R, Botnen A, Gandhi A, Maire P, Barbaut X, Bleyzac N, and Bondareva I: Optimizing Individualized Dosage Regimens of Potentially Toxic Drugs, in Pharmacokinetic Applications in Drug Development, ed by Rajesh Krishna, Ph.D., Kluwer Academic/Plenum Publishers, pp 477–528, 2003.

the outgrowth by about one day. Both analyses correlated well with the patient's clinical relapse at that time and with her development of septic shock.

Fig. 10.16 shows her second phase, that of acute sepsis. There was essentially no carry-over of drug from the last dose shown in Figs. 10.13 and 10.14 to the patient's next dose, which was given at time zero in Fig. 10.16. Fig. 10.16 shows the many serum concentrations measured during this second phase of her hospital course. It also shows the results of NP Bayesian fitting but not the IMM fitting. During this time, her serum creatinine rose from 0.7 mg/dL to 3.7 mg/dL.

It took about two days, as new serum concentrations were obtained, for ward personnel to react fully to her suddenly much increased volume of distribution (from 0.18 before her sepsis, in Figs. 10.13–10.15, to 0.51 L/kg during her sepsis) and her much decreased renal function to give her the much larger doses required to achieve effective peak serum concentrations. Note also that her trough concentrations rose from about 0.3 to 2 μg/mL during this time, so that the time that her serum concentrations were above the MIC of her organism was also greatly increased.

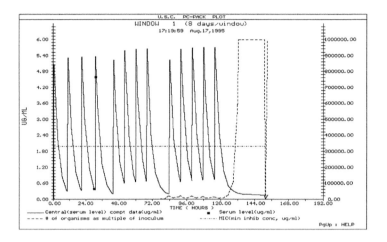

FIGURE 10.14

Patient receiving tobramycin, before becoming septic. Measured serum concentrations (small solid rectangles) and her individualized Bayesian fitted model for this part of her history. Solid line and left-hand scale show fitted serum drug concentrations. Dashed line and right-hand scale indicate relative numbers of organisms. The plot always begins with 1.0 relative units of organism. Horizontal dashed line shows the patient's MIC of 2 μg/mL.

Reproduced with permission from Jelliffe R, Schumitzky A, Leary R, Botnen A, Gandhi A, Maire P, Barbaut X, Bleyzac N, and Bondareva I: Optimizing Individualized Dosage Regimens of Potentially Toxic Drugs, in Pharmacokinetic Applications in Drug Development, ed by Rajesh Krishna, Ph.D., Kluwer Academic/Plenum Publishers, pp 477–528, 2003.

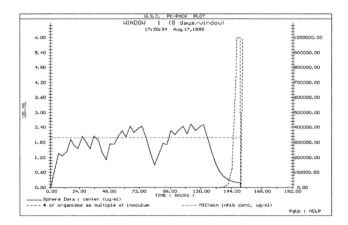

FIGURE 10.15

Graph of killing effect found with the model simulating the PAE of about 6 h. Solid line and left-hand scale indicate drug concentrations in the microorganism simulating the 6-h postantibiotic effect. Dashed line and right-hand scale indicate relative numbers of organisms. The plot always begins with 1.0 relative units of organism, as shown on the right-hand scale. Horizontal dashed line shows the patient's MIC of 2 μg/mL.

Reproduced with permission from Jelliffe R, Schumitzky A, Leary R, Botnen A, Gandhi A, Maire P, Barbaut X, Bleyzac N, and Bondareva I: Optimizing Individualized Dosage Regimens of Potentially Toxic Drugs, in Pharmacokinetic Applications in Drug Development, ed by Rajesh Krishna, Ph.D., Kluwer Academic/Plenum Publishers, pp 477–528, 2003.

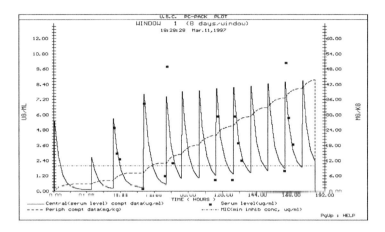

FIGURE 10.16

Plot of serum and peripheral compartment concentrations during the time of the patient's sepsis and her recovery. Small solid rectangles indicate measured serum concentrations. Solid line and left-hand scale indicate fitted serum concentrations. Dashed line and right-hand scale indicate peripheral compartment concentrations, also fitted from the serum data. Horizontal dashed line shows the patient's MIC of 2 μg/mL.

Reproduced with permission from Jelliffe R, Schumitzky A, Leary R, Botnen A, Gandhi A, Maire P, Barbaut X, Bleyzac N, and Bondareva I: Optimizing Individualized Dosage Regimens of Potentially Toxic Drugs, in Pharmacokinetic Applications in Drug Development, ed by Rajesh Krishna, Ph.D., Kluwer Academic/Plenum Publishers, pp 477–528, 2003.

Fig. 10.17 then shows her computed bacterial growth and kill based on the input from the reconstructed (fitted) serum concentration profile during this time, without any aid from any simulated PAE. The organisms grow out of control in the first two days, correlating with the patient's sepsis and the time required for ward personnel to react and adjust her dosage sharply upward. As higher and more effective concentrations were achieved, however, killing could finally be seen at about the sixth day in this figure and appeared to be effective after that. The behavior of this model correlated quite well with the patient's subsequent clinical recovery and discharge home.

Fig. 10.18 shows the same events but now with the diffusion model of the small microorganism with the simulated 6-h PAE. Concentrations in the center of the simulated microorganism do not exceed the MIC until almost 72 h, with the fourth peak in concentration. Significant killing can be seen to begin about a day earlier in this figure, at about 110 h here compared to about 130 h in Fig. 10.17, and appeared to be effective after that.

In general, models of bacterial growth and kill let one incorporate known in vitro data of the logarithmic growth rate of the organism and the maximum kill rate achieved with an antibiotic, integrate it with data of the MIC of each individual patient's organism, and model its growth and kill in units of relative numbers of organisms. These Zhi and Hill models correlated well in this patient with her unexpected relapse from having what had seemed to be an apparently satisfactory response to therapy to becoming a seriously ill patient with septic shock and then with her subsequent recovery later on as effective serum concentrations were eventually achieved and maintained. They give a much richer picture of the clinical events than do the more traditional indices of kill such as peak/MIC and AUC/MIC ratios.

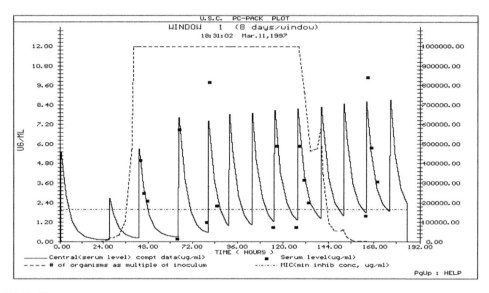

FIGURE 10.17

Plot of the effect on growth and kill using input from the serum concentration profile. The organisms grow out of control when serum concentrations were low at the left but are killed again when they become higher. These events correlated well with the patient's relapse at the beginning of the plot, at the left, and with her recovery about one week later. Small solid rectangles indicate measured serum concentrations. Solid line and left-hand scale indicate estimated serum concentrations after fitting to her data. Dashed line and right-hand scale indicate calculated relative numbers of organisms, with 1.0 relative unit present at the start of therapy. Horizontal dashed line shows the patient's MIC of 2 μg/mL.

Reproduced with permission from Jelliffe R, Schumitzky A, Leary R, Botnen A, Gandhi A, Maire P, Barbaut X, Bleyzac N, and Bondareva I: Optimizing Individualized Dosage Regimens of Potentially Toxic Drugs, in Pharmacokinetic Applications in Drug Development, ed by Rajesh Krishna, Ph.D., Kluwer Academic/Plenum Publishers, pp 477-528, 2003.

10.5.1 FURTHER ANALYSIS OF THE MODEL

However, there are several ways in which the Zhi−Hill model is not realistic. It does not describe the decline of bacterial growth rate seen over time as substrates decline, reaching a maximum number of organisms, as found by Mouton, Vinks, and Punt [10]. In the present model, the organisms are always assumed to be in their logarithmic, most virulent growth phase. In addition, the model does not account for the increase in bacterial resistance commonly found over time due to the emergence of resistant organisms. However, one can use clinical judgment to estimate the maximum possible MIC that the emerging resistant organisms might reach, enter this at the beginning of the analysis, and examine the behavior of the model. Lastly in this model, the growth is only suppressed. The organisms are not really killed in the model, and whatever numbers of organisms are still alive are still in their most virulent, logarithmic growth phase, always trying to emerge again.

When set up this way, the model becomes a useful example of a "worst case" scenario, with the presumed more resistant organisms being so from the very beginning of therapy, and with the

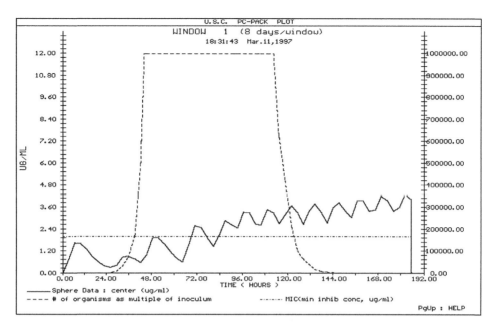

FIGURE 10.18

Plot of the effect on organism growth and kill using input from the center of the organism, with its computed concentrations in its center as input to the effect model. The postantibiotic effect (PAE) helps somewhat to delay the relapse and augment the kill. Solid line and left-hand scale indicate computed concentrations in center of microorganism simulating the PAE. Dashed line and right-hand scale indicate relative numbers of organisms, with 1.0 relative unit present at the start of therapy. Horizontal dashed line shows the patient's MIC of 2 μg/mL.

Reproduced with permission from Jelliffe R, Schumitzky A, Leary R, Botnen A, Gandhi A, Maire P, Barbaut X, Bleyzac N, and Bondareva I: Optimizing Individualized Dosage Regimens of Potentially Toxic Drugs, in Pharmacokinetic Applications in Drug Development, ed by Rajesh Krishna, Ph.D., Kluwer Academic/Plenum Publishers, pp 477–528, 2003.

logarithmic growth rate always being in effect, never slackening. If a given dosage regimen generating a certain serum concentration profile can kill well using this model, one might expect it to do well clinically, where the growth rate may (but may not) slacken with time and may (but may well not—who dares trust that clinically for a patient?) reach a maximum number of organisms, and the resistant organisms emerge more slowly with time.

Models of this type are easy to make from in vitro data. They provide rich and dynamic new ways to perceive, analyze, and evaluate the efficacy of antibiotic therapy. Similar approaches may also be useful in analyzing therapy of patients with AIDS, using the PCR assays, and of those with cancer.

ACKNOWLEDGEMENTS

Many thanks to Dr. David Bayard for his help with writing the various equations.

REFERENCES

[1] Maire P, Barbaut X, Vergnaud JM, El Brouzi M, Confesson M, Pivot C, et al. Computation of drug concentrations in endocardial vegetations in patients during antibiotic therapy. Int J Biomed Comput 1994;36:77−85.

[2] Bayer A, Crowell D, Yih J, Bradley D, Norman D. Comparative pharmacokinetics and pharmacodynamics of amikacin and ceftazidime in tricuspid and aortic vegetations in experimental *Pseudomonas* endocarditis. J Infect Dis 1988;158:355−9.

[3] Bayer A, Crowell D, Nast C, Norman D, Borelli R. Intravegetation antimicrobial distribution in aortic endocarditis analyzed by computer-generated model: implications for treatment. Chest 1990;97:611−17.

[4] The BestDose clinical software is freely available for evaluation at <www.lapk.org>.

[5] Jelliffe R. Estimation of creatinine clearance in patients with unstable renal function, without a urine specimen. Am J Nephrol 2002;22:320−4.

[6] Zhi J, Nightingale CH, Quintiliani R. Microbial pharmacodynamics of piperacillin in neutropenic mice of systemic infection due to *Pseudomonas aeruginosa*. J Pharmacokinet Biopharm 1988;4:355−75.

[7] Schumitzky A. personal communication.

[8] Bouvier D'Ivoire M, Maire P. Dosage regimens of antibacterials: implications of a pharmacokinetic/pharmacodynamic model. Drug Invest 1996;11:229−39.

[9] Craig W, Ebert S. Killing and regrowth of bacteria in vitro: a review. Scand J Infect Dis Suppl 1991;74:63−70.

[10] Mouton J, Vinks AATMM, Punt NC. Pharmacokinetic-pharmacodynamic modeling of ceftazidime during continuous and intermittent infusion. Chapter 6, pp. 95−110, in the PhD Thesis of Vinks AATMM: Strategies for Pharmacokinetic Optimization of Continuous Infusion Therapy of Ceftazidime and Aztreonam in Patients with Cystic Fibrosis, November, 1996.

INDIVIDUALIZING DIGOXIN THERAPY

11

R. Jelliffe

CHAPTER OUTLINE

11.1 INTRODUCTION

Digitalis compounds have been used for the management of congestive heart failure since its introduction in the late 1700s by William Withering. Since about 1960, digoxin has become the major agent in this class, and this is what we will discuss here. It has always appeared to me to be a mysterious drug that somehow had to be given "just right" to obtain clinical benefit and avoid toxicity. It had the irritating property that it might suddenly cumulate in the patient and cause toxicity for no apparent reason.

Digoxin has traditionally been given without recourse to any pharmacokinetic (PK) model, usually in the form of a loading dose, as advocated by Harry Gold many years ago, and then of a maintenance dose, intended to maintain the amount of drug originally placed in the body with the loading dose. Since the 1970s, serum concentrations have been measured, and their results have been generally interpreted

Individualized Drug Therapy for Patients. DOI: http://dx.doi.org/10.1016/B978-0-12-803348-7.00011-3

as being in a subtherapeutic, therapeutic, or toxic range, followed by dosage adjustments based on clinical intuition without any PK guidance, usually still in the form of other standardized dosages.

The usual therapeutic range of serum digoxin concentrations has been said to be from about 0.5 to 2 ng/mL. The usual daily maintenance dose has ranged from 125 to 500 μg/day or more in the past, though more recently, it has been reduced to below 125 to about 250 μg/day. About two-thirds to three-quarters of the daily excretion of the drug is by the renal route, and it has been customary to reduce the dose in the presence of renal impairment [1,2]. Nevertheless, the use of therapeutic drug monitoring (TDM) and only the raw data of serum digoxin concentrations has been a frustrating experience for many cardiologists, who have not found useful correlations between serum concentrations and clinical behavior, so that dosage has generally continued to be basically one dose fits all, with relatively little attention to serum concentrations.

Further, despite the advances in quantitative pharmacokinetically oriented approaches to therapy in the last 60 years, medical schools have resisted them, and pharmacokinetics has not been incorporated into the education of physicians in any clinically meaningful way. Physicians still usually look to the package insert for whatever drug they use and follow the one-size-fits-all approach promoted so strongly by the pharmaceutical industry that it is usually accepted by the untrained physicians without any further thought. There have been some categorical adjustments of dosage to renal function, but again, with little thought of a specific therapeutic target, and no real thought of the dosage as anything other than an approved ritual behavior rather than optimal control of the model of drug behavior in a given patient to achieve and maintain a chosen target goal. Maximally precise control of a system is widely used in the aerospace community for flight and spacecraft control systems. Now the same maximally precise control techniques can be brought to the area of patient care as a significant improvement over one-size-fits-all dosage rituals without any specifically stated target goal.

Because of this, the dosage of digoxin has remained most imprecise. This is well seen in many studies that have examined the use of digoxin in various populations of patients and not infrequently found that mortality may be increased. Because of this, the use of digoxin has often become controversial in many settings, and physicians have become less and less inclined to use it, as one size fits all is the only way they have known how to give it.

11.2 THE POPULATION MODEL OF DIGOXIN

What we now call a population pharmacokinetic/pharmacodynamic (PK/PD) model describing the behavior of digoxin in adult subjects was originally developed by Reuning et al. in 1973 [3]. Nobody seems to have paid any attention to their important work. It described the two-compartment behavior of digoxin, the lack of correlation of effect with serum concentrations but the close correlation of the observed inotropic effect of digoxin with the calculated amount of drug present in the peripheral, nonserum compartment of the model of the drug. It was revised for clinical use in [2]. Those model parameter distributions became well suited for use in developing maximally precise digoxin dosage regimens, using the method of multiple model (MM) dosage design. This model has permitted improved understanding of the clinical behavior of digoxin in patients and optimally precise management of digoxin therapy [4]. It is diagrammed in Fig. 11.1.

Fig. 11.2 shows the basic relationship between the serum concentrations after an intravenous (IV) dose of digoxin, the calculated amounts in both the central (serum) and the peripheral (nonserum = everything else) compartments, and the inotropic response to the drug.

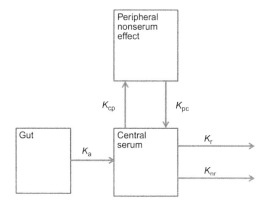

FIGURE 11.1

Diagram of the population model of digoxin. K_a = rate constant for absorption. K_{cp} = rate constant for distribution from serum to peripheral compartment. K_{cp} = rate constant from peripheral back to serum compartment. The overall rate constant for elimination represents the sum of K_r, the renal component, described per unit of creatinine clearance, and K_{nr}, the nonrenal component of elimination.

Reproduced with permission from Jelliffe R, Milman M, Schumitzky A, Bayard D, and Van Guilder M: A Two-Compartment Population Pharmacokinetic — Pharmacodynamic Model of Digoxin in Adults, with Implications for Dosage. Therap. Drug Monit. 2014 Jan 31 (epub ahead of print).

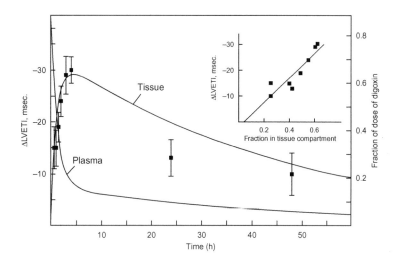

FIGURE 11.2

Comparison of the inotropic effect of digoxin on left ventricular ejection time index (ΔLVETI) as a function of time after a single intravenous dose of digoxin with computer-simulated curves (−) for the time course of digoxin in the central (plasma) and peripheral (tissue) compartments. Reproduced from Reuning R, Sams R, Notari R. Role of pharmacokinetics in drug dosage adjustment. 1. Pharmacologic effects, kinetics, and apparent volume of distribution of digoxin. J Clin Pharmacol 1973;13:127−41 with permission.

Reproduced with permission from Reuning R, Sams R, and Notari R: Role of Pharmacokinetics in Drug Dosage Adjustment. 1. Pharmacologic Effects, Kinetics, and Apparent Volume of Distribution of Digoxin. J. Clin. Pharmacol. 1973; 13: 127−141.

One can see that the effect clearly does not correlate with the serum concentrations. The effect increases while the serum concentrations fall as the drug is distributed from the serum to the peripheral compartment and is equilibrated, after which the drug is excreted.

11.3 IMPLICATIONS FOR DOSAGE

Using this model, if one considers a 65-year-old man, 70 in. tall, weighing 70 kg, who has a serum creatinine of 1 mg/dL, his estimated creatinine clearance (CCr) [5] is 69.14 mL/min/1.73 M^2. To develop an initial oral loading and daily maintenance digoxin dosage regimen to achieve and maintain a desired trough serum concentration of 0.9 ng/mL (a common target goal for a patient in congestive heart failure with regular sinus rhythm (RSR)), the ideal dosage regimen is a total loading dose of 1027 μg, given in 3 parts 6 h apart, checking for effect and toxicity before giving each next part, followed by 261 μg for the second day, decreasing gradually (due to the two-compartment behavior of the drug) to 251 μg for the eighth day. Each dose is actually a loading dose, as each dose is designed to take the model from the initial state at the time the dose is given, to that of the desired target.

Fig. 11.3A shows the calculated serum concentrations resulting from this regimen. The predicted weighted average peak serum concentration is 2.4 ng/mL at the first dose (but only if the total loading dose is given all at once—less if given in parts), and ranges from 1.6 to 3.5 ng/mL. The peak serum concentration occurs about 1.5–1.75 h after an oral dose or at the end of an intravenous infusion. After the first of the daily oral maintenance doses, starting on the second day, the predicted weighted average peak serum concentration is 1.49 ng/mL, ranging from 1 to 2.3 ng/mL. At the eighth day, the predicted peak weighted average serum concentration is 1.4 ng/mL, ranging from 0.9 to 2.2 ng/mL. On this ideal and maximally precise dosage regimen, all weighted average predicted trough serum concentrations are exactly 0.9 ng/mL, and the distribution ranges from 0.6 to 1.4 ng/mL.

Fig. 11.3B shows the calculated peripheral compartment concentrations over the same time period of initial therapy. Note that the concentrations in the peripheral effect compartment do not correlate with serum concentrations, as they rise when the serum concentrations are falling sharply due to distribution from the central to the peripheral compartment.

The predicted weighted average peak concentration in the peripheral compartment is 6.4 μg/kg (again, only if the total loading dose is given as a single dose rather than in three increments as described above). This peak occurs about 7 h after the first oral dose and ranges from 5.4 to 7.3 μg/kg. The predicted peripheral compartment concentrations parallel the inotropic effect of the drug [3]. The average computed peripheral compartment concentrations then fall to 5.6 μg/kg at the end of the first dose. The peaks then gradually rise to a weighted average of 6.8 μg/kg on the eighth day and range from about 3.8 to 10.7 μg/kg. The predicted peripheral trough concentrations average 5.7 μg/kg and range from 2.8 to 9.6 μg/kg at that time.

The weighted average peak peripheral concentrations of 6.8 μg/kg of body weight (reached about 7 h after each oral dose) correlate quite well with trough serum concentrations of 0.9 ng/mL 24 h after each dose, once a final steady state has been reached.

Once the ideal dosage regimen is known, it can be reasonably well approximated by a more practical one, in this case of a total loading dose of 1 mg, given as 500 μg initially, followed by 250 μg at 6 h, by another 250 μg at 12 h, checking for toxicity before giving the next part, then followed by 250 μg daily for maintenance thereafter.

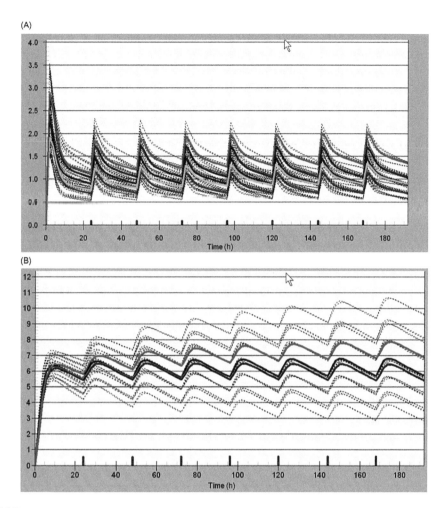

FIGURE 11.3

(A) Estimated weighed average serum digoxin concentrations (central dark line) resulting from the ideal dosage regimen targeted to hit a trough serum concentration of 0.9 ng/mL for the patient described above. Other lines represent the other predictions generated by the 64 support points in the population model. Horizontal axis indicates hours into the regimen. Vertical axis indicates serum concentrations (ng/mL). In this figure, the variability is primarily due to the variability of the volume of distribution of the central (serum) compartment, the rates of distribution from central to peripheral compartment and back again, and in both renal and nonrenal elimination. (B) Calculated peripheral compartment concentrations resulting from the ideal regimen described above. Weighted average prediction is a central dark line. Other lines represent the predictions generated by the 64 support points of the population model. Horizontal axis indicates hours into the regimen. Vertical axis indicates peripheral concentrations in μg/kg. In this figure, the variability is primarily due to that of the rates of distribution from central to peripheral compartment and back again, and from that of both renal and nonrenal elimination.

Reproduced with permission from Jelliffe R, Milman M, Schumitzky A, Bayard D, and Van Guilder M: A Two-Compartment Population Pharmacokinetic – Pharmacodynamic Model of Digoxin in Adults, with Implications for Dosage. Therap. Drug Monit. 2014 Jan 31 (epub ahead of print).

Thus, in the process of developing a dosage regimen to achieve and maintain a target trough serum concentration of 0.9 ng/mL, we are also achieving and maintaining a peak concentration in the peripheral compartment of not quite 7 μg of digoxin/kg of body weight. Trough serum concentrations of 0.9−1.0 ng/mL are achieved when we develop regimens to achieve peaks of 6.8−7.0 μg/kg in the peripheral compartment once a steady state has been reached (about 8 days with normal renal function, about 3 weeks in essentially anephric patients). Further details of the relations between dosage and serum and peripheral concentrations are given in [1,4].

11.4 ADJUSTING INITIAL DOSAGE TO BODY WEIGHT AND RENAL FUNCTION

Heavier patients require bigger doses, and smaller patients need smaller ones. Patients with reduced renal function will also require smaller maintenance doses but not loading doses. To illustrate this point, the model suggests that for the same target serum concentration goal for a patient similar to the one above, but having very reduced renal function with a serum creatinine of 5 mg/dL and a CCr of only 11 mL/min/1.73 M^2 [5], an ideal loading dose of 864 μg (again divided into 3 parts, each 6 h apart) will probably be required, followed by 138 μg on the second day, tapering down to 132 μg on the eighth day. Here, because of the smaller maintenance dose, the weighted average peak serum concentration is only 1.2 ng/mL in order to result in 0.9 ng/mL at the trough. In addition, somewhat lower peak concentrations are achieved in the peripheral compartment, only an average of 6 μg/kg on day 8, ranging from 3.5 to 8.4 μg/kg.

A practical approximation of this ideal regimen can be represented by a total loading dose of 875 μg (7 tablets of 125 μg each) given, eg, as 4, 2, and 1 tablet at time 0, 6, and 12 h into the regimen (again checking for toxicity before giving each next dose), followed by 125 μg daily thereafter. The results of this modified regimen are shown in Figs. 11.4A and B.

11.5 VARIABILITY IN RESPONSE: THE NEED FOR MONITORING SERUM CONCENTRATIONS AND DOSAGE ADJUSTMENT

The figures presented here show the usefulness of this model in planning initial dosage regimens of digoxin for individual patients, adjusted to their body weight and renal function. They also clearly show the wide variability in the responses of patients from whom this population model was developed. Population models of drug behavior all have diversity in them because they are made from a population.

This is why one needs to learn about each patient as an individual as soon as possible after implementing the first dose. This is best done by measuring serum digoxin concentrations, making an individualized model of the behavior of the drug in that particular patient, and, especially, correlating the plots and all other data with the patient's clinical response. This response is evaluated, and one then decides upon a specific target goal to be achieved, followed by developing the dosage regimen to achieve it with maximal precision.

(A)

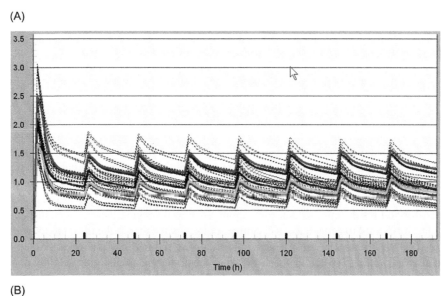

(B)

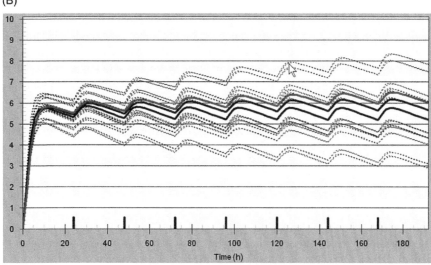

FIGURE 11.4

(A) Estimated serum digoxin concentrations (weighted average and ranges) from the modified dosage regimen of 875 μg in three parts for the loading dose, followed by 125 μg daily thereafter. The weighted average trough concentration is 0.86 ng/mL at the eighth day. Lines and axes as in Fig. 11.3A. (B) Estimated peripheral compartment concentrations on the dosage regimen described in Fig. 11.3A. Lines and axes as in Fig. 11.3B.

Reproduced with permission from Jelliffe R, Milman M, Schumitzky A, Bayard D, and Van Guilder M: A Two-Compartment Population Pharmacokinetic – Pharmacodynamic Model of Digoxin in Adults, with Implications for Dosage. Therap. Drug Monit. 2014 Jan 31 (epub ahead of print).

11.5.1 PROTOCOLS FOR MONITORING SERUM CONCENTRATIONS

It has become customary to wait for a steady state and then to check what one has done by obtaining a sample, usually at the trough, just before a subsequent dose to be given. The reasoning behind this strategy, which at first seems natural enough, to our knowledge has never been rigorously stated or justified. It is likely that the policy comes from the old and now obsolete method of using linear regression to fit the logarithms of the serum concentrations. That method only works for a one-compartment model in a steady-state situation and is not nearly as capable as more modern Bayesian methods (see Chapter 7: Monitoring the Patient: Making Individual Models) to make an individualized pharmacokinetic model of drug behavior in each patient.

Bayesian methods will work with only a single serum sample. However, the quality and precision of a result obtained from only a single measurement is suboptimal. It is probably adequate for monitoring stable patients with sinus rhythm in stable situations and for making reasonable adjustments to the dose.

However, for best results in more acute situations, such as managing patients with atrial fibrillation (AF) or flutter, it is useful to get at least one sample for each parameter in the drug model one wishes to estimate [6]. The most basic pair consists generally of a peak serum digoxin concentration taken about 1 h 45 min after an oral dose (when the peak serum concentration is usually reached after an oral dose) and a trough before a subsequent dose. There is no need to wait at least 6 h after a dose before getting a serum sample, as is commonly supposed. That also is an outmoded idea left over from using the method of linear regression on the logarithms of the serum concentrations. In addition, see Chapter 8: Monitoring Each Patient Optimally: When to Obtain the Best Samples for Therapeutic Drug Monitoring.

Further, there is no need to wait for a steady state or for distribution of the drug in the body to be complete before getting a serum sample. Learn about the patient as soon as possible. Start with the first dose. There is no need to keep the patient at risk by not learning his response immediately with the very first dose. In addition, if needed, one might also consider getting a serum digoxin sample a half-hour after an oral dose (to best estimate the rate constant for absorption after an oral dose) and at 5 h after an intravenous dose when the peak effect is usually reached [2] or at 7 h after an oral dose, to best estimate the rate constant from the peripheral back to the serum compartment. The samples do not have to be all in the same dose interval but can well be, as you want to learn each patient's response as soon as possible. As one acquires such data, supplemented with other similarly planned samples as clinically indicated, one can analyze the patient's model as the sample results become available, make the patient's model, compare the behavior of the model with the patient's clinical behavior, and choose a therapeutic target goal based on your assessment of the patient's need for the drug and the risk of toxicity that appears reasonable to accept in order to get the hoped-for benefit of the drug. One then can develop the MM dosage regimen to hit the target goal with maximum precision (minimum expected weighted squared error).

11.6 THE VERY WIDE SPECTRUM OF SERUM DIGOXIN CONCENTRATIONS AND PATIENT RESPONSES

Despite the commonly used therapeutic range of serum concentrations from about 0.5 to 2 ng/mL, patients have an extremely great variability in their clinical response to the drug. I have seen data of a patient who required a dose of 500 µg of digoxin three times daily to keep his ventricular rate controlled below 80/min. His serum digoxin concentration was 8 ng/mL. I have a colleague with a similar patient who required a concentration of 6 ng/mL to obtain a similar response. Doherty [7] published data of serum digoxin concentrations in toxic and nontoxic patients. The highest value was 6.5 ng/mL, and it was in a nontoxic patient. There was an extremely great overlap in serum concentrations between patients with and without toxicity, so that a serum concentration clearly by itself cannot discriminate between toxic and nontoxic patients. Moreover, it is the patient who gets toxic. There are actually no toxic serum concentrations, only toxic patients who have a very wide range of serum concentrations [7]. However, there was a definite increased incidence and therefore risk of toxicity with increased serum concentrations.

In the area of infectious diseases, we are well aware of organisms that have extremely variable responses to antibiotics, with wide ranges of minimum inhibitory concentration (MIC). We tailor our dosage to achieve serum concentrations adequate to kill them at concentrations that can be achieved without toxicity. Otherwise the organism is thought to have an MIC that is too high and is termed resistant. What we need to realize is that *all patients* very likely have much the same great variation in their responses and sensitivity to drugs, just as bacteria do. We do TDM to model the drug in each patient, but the patient, not the serum concentration, is always the true guide to successful individualized therapy.

11.7 MANAGEMENT OF PATIENTS WITH ATRIAL FIBRILLATION AND FLUTTER

Many patients are stable and need only a regimen to achieve and maintain a modest stable target serum concentration goal. However, other patents, especially those with atrial fibrillation (AF) or flutter, require judicious titration with incremental doses of digoxin to control ventricular rate or convert them to regular sinus rhythm (RSR) [4]. This can be done. Digoxin can and does convert patients with AF to sinus rhythm, and it can maintain them there for at least 2 weeks, despite the clinical impression otherwise [4]. The BestDose clinical software provides crucial guidance by providing us with models of the behavior of digoxin in both the serum and the peripheral compartments, and the patient's clinical behavior is best correlated with concentrations in the peripheral compartment.

If one is starting to titrate a patient with new-onset AF and expects perhaps to give a total of three incremental doses during this process about 6 h apart (thus waiting to see the full effect of each intravenous dose before committing the patient to the next dose), a full D-optimal sampling strategy, based on the population model described here, with normal renal function, might consist of five samples, one for each model parameter. The five D-optimal times for this model, in the above dosage scenario, are at 24 min after the first dose, 2 h 12 min after the first dose, 5 h 6 min after the first dose, 6 h after the second dose (just before the third dose), and then at 12 h after the third part of the loading dose (24 h from the start of the process). At present, this strategy appears to be the best one can suggest for this process. One should always learn the behavior of the drug in the patient in the most rapid and informative way currently known. Especially in intensive care unit settings, we usually do not get enough TDM samples to understand the process well and control it optimally. Current policies and protocols for TDM are extremely sparse, suboptimal, and poorly informative in helping us understand what is really going on with the drug in the patient. The pharmacy and the laboratory get stuck with the increased cost of this. Despite studies showing the effectiveness of TDM to improve care and shorten hospital stays [8], the administrators are not generally aware of this yet.

Patients with AF or atrial flutter usually require larger doses, and the serum concentrations do not reflect their rapidly changing clinical behavior, as shown by this model. While the commonly accepted therapeutic range of serum digoxin concentrations is usually from about 0.5 to 2 ng/mL, it is also clear that patients with AF who have good atrioventricular conduction require serum concentrations of about 2 ng/mL [9]. Others have described the inadequacy of serum concentrations in the therapeutic range to control ventricular rate adequately in patients with AF [10,11]. It thus appears that patients with AF or atrial flutter may well require a higher general target therapeutic range of serum concentrations, probably somewhere from 1.5 to perhaps 2.4 ng/mL. A good part of the problem is that when one wishes to control patients in such acute clinical situations, since their clinical behavior at a particular time does not correlate directly with measured serum concentrations, many clinicians have come to believe that digoxin serum level monitoring is not useful.

When one only looks at the raw data of the measured serum concentrations, they seem to be quite right. However, as shown by this model, it is really the concentrations in the peripheral effect compartment that correlate with clinical response in these rapidly changing situations, rather than the serum concentrations themselves. Nevertheless, it is the measured serum concentrations, coupled with the use of models of this type, that are required to calculate and evaluate the complex and otherwise incomprehensible relationships between the doses given, the serum concentrations, and the resulting concentrations in the peripheral effect compartment in order to correlate everything with the patient's overall clinical response. All this is needed to develop the specific dosage regimens required to achieve and maintain desired target concentrations in either the serum or the peripheral effect compartment. Peripheral compartment peak target goals of $6-8\ \mu g/kg$ appear appropriate for most patients with congestive failure and RSR, while higher peripheral concentrations ($9-18\ \mu g/kg$) are often needed to achieve and maintain good rate control or conversion in patients with AF or atrial flutter [4].

For patients with AF or atrial flutter, after one has titrated the patient with incremental doses of digoxin and achieved a desired clinical goal such as either good rate control or conversion to RSR, the really difficult and crucial task is then to plan the clinical next move: to come up with the correct maintenance dosage regimen that keeps the patient in the clinical state one has successfully achieved. Without guidance by models, this is usually impossible. That has been the clinical problem.

11.8 AN ILLUSTRATIVE PATIENT

A 92-year-old woman was coming to the end of her life because of an inoperable transitional cell carcinoma of the bladder which had obstructed her ureters and produced severe renal failure, with a serum creatinine of 8 mg/dL. She had stopped taking food or medicines by mouth. She was getting ready to die. One day she became acutely dyspneic, with acute pulmonary edema, wet rales halfway up both her posterior lung fields, and new-onset rapid AF with a ventricular rate of 170/min. She was in great distress. She was 66 in. tall and weighed 75.75 kg. Her estimated CCr was only 3.9 mL/min/ 1.73 M^2 as her serum creatinine was 8 mg/dL [5].

She was given oxygen, diuretics, and an initial dose of 500 μg of digoxin intravenously. After 3 h 20 min, her ventricular rate had fallen to 135/min. She was feeling a bit better, and a dose of

250 µg was given intravenously. Shortly after, however, she developed atrial flutter with 2:1 AV block, and her ventricular rate actually increased from 135 to 150 per minute. This was a clinical puzzle, as it raised the question of digoxin toxicity. Because of this, she was watched and monitored closely. After 7 h, she reverted to AF, with larger fibrillatory waves on her electrocardiogram (EKG) than before. Such increases in the size of the fibrillatory waves in the EKG are commonly seen while titrating AF patients with digoxin. It seemed clinically that she may have developed her flutter as larger portions of her atrial myocardium were participating in atrial depolarization, and this was still evident now, with her larger fibrillatory waves than at the beginning. It might be, it seemed, that a bit more digoxin might further facilitate this process. If so, it might bring about sinus rhythm if the entire atrial myocardium should participate in depolarization once again. Because of this, and because she was again in AF with a still inadequately controlled ventricular rate, she was given another dose of 250 µg intravenously. After 1 h and 15 min, she converted to RSR at 110/min. At this time, her clinical situation was closely analyzed.

The clinical task then was to develop a subsequent dosage regimen to keep her in her newfound sinus rhythm, and to do this in a patient with profound renal insufficiency. Can one do this by intuition and traditional clinical judgment? Very doubtful. The models and software described here provided the key to successful therapy in this otherwise extremely difficult patient.

Fig. 11.5A shows the calculated serum digoxin concentrations over time, using the population model for digoxin. During the first 12 h, her weighted average serum concentrations are shown as they were predicted to be during her period of clinical titration. She converted to sinus rhythm at 13 h into the figure. The figure also shows the subsequent predictions of her serum concentrations on the dosage regimen she then received. There is no clear correlation between this plot of her estimated serum concentrations and her clinical response.

Fig. 11.5B shows the predicted weighted average concentrations in her peripheral nonserum compartment. In contrast to her serum concentrations, her peripheral concentrations correlate quite well with her clinical response. They rose steadily during the process of her clinical titration, and she converted when they were about 9.3 µg/kg.

Now the clinical question was what dosage regimen to place her on to keep her in the sinus rhythm that had been achieved. Using the older USC*PACK software [10] and the clinical model of digoxin described here, her data and doses were entered into the program. As shown in Fig. 11.5A, the profile of her predicted serum concentrations was not helpful in understanding what was going on. However, the profile of her predicted peripheral concentrations in Fig. 11.5B correlated very well with the evolution of her clinical status. Her ventricular rate dropped as the peripheral compartment concentrations rose with the doses of titration, and she converted to sinus rhythm when her weighted average predicted peripheral concentration was about 9.3 µg/kg. Based on this good correlation of the model with her clinical behavior, a target peripheral concentration of 9.5 µg/kg was chosen, and the regimen was developed to achieve and maintain that peripheral peak target goal. The ideal regimen was 141 µg/day, difficult to give on a daily basis. However, thinking in weekly terms, the total weekly maintenance dose was 141 times 7, or 987 µg/week. This was approximated by a weekly dose of 1000 µg/week, or 8 units of 125 µg intravenously per week, each infused over 15 min. Based on this, a daily dose of 125 µg was given for 3 days, then a single dose of 250 µg the next day, followed by 125 µg daily for the remainder of the week, and so on. On this regimen, her peripheral compartment concentration was maintained at close to the desired target value, as shown. The patient remained in sinus rhythm for the next 2 weeks of her life until

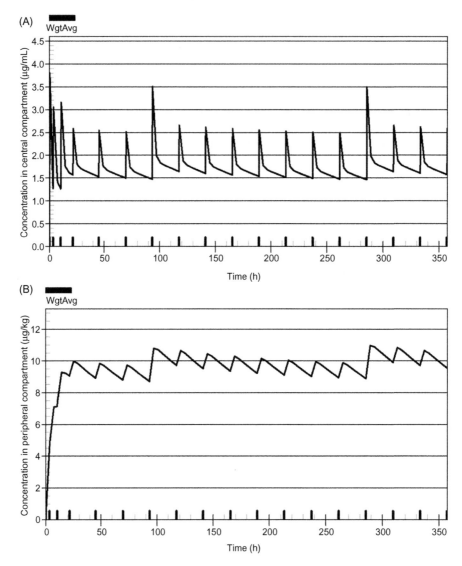

FIGURE 11.5

(A) Predicted serum concentrations in a 92-year-old female patient with AF. Conversion to regular sinus rhythm occurred at 13 h into the regimen. Horizontal axis = time into regimen. Vertical axis = serum digoxin, ng/mL. Dark line = weighted average predicted serum digoxin, ng/mL. (B) Predicted peripheral compartment concentrations in the same patient. Conversion to regular sinus rhythm occurred at 13 h into the regimen when the weighted average concentration was 9.3 μg/kg, ranging from 8 to 10.5 μg/kg. Horizontal axis = time into regimen. Vertical axis = predicted peripheral compartment digoxin concentrations.

Reproduced with permission from Jelliffe R: The Role of Digitalis Pharmacokinetics in Converting Atrial Fibrillation and Flutter to Regular Sinus Rhythm. Clinical Pharmacokinetics 2014: 53:397–407.

she died of a pneumonia. No evidence of digitalis toxicity was present at any time. In this particular woman, no serum concentrations were measured.

11.9 ANOTHER PATIENT WHO CONVERTED THREE TIMES BUT RELAPSED

Another patient, also described elsewhere [4], developed AF and was converted to RSR three times before we were consulted by telephone and developed a regimen for him. Three serum concentrations had been measured. By themselves, they were not at all useful. However, coupled with the model described here, they contributed significantly to a good understanding of his clinical situation and to the subsequent dosage regimen required to maintain him in sinus rhythm.

Briefly, he had entered the hospital in RSR. At about 400 h into the regimen (see Figs. 11.6A and B), he missed a dose and went into rapid AF. He was titrated with four doses of 250 μg of digoxin intravenously and converted to RSR.

He then was placed back on his original maintenance dose of 250 μg/day. He excreted the extra digoxin he had been given and went back into AF at about 480 h into the regimen. A serum digoxin concentration taken when he was in AF was 1.0 ng/mL, just slightly before 500 h into the regimen.

He was then given two doses of 250 μg intravenously and converted once again to RSR. A serum digoxin concentration at this time, in RSR, surprisingly was also 1.0 ng/mL, exactly the same as when he had been in AF.

How can a patient be in AF at one time and in RSR at another and have exactly the same serum concentration? Two reasons for this stand out. First, the patient was not at all in the usual steady state with either sample in order to permit such conventional interpretations of the relationship between serum concentrations and clinical behavior. In addition, the samples were not drawn at the same time after the dose.

They continued to watch the patient and again placed him back on his original maintenance dose of 250 μg/day. He again went back into AF at about 590 h into the regimen. He was again titrated with digoxin and once again converted to RSR. Another serum digoxin, obtained at about 600 h into the regimen when he was in RSR, was 1.2 ng/mL.

One can see here the extremely poor correlation between the patient's clinical behavior and the raw data of his serum digoxin concentrations. He was in AF at 1.0 ng/mL and in RSR at 1.0 and 1.2 ng/mL. This is the problem cardiologists have with the usual way digoxin is given and monitored, and only the raw data is seen.

Now let us see if the model can be of any help to us (and them). Note that the profile of the serum concentrations over time in Fig. 11.6A is quite uninformative. This is because, as shown by the work of Reuning et al. [3] and our population model based on it [2], that the real relationship to clinical behavior is with the computed concentrations in the peripheral nonserum compartment. If we now look at Fig. 11.6B, we can see clearly that the patient first went into AF when his peripheral digoxin concentrations were quite low, a little less than 3 μg/kg. After the first course of IV titration, they rose to about 11 μg/kg when he converted to RSR. Then he went back into AF again when they fell to about 8.5 μg/kg. He then converted again as they rose to about 11 μg/kg with the second course of titration, and he reverted back to AF again when they fell to about 7 μg/kg. The last course of titration took his peripheral concentrations to over 13 μg/kg. However, he relapsed

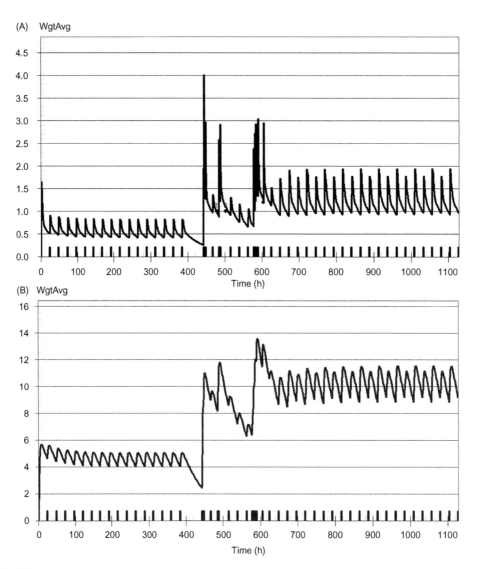

FIGURE 11.6

(A) Time course of estimated and measured serum digoxin concentrations in this patient. Horizontal axis = time into regimen. Vertical axis = serum concentration (ng/mL). Solid line = weighted average estimated serum concentration. Three dots represent the measured concentrations of 1, 1, and 1.2 ng/mL at about 475, 500, and 605 h into the regimen, respectively. (B) Time course of estimated peripheral (nonserum) compartment digoxin concentrations in this patient. Horizontal axis = time into regimen. Vertical axis = peripheral compartment concentration (μg/kg). Solid line = weighted average estimated concentration.

Reproduced with permission from Jelliffe R: The Role of Digitalis Pharmacokinetics in Converting Atrial Fibrillation and Flutter to Regular Sinus Rhythm. Clinical Pharmacokinetics 2014: 53:397–407.

again when they fell below 10 μg/kg. There is thus very clear correlation between the computed concentrations in his peripheral compartment and his clinical behavior.

Based on this, it was decided to choose a peak peripheral compartment target goal of 11.5 μg/kg and to develop an oral regimen to achieve and maintain this target peak, 7 h after each oral dose. The ideal regimen was 571 μg/day. Many cardiologists would not give what is felt by so many to be a high dose. However, Dr. William Nicholson, whose patient this was, had spent several years as a medical student and resident working in our laboratory. We approximated this ideal regimen as 500 and 625 μg on alternate days.

On this regimen, the patient remained in sinus rhythm, whereas the prior week of intense effort had been unsuccessful. He was able to leave the hospital in RSR, and when seen 2 weeks later in the clinic, still on this regimen, he was still in RSR. Unfortunately, a serum concentration was not obtained at that time.

11.10 ANOTHER CASE—A VERY LARGE, HEAVY PATIENT WHO DID NOT CONVERT

A 41-year-old man, 71 in. tall, weighing 300 lb (118 kg) was in chronic AF. His serum creatinine initially was 0.6 mg/dL. It rose to 1.4 mg/dL and then fell later to 0.8 mg/dL. His estimated CCr began with a very high value of 205 mL/min/1.73 M^2. It then fell to 75 and rose again to 155 mL/min/1.73 M^2 [5]. His ventriclar rate was about 130/min throughout, and there was little change during his therapy.

Oral digoxin dosage began at 250 μg/day but rose to 500 and 875 μg/day in divided doses, checking clinically before each next dose, and to 1250 μg/day one day, followed by 1000 μg/day, checking before each dose, in an attempt to control his ventricular rate or possibly to convert him to sinus rhythm. At this point, others involved in his care did not wish to keep up these doses, even though 1000 mcg/day for a 300-lb man is equivalent to 500 mcg/day for a 150-lb person.

He had 10 serum concentrations that ranged from 0.9 to 2.7 ng/mL and averaged about 2 ng/mL. When his data were fitted, the hybrid Bayesian procedure in the BestDose clinical software [12] and see Chapter 7, was used, which can reach out beyond the stated parameter ranges of the original population model, which was developed for patients not so heavy. A reasonable fit was obtained, as shown in Fig. 11.7A.

On the other hand, his peripheral compartment concentrations reached only about 6 μg/kg, as shown in Fig. 11.7B. This very heavy patient's clinical behavior correlated well with other patients in the literature whose clinical response concerning conversion to sinus rhythm was not significantly different from placebo [4].

11.11 RATIOS BETWEEN CENTRAL AND PERIPHERAL COMPARTMENTS

It is also noteworthy that while his many serum concentrations were in the range of about 1−2.5 ng/mL and averaged about 2 ng/mL, his peripheral compartment concentrations were quite low, only about 6 μg/kg, where the effect to convert AF is no better than placebo [4]. It may well be that each patient may have his own relationship or ratio of concentrations between the central and peripheral compartments.

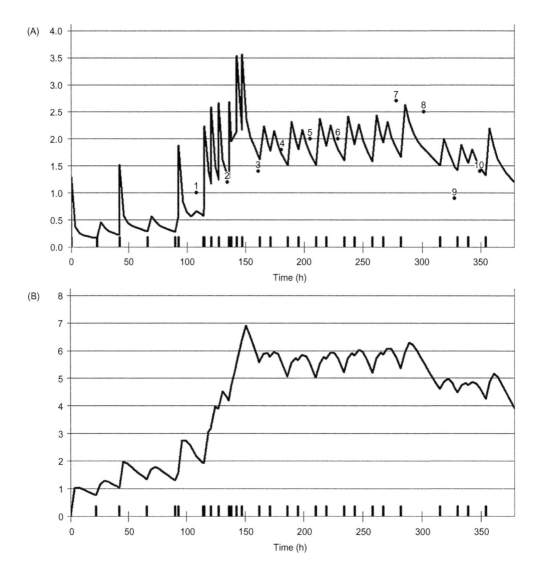

FIGURE 11.7

(A) Time course of estimated weighted and measured serum digoxin concentrations in this patient. Horizontal axis = time into regimen. Vertical axis = serum concentration (ng/mL). Solid line = weighted average estimated serum concentration. The dots represent the measured serum digoxin concentrations. (B) Time course of estimated average peripheral (nonserum) compartment digoxin concentrations in this patient. Horizontal axis = time into regimen. Vertical axis = peripheral compartment concentration (μg/kg). Solid line = weighted average estimated concentration.

Reproduced with permission from Jelliffe R: The Role of Digitalis Pharmacokinetics in Converting Atrial Fibrillation and Flutter to Regular Sinus Rhythm. Clinical Pharmacokinetics 2014: 53:397–407.

11.12 **THE EFFECT OF SERUM POTASSIUM**

Digoxin competes with potassium for binding sites on Na−K-ATPase. It is well known that hypo-kalemia predisposes to digitalis toxicity and that hyperkalemia may perhaps be protective. Studies of serum potassium concentrations in patients with digitalis toxicity, however, have not been shown to be significantly different from those in patients without toxicity.

In [13], using a much earlier and more primitive one-compartment model of digoxin [14], in which a total body concentration of 10 µg/kg was approximately equivalent to 7 µg/kg in the peripheral compartment using the present model, 46 patients who had no evidence of toxicity were studied. Their computed total body glycoside concentration, using that earlier model, averaged 15.4 + 6.3 µg/kg. This is approximately equivalent to 10.8 µg/kg using the present model. Their serum potassium averaged 4.6 ± 0.7 mEq/L.

In contrast, 33 patients were seen who were toxic. Their computed total body digoxin concentrations averaged 19.3 ± 10.0 µg/kg, approximately equivalent to 13.4 µg/kg with the present model. Their average serum potassium was almost identical at 4.7 ± 0.9 mEq/L. Thus, their computed total body glycoside concentrations were significantly higher than in those without toxicity, but their serum potassium was not.

However, in the 33 toxic patients, each patient's computed total body glycoside concentration correlated very well with his serum potassium concentrations. A significant relationship was found, as shown in Fig. 11.8. Patients with low serum potassium had lower computed body digoxin concentrations when

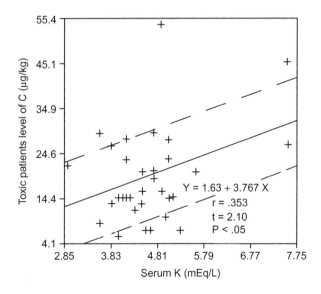

FIGURE 11.8

Relationship between computed total body glycoside concentration (level of C, vertical) using an earlier model (see text) and serum potassium concentrations (serum K, horizontal), in patients with digitalis toxicity.

Reproduced with permission from Jelliffe RW: Reduction of Digitalis Toxicity by Computer-Assisted Digitalis Dosage Programs: Quantitative Relationship to Serum Potassium. Fed Proc, 30(2): 284, 1971. Federation of American Societies for Experimental Biology, Chicago, Illinois, April 13, 1971.

they became toxic, while those with higher serum potassium became toxic only at higher computed digoxin concentrations. It thus appears, from the relationship shown in Fig. 11.8, that patients with a serum potassium of 3.0 mEq/L may well become toxic at about half the peripheral body concentrations as when serum K is 5 mEq/L, using the 2 compartment model described here. This data may provide a rough guide to the adjustment of initial target peripheral compartment goals in the presence of high, and especially of low, serum potassium concentrations until the electrolyte abnormality can be corrected.

11.13 A VERY RELEVANT PATIENT

The following patient, seen back in the mid-1970s, had a history of exertional dyspnea. He actually had chronic obstructive pulmonary disease and emphysema. Because he was dyspneic, he was given digitalis leaf by his physician. He eventually became depressed and attempted suicide by taking 43 tablets of digitalis leaf 0.1 g (each equivalent to about 0.1 mg of digitoxin, the main glycoside in digitalis leaf). When he was brought to the hospital, he was very obtunded and difficult to arouse. His physical examination was remarkable for evidence of chronic obstructive pulmonary disease and emphysema. His vital signs were within normal limits. His EKG showed sinus rhythm and ST-T-wave changes consistent with digitalis effect.

His serum potassium was 8 mEq/L. It is said that in patients with acute digitalis toxicity their half-time is shorter than usual. The usual half-time of digitoxin is 6 days in patients with normal renal function and about 9 days if renal function is severely impaired.

His initial serum digitoxin concentration, measured by a method of enzymatic isotope displacement that assayed all biologically active digitalis compounds [15], was expressed as 240 ng/mL of digitoxin, extremely high. He was given supportive therapy, and dialysis was not done, as it was felt that his elevated serum potassium was probably due to his severe digitalis intoxication.

As shown in Fig. 11.9, in the next day and a half, his serum potassium fell remarkably to 4.1 mEq/L, and his serum digitoxin also fell fully by half to 120 ng/mL. His EKG now showed a prolonged PR interval and increased ST-T changes of increased digitalis effect. Digitalis toxicity was clearly present. His initial electroencephalogram (EEG) showed diffuse slow-wave changes consistent with hypercalcemia, although his serum calcium was within normal limits.

At this time, vigorous potassium replacement therapy was begun, and in the next day and a half, it rose from 4.1 to 5.9 mEq/L. At the same time, his serum digitoxin rose from 120 to 230 ng/mL However, his EKG improved, with less digitalis effect and a PR interval that was normal once more, as the digitalis came off his cell membranes and out into the serum once again. What is in the serum never is toxic unless it gets out of the serum and bound to the cell membranes.

All these changes mirror in this patient's clinical situation what is known in vitro about the mechanism of action of digitalis compounds to compete with potassium for binding sites on the Na−K-ATPase on cell membranes. Digitalis interferes with potassium uptake by the cell, and potassium tends to remain in the serum. The sodium then exchanges with calcium by the Na−Ca-APTase, which then makes calcium more available within the cell, thus producing the inotropic effect and probably also all the other manifestations of digitalis toxicity that can also be seen with hypercalcemia, including the diffuse slow wave changes on the EEG. In my opinion, the visual symptoms may well be produced by retinal cells that fire several times instead of only once (retinal extrasystoles!), thus facilitating the formation of afterimages in the retina.

His potassium was excreted much more rapidly than was his digitoxin, which then became more tightly bound to his cell membranes, causing the rapid fall in his serum digitoxin concentrations and the increased digitalis effect of toxic first-degree AV block and increased ST-T changes of digitalis effect on his EKG, and slow waves on his EEG. Replacement of his potassium to high-normal concentrations was effective in helping to get the digitoxin off his cell membranes and back out into his serum again where it would do no further harm, as his potassium stores had been replaced. His EKG and EEG both improved, with a normal PR interval, less digitalis effect on his EKG, and disappearance of the abnormal slow-wave activity on his EEG. After that, his clinical condition became much more stable. His serum potassium remained about 5 mEq/L, he gradually excreted his digitoxin, and he was discharged on the 12th day with a serum digitoxin concentration of 35 ng/mL for further outpatient care and support (Fig. 11.9).

This patient's clinical course reflects the competition between digitalis and potassium just as it is known to occur in vitro. It also illustrates the wide variation between serum concentrations and clinical status that are dependent on many other factors and makes the patient, and not some arbitrary therapeutic range developed by a committee of people who have never seen a particular

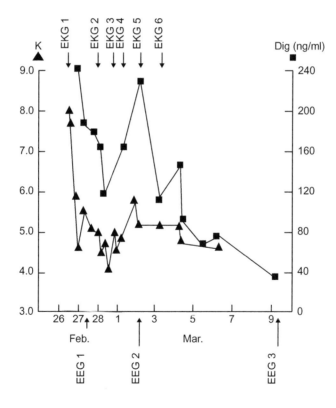

FIGURE 11.9

Data of patient in severe digitalis intoxication with initial severe hyperkalemia. Horizontal axis = dates and times of events. Left vertical axis = serum potassium (mEq/L). Right vertical axis = serum digitoxin concentration (ng/mL). Solid triangles = serum potassium concentration over time. Solid squares = serum digitoxin over time. EKG = various electrocardiograms over time. EEG = various electroencephalograms over time.

patient, be the final arbiter of therapy. Patients, by their clinical behavior, tell us what they like and do not like. The clinician's job is to use the drug, the PK/PD model of its behavior, and the serum concentration data, to hold it up to the patient as a mirror to his clinical status, to help us select a target therapeutic goal of a serum or peripheral compartment concentration that is felt to be appropriate to that patient's need, and to use the clinical software to develop the maximally precise regimen to achieve that selected goal. As always, this will be followed by subsequent reappraisal, further serum concentrations, and dosage adjustments as clinically indicated.

REFERENCES

[1] Jelliffe R. Some comments and suggestions concerning population pharmacokinetic modeling, especially of digoxin, and its relation to clinical therapy. Ther Drug Monit 2012;34:368−77.

[2] Jelliffe R, Milman M, Schumitzky A, Bayard D, Van Guilder M. A two-compartment population pharmacokinetic−pharmacodynamic model of digoxin in adults, with implications for dosage. Ther Drug Monit 2014;36(3):387−93 (epub ahead of print).

[3] Reuning R, Sams R, Notari R. Role of pharmacokinetics in drug dosage adjustment. 1. Pharmacologic effects, kinetics, and apparent volume of distribution of digoxin. J Clin Pharmacol 1973;13:127−41.

[4] Jelliffe R. The role of digitalis pharmacokinetics in converting atrial fibrillation and flutter to regular sinus rhythm. Clin Pharmacokinet 2014;53:397−407. Available from: http://dx.doi.org/10.1007/s40262-014-0141-6.

[5] Jelliffe R. Estimation of creatinine clearance in patients with unstable renal function, without a urine specimen. Am J Nephrol 2002;22:320−4.

[6] D'Argenio D. Optimal sampling times for pharmacokinetic experiments. J Pharmacokin Biopharmaceut 1981;9:739−56.

[7] Doherty J. Digitalis glycosides − pharmacokinetics and their clinical implications. Ann Int Med 1973;79:229−38.

[8] van Lent-Evers N, Mathot R, Geus W, van Hout B, Vinks A. Impact of goal-oriented and model-based clinical pharmacokinetic dosing of aminoglycosides on clinical outcome: a cost-effectiveness analysis. Ther Drug Monit 1999;221:63−73.

[9] Chamberlain D, White R, Howard M, Smith T. Plasma digoxin concentrations in patients with atrial fibrillation. Br Med J 1970;3:429−32.

[10] Jelliffe RW. The USC*PACK PC programs for population pharmacokinetic modeling, modeling of large kinetic/dynamic systems, and adaptive control of drug dosage regimens. Presented at the 15th annual symposium on computer applications in medical care. Washington DC; November 17−20, 1991. pp. 922−3.

[11] Goldman S, Probst P, Selzer A, Cohn K. Inefficacy of "therapeutic" serum levels of digoxin in controlling the ventricular rate in atrial fibrillation. Am J Cardiol 1975;35:651−5.

[12] The BestDose clinical software is available for free evaluation at <www.lapk.org>.

[13] Jelliffe R. Effect of serum potassium level upon risk of digitalis toxicity. Ann Int Med 1973;78:821.

[14] Jelliffe RW. An improved method of digoxin therapy. Ann Int Med 1968;69:703−17.

[15] Brooker G, Jelliffe RW. Serum cardiac glycoside assay based upon displacement of 3H ouabain from Na-K ATPase. Circulation 1972;45:20−36.

CLINICAL APPLICATIONS OF INDIVIDUALIZED THERAPY

OPTIMIZING SINGLE-DRUG ANTIBACTERIAL AND ANTIFUNGAL THERAPY

12

M. Neely and R. Jelliffe

CHAPTER OUTLINE

12.1 INTRODUCTION

Antimicrobial drugs interfere with the life cycle of an organism in various ways. To alter the life cycle, all antimicrobials must bind to a cellular target. Binding of the drug to its target results in alteration of the normal function of the bacterium or fungus, leading to either inhibition of growth or cell death. In addition to the ability of an antimicrobial agent to reach its target site of action (ie, the receptor), the drug must also possess sufficient affinity for its receptor, and it must achieve a sufficient concentration to affect organism function. These pharmacologic characteristics are the primary determinants of antimicrobial activity.

Individualized Drug Therapy for Patients. DOI: http://dx.doi.org/10.1016/B978-0-12-803348-7.00012-5

Unfortunately, because the interaction between drug and "bug" receptors occurs on a microscopic scale, we cannot directly quantify these effects in patients. Moreover, infection eradication is the desired ultimate outcome, but this is typically delayed by days to weeks after initiation of therapy, and we do not want to wait that long to discover that we chose the wrong drug or dose. As such, we must use surrogate markers in an attempt to reflect the crucial cellular interactions and to predict our desired outcome. These surrogate markers are ideally easily measured, and they substitute for the truly desired outcome, which is eradication of infection.

12.2 MINIMUM INHIBITORY CONCENTRATION

For antibacterials and antifungals, the most commonly used efficacy surrogate is the in vitro minimum inhibitory concentration (MIC). The MIC is a direct measure of in vitro drug potency and an indirect measure of in vivo activity. However, MIC itself does not provide sufficient information on the temporal pattern of exposure of an organism to antimicrobial agents or the antimicrobial concentration that must be achieved relative to the MIC to ensure a sufficient therapeutic response.

Consideration of the laboratory procedures involved in the determination of MICs raises additional questions about MIC alone as a primary surrogate for clinical antimicrobial activity. First, measurements of MIC are obtained in bacterial growth media that are devoid of protein, which may have implications for agents that are highly bound to plasma proteins (for example, >70% bound). Thus, antibiotic concentrations used to determine MICs represent 100% free active drug. Similar concentrations of free drug at the anatomic site(s) of infection may not be achievable clinically because of extensive protein binding, drug molecular weight, and degree of ionization at pathophysiologic pH.

12.3 BREAKPOINTS

Breakpoints are an attempt to overcome some of these limitations by providing a clinical context in which to interpret MICs. A breakpoint is a reference MIC above which sufficient drug concentrations are unlikely to be achieved in patients (resistance breakpoint) or unlikely with standard dosing (intermediate breakpoint). Of course, a breakpoint is based on average drug kinetic behavior integrated with clinical response measured in a population. There is little in the way of individualization in the concept of a breakpoint. Second, measuring MICs usually involves maintaining a constant concentration of free drug for a standard period (generally 24 h). Such a constant concentration simulates a continuous infusion of antibiotic whereas clinically, antibiotics are usually administered intermittently, which results in peaks and troughs rather than constant concentrations. Third, MICs are measured on a standard inoculum of bacteria or fungi that may or may not reflect the actual density of bacteria present at the site of infection. Fourth, measured MICs are considered acceptable if day-to-day variability is ≤two-fold. However, two-fold above and below the "truth" means a four-fold difference is possible. Fifth, MICs from different methods may vary by at least two-fold. Finally, the laboratory procedures used to determine the MIC do not account for the antimicrobial activity of various host defenses, including immunoglobulins and leukocytes.

Despite all these limitations, the MIC is still the foundation for antimicrobial therapy against bacteria and fungi. Intuitively, it is important to select an antibiotic with demonstrated activity against the pathogen, and in vitro susceptibility testing is especially valuable in identifying antimicrobial agents that will be ineffective in eradicating the pathogen. That is, MIC is a better predictor of failure than success, because there are many factors other than a low MIC (high drug potency) that contribute to the likelihood of infection eradication. However, a very high MIC far above an established breakpoint suggests that success is unlikely with a given drug, because a safe but effective exposure will be hard to obtain. On the other hand, a pathogen can appear susceptible to a particular agent from in vitro testing (ie, low MIC), yet information is lacking on the ability of the agent to achieve the necessary concentrations for a sufficient period at the site of infection to eradicate the pathogen. The time course of the drug must be integrated with the concentration at the receptor site to reflect the in vivo antibiotic-bacteria interaction adequately [1].

12.4 **THE APPROACH**

In this chapter, we consider dose and plasma exposure as important variables that can be controlled in individual patients to improve the chance of successful clinical outcomes from an infection with bacteria or fungi. As a result of the differences in the mechanisms by which antibiotics kill these organisms and the position of safely achievable concentrations on the concentration-response curve, specific pharmacokinetic and dynamic (PK/PD) properties can be correlated with efficacy. These are shown in Fig. 12.1. They include drugs whose efficacy is linked to (1) the percent time above the MIC within a dosing interval ($\%T > MIC$); (2) the ratio of peak concentration to MIC (Peak: MIC); and (3) the ratio of the area under the time-concentration curve to MIC (AUC/MIC). For all of these relationships, free drug (ie, not protein-bound) concentrations are the active form of the drug. However, in clinical practice, routine measurement of free drug concentrations is not typical due to increased complexity and cost of the assays. Therefore, even though there is variability in protein binding for a given drug between patients, total drug concentration is used most often.

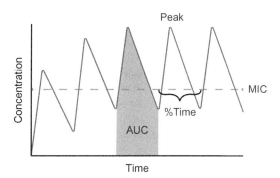

FIGURE 12.1

Differing pharmacokinetic-pharmacodynamic surrogate endpoints to predict antimicrobial efficacy.

Fig. 12.2 explains in more basic pharmacologic terms why drugs display these patterns of activity. The first pattern is for drugs that have minimal postantibiotic effect (PAE); that is, ongoing killing after serum concentrations have dropped below the MIC. The activity of these drugs depends on the duration of time that the antibiotic concentration exceeds the MIC ($\%T > MIC$). Because of the limited PAE, as soon as drug concentrations drop below the MIC, the organism can begin to regrow. Also, because clinical concentrations are near the upper, flat portion of the concentration-response curve, for these antibiotics, saturation of the organism killing rate is observed at certain multiples of the MIC, usually two to four times, and antibiotic concentrations exceeding this level do not generally achieve any greater killing rate. Clearly, the duration that the antibiotic concentration exceeds the MIC of the pathogen is influenced by several factors, including the dosing interval, the pathogen, and the site of infection. Drugs that demonstrate this type of PK/PD relationship are referred to as *time-dependent*. Some refer to this class as concentration-independent antibiotics, but this term is not as preferable because all antibiotics require a minimal concentration for efficacy and therefore cannot be fully independent of concentration. Examples of drugs that exhibit time-dependent killing include all the β-lactams (see Table 12.1).

In contrast, a second pattern of bacterial killing has been characterized for drugs that have concentrations in the steeper portion of the concentration-response curve and have some degree of PAE. The killing ability of agents in this group depends on the *peak concentration to MIC (peak/MIC)* within the dosing interval. In other words, the higher the antibiotic peak concentration, the greater the kill. Agents that demonstrate this type of PK/PD interface are referred to as *concentration-dependent* or *peak-dependent* antibiotics and include aminoglycosides and fluoroquinolones.

A third class of drugs also have a PAE, but lie near the upper portion of the concentration-response curve, such that it is simply the *area under the time-concentration curve (AUC) to MIC (AUC/MIC)* ratio that best describes activity. These are also called time-dependent drugs, but the moderate PAE makes the choice of dose interval less critical than the time-dependent drugs with little to no PAE. Examples include vancomycin and azithromycin.

The clinical challenge relative to the PK/PD properties of $\%T > MIC$ and peak/MIC or AUC/MIC is determining the target goal for each that correlates with response. These are also summarized in Table 12.1.

12.4.1 PHARMACOKINETIC AND PHARMACODYNAMIC RELATIONSHIPS

The superior ability to predict infection cure by using integrated PK/PD characteristics rather than MIC alone helps standardize antimicrobial dosing in clinical trials and assists in guiding antimicrobial therapy for individual patients. Furthermore, providing adequate amounts of antibiotic for sufficient periods via optimal dosing based on PK/PD properties may also decrease the rate and extent of organism resistance. One example of the application of PK/PD principles to antibiotic dosing is the current wide acceptance of once-daily aminoglycoside dosing for the treatment of systemic infections. An appreciation of the PK/PD characteristics of aminoglycosides, combined with a better understanding of their safety profiles, led to a once-daily dosing of aminoglycosides that can take advantage of the concentration-dependent killing characteristics of this class of antibiotics [16]. However, combining models of the kinetic behavior of aminoglycosides and bacterial growth and kill suggests that in the absence of immune function, bacterial regrowth could occur at the end of a prolonged dosing interval.

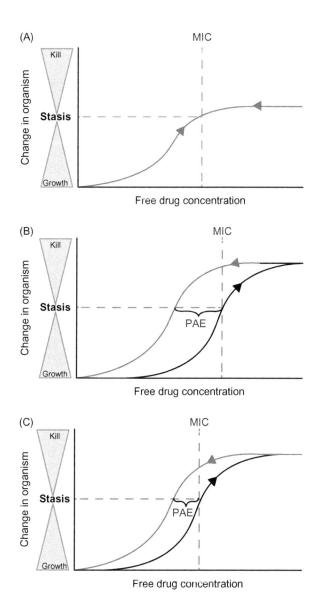

FIGURE 12.2

Basic pharmacologic reasons for differing pharmacokinetic-pharmacodynamic associations. (A) As soon as drug concentration falls below MIC, organism growth resumes. This is typical of a time-dependent drug. (B) Peak-dependent drug, which is caused by a negative hysteresis loop, whereby free drug concentration increases and effect increases along the lower curve, rising above the MIC and causing net loss of organism. Free drug concentration decreases, with effect also decreasing, but along the upper curve. When concentration first falls below MIC, the effect is still in the net organism loss state. (C) This pattern is a combination of (A and B).

Table 12.1 Classification of Selected Antibacterials Based on Their Pattern of Antimicrobial Activity

Pattern	Drug	Target
Peak/MIC Concentration-dependent killing, prolonged postantibiotic effects	Aminoglycosides	10
	Daptomycin [4]	100 (*Staphylococcus aureus*)
		36 (*Streptococcus pneumoniae*)
		0.25 (*Enterococcus faecium*)
	Fluoroquinolones	10
	Metronidazole	?
Time > MIC Time-dependent killing, minimal postantibiotic effects	Carbapenems, Aztreonam	>20−40%
	Cephalosporins	>20−40%
	Penicillins	>40−60%
AUC/MIC Time-dependent killing, moderate to prolonged persistent antibiotic effects	Azithromycin	25 [5]
	Clindamycin	?
	Telithromycin	3 [6]
	Dalbavancin [7]	1000 (*S. aureus*)
		100 (*S. species*)
	Linezolid	80 (or trough $>1 \times$ MIC) [8]
	Metronidazole	70 [9]
	Macrolides	30 [10,11]
	Quinupristin/Dalfopristin	?
	Telavancin	219 [12]
	Tetracyclines	10
	Tigecycline	18 (Gram-positive) [13]
		7 (Gram-negative) [14]
	Vancomycin	400 (trough $\sim 8 \times$ MIC) [15]

AUC, area under the time-concentration curve; MIC, minimum inhibitory concentration.
Source: *Data are from Levison ME. Pharmacodynamics of antibacterial drugs. Infect Dis Clin North Am 2000;14:281−91; Nightingale CH, Ambrose PG, Drusano GL, Murakawa T. Antimicrobial pharmacodynamics in theory and clinical practice. 2nd ed. Informa Healthcare; 2007. unless otherwise noted.*

Moreover, in patients with a poor clinical response, an understanding of a particular drug's PK/PD characteristics allows the clinician rationally to assess the potential contribution of suboptimal dosing and to develop an effective, alternative regimen. In their assessment of published data, Craig and Andes demonstrated that the $\%T >$ MIC for β-lactam antibiotics predicted bacteriologic efficacy with accuracy similar to that of the ratio of middle-ear fluid concentration to MIC [17]. Moreover, when the $\%T >$ MIC exceeded 40−50% of the dosing interval, bacteriologic and clinical cure was achieved in 80−85% of the patients studied. Although most of the *Streptococcus pneumoniae* isolates in these studies were susceptible to penicillin, the same principles apply in an era of increasing resistance. For example, conventional amoxicillin dosing (13.3 mg/kg per dose three times daily) would be expected to exceed the target $\%T >$ MIC for penicillin-susceptible and penicillin-intermediate *Str. pneumoniae*, whereas higher doses (45−50 mg/kg per dose twice daily) are often required to achieve the target $\%T > MIC$ for more resistant isolates. Note that it is not the increased dose of amoxicillin per se that correlates with increased efficacy but the longer $\%T > MIC$ afforded by higher concentrations. As an extension of this work, much attention has been paid recently to modeling improved efficacy of prolonged infusion of β-lactams against resistant gram-negative organisms [18], with improved clinical cure in critically ill adults, but no difference in survival [19]. In general, prospective studies are as yet lacking [20]. Similarly, for vancomycin, there are many studies showing a retrospective correlation between AUC/MIC and efficacy, but as yet no prospective studies save our own, which we discuss later in this chapter [21−25].

An awareness of PK/PD characteristics also permits more sophisticated interpretation of the breakpoints for in vitro susceptibility. Frequently, clinical laboratories do not report actual MICs for drugs against cultured pathogens but assign descriptive categories of "susceptible," "intermediate," or "resistant" to the organism based on defined guidelines for interpreting MICs. As we have mentioned already, in general, these guidelines are derived from the likelihood of bacteriologic success relative to the MIC of the infecting organism and the projected achievable *serum* concentration of antibiotic. A major exception is the breakpoint reporting for *Str. pneumoniae*, which is based on projected achievable central nervous system concentrations. Thus, if the infection is in an anatomic location other than that for which the breakpoints were derived, the breakpoints may be less relevant.

Maximizing desirable PD outcomes plus minimizing undesirable adverse effects necessarily requires the ability to quantify such endpoints. Furthermore, an objective index variable must be identified to which therapy can be linked to achieve the therapeutic goals.

12.5 ANTIFUNGAL AGENTS

Although our knowledge of PK/PD relationships for other antimicrobial agents (eg, antifungal, antiviral, antimycobacterial) is not yet as advanced as for antibacterial agents, some progress has been made.

Antifungal MICs are determined most reliably for yeasts (eg, *Candida* and *Cryptococcus*). The value of MICs lies in the assignment of susceptibility breakpoints: drug concentrations above which the isolate is considered resistant and below which it is considered susceptible. These breakpoints allow clinicians to choose appropriate antimicrobial therapy.

The Clinical Laboratory Standards Institute and the European Committee on Antimicrobial Susceptibility Testing have established breakpoints for azoles, echinocandins, and flucytosine against *Candida* spp. Although methods for MIC testing are standardized, breakpoints for filamentous fungal infections, such as with *Aspergillus*, still do not exist, and will be very difficult to generate now that combination therapy is widely employed for *Aspergillus* and other filamentous fungal infections. We are only in the early stages of understanding optimal PK-based dosing of antifungal drugs, and Table 12.2 shows the hypothesized relationships and dosing implications.

12.6 USE OF THERAPEUTIC DRUG MANAGEMENT AND MULTIPLE MODEL BAYESIAN ADAPTIVE CONTROL OF DOSAGE REGIMENS

We now turn to examples of patients whose infections were managed with careful attention to antimicrobial serum concentrations, and management of dosages according to principles discussed throughout this book: nonparametric population modeling and multiple model Bayesian adaptive control.

Table 12.2 Proposed Pharmacokinetic–Pharmacodynamic (PK–PD) Relationships for Antifungal Drugs

Drug	PK-PD Relationship	Notes
Amphotericin B	Peak/MIC?	Single, large daily doses are more effective than smaller, frequent doses; the dosage is limited by toxicity to a maximum of 1.5 mg/kg per day
Lipid amphotericin B (AmBisome, Abelcet, Amphotec)	Peak/MIC?	As previous, but the pharmacokinetics of the three preparations are different and more studies are required to determine whether PD differences also exist. Lower toxicity in general permits a higher dosing of 5 mg/kg per day, and tolerability up to 15 mg/kg per day (AmBisome [26]) and 10 mg/kg per day (Abelcet [27]) has been reported, but added efficacy at the higher doses has not been demonstrated and may result in increased nephrotoxicity [28]
Fluconazole	AUC/MIC	Optimal dosing is 6 mg/kg per day IV/PO for susceptible isolates, 12 mg/kg per day for dose-dependent isolates. A loading dose of 25 mg/kg on Day One should be strongly considered in infants [29]. Doses >12 mg/kg offer unproven additional benefit and increase the risk of toxicity. A dose/MIC ratio of >50 or AUC/MIC ratio of >25 have been suggested as targets [30]
Itraconazole	AUC/MIC	Target trough concentrations of >0.5 mg/L are recommended [31]
Posaconazole	AUC/MIC	Concentrations demonstrate a great deal of inter-patient variability; in two pivotal Phase 3 studies analyzed by the FDA, a plasma concentration of >0.35 mg/L 3–5 h after dosing on Day Two, was predictive of a concentration of >0.70 mg/L at the same time on Day Seven, which was associated with *prevention* of invasive fungal infections [31]. Another study reported best *treatment* outcomes with average concentrations of >1.25 mg/L [32]. In practice such concentrations are difficult to achieve in children with the suspension; [33] however, the newer delayed release tablet formulation (approved for ≥13 years of age) has greatly enhanced absorption and such concentrations are easier to obtain
Voriconazole	AUC/MIC	Target trough concentrations of >1.0 mg/L have been associated with survival benefit in children [34]
Flucytosine	T > MIC	In vitro data suggest that peak efficacy occurs at a serum concentration-MIC ratio of 4:1. No data exist on the most effective duration of serum concentration above the MIC. If toxicity is problematic (typically with peak >100 mg/L), smaller, more frequent doses or even continuous infusion may be more effective, but human data are lacking. Usual peaks are 30–100 mg/L [35]
Echinocandins (caspofungin, micafungin, anidulafungin)	AUC/MIC	Clinical data are lacking, but in vitro and animal models suggest for *Candida* species, a free drug AUC/MIC ratio of 5–20 (high end for *Candida albicans*, lower for *Candida parapsilosis*) may be adequate [36], which is an AUC/MIC ratio of 3000 in patients [37]. For *Aspergillus* species, the target is a free C_{max}/MEC ratio of about 10 [38]

MIC, minimum inhibitory concentration; MEC, minimum effective concentration, which is the minimum amount of drug to cause transition to a compact, rounded hyphal form.

The first drug that we will consider is vancomycin. Optimal vancomycin dosing remains a challenge. Vancomycin is the mainstay of treatment for many serious gram-positive bacterial infections and has been used for over 60 years. A consensus review published in 2009 by the Infectious Diseases Society of America, the American Society of Health-System Pharmacists, and the Society of Infectious Diseases Pharmacists recommends a target ratio of ≥400 for vancomycin 24-h AUC/MIC [15]. Several subsequent studies have supported this recommendation [21,23,24,39]. According to the consensus review, in adults, for an organism with an MIC of 1 mg/L, this ratio corresponds to trough concentrations of 15−20 mg/L for most patients. However, the recommended dosing is not actually based on the MIC. Rather, based on the increased risk of morbidity or mortality from complicated infections such as bacteremia, endocarditis, osteomyelitis, meningitis, and hospital-acquired pneumonia caused by *Staphylococcus aureus*, total trough serum vancomycin concentrations of 15−20 mg/L are recommended regardless of the actual MIC, as long as it is <2 mg/L.

The guidelines emphasize trough monitoring because of the stated difficulty to calculate an AUC in clinical practice. Without a population modeling approach, one must have at least two measured drug concentrations to estimate an AUC. Furthermore, because the target AUC or trough is based on steady-state conditions, one must wait 4−5 half-lives for this condition to occur. The usual half-life in adults with normal renal function is 4−5 h, meaning steady state is about 97% achieved after 24 h. Since adults are usually dosed twice daily, the recommended first trough is just prior to the fourth dose. If one were to estimate AUC by also obtaining a peak concentration, it would usually be done *after* the fourth dose for convenience. Even though this is not in the same interval as the trough prior to the fourth dose, there is an assumption of superimposability; that is, that the peak after one dose is the same as after any other dose at steady state. Again, the same requirement for steady state is also present even for trough-only monitoring, when pharmacometric tools are not used.

12.7 PROBLEMS WITH TROUGH-ONLY SAMPLING

Of course, with trough-only monitoring, it becomes very difficult to estimate the true half-life in an individual patient. Therefore one does not truly know when steady state has been achieved. In addition, the trough is not a very good estimator of AUC [40]. Remember that the trough concentration is the least informative sample, as many possible time-concentration curves can all pass through or very near the same trough concentration, as shown in Fig. 12.3, using our population model of vancomycin [40] as the basis for simulated profiles of differing AUCs, but with the same trough concentrations.

Another major problem with trough monitoring, then, is that many patients will have a perfectly adequate vancomycin AUC even without a trough of 15−20 mg/L. In fact, targeting such elevated troughs is frequently difficult with standard dosing and increases the risk of nephrotoxicity [41−44].

12.8 AN ILLUSTRATIVE PATIENT

Our patient was a 7-year-old boy, weighing 25 kg, who had a resection of a cerebellar tumor. Unfortunately, he developed an infection in the surgical site with methicillin-resistant *S. aureus* (MRSA).

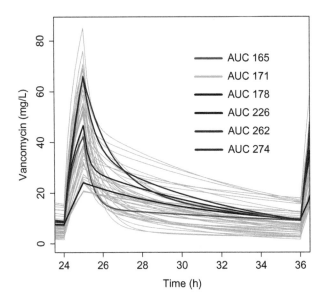

FIGURE 12.3

50 simulated time-concentration profiles for vancomycin. Profiles with differing areas under the curve (AUC), yet with the same trough concentration, are highlighted in color.

Cultures from the cerebrospinal fluid coming from his surgical drain were repeatedly positive for MRSA, with a measured MIC of 0.5 mg/L, and he had daily fevers up to 40°C. His primary team continued to increase the dose of vancomycin based on repeatedly low trough concentrations <10 mg/L. Despite the package insert dose for children of 40 mg/kg/dose intravenously divided every 6–12 h, the standard pediatric dose in children <12 years of age is 15 mg/kg/dose intravenously every 6 h. This patient was receiving 20 mg/kg/dose (500 mg) with a trough concentration of 7.7 mg/L when M.N. was called to assist. The patient's dose was double that in the package insert, and his trough concentrations were still inadequate by the recommended criterion, which is a target of 15–20 mg/L based on an infection in the central nervous system.

The first thing we did was to fit his vancomycin dosing history, weight, serum creatinines, and vancomycin measured concentrations to the population model for vancomycin that is included with BestDose. Of course, it is imperative to have a fit that one "trusts" before accepting any dose recommendations that BestDose produces. The fit of our patient's data is shown in Fig. 12.4A. Concentrations #1 (−5%), #2 (−19%), and #4 (6%) are quite well predicted, but Concentration #3 is relatively poorly predicted, with a −30% error for the weighted mean prediction of 30.9 mg/L versus the measured concentration of 45 mg/L. While the figure suggests that the fitted peak value is about 35 mg/L, the actual numerical value at the time the sample was drawn was 30.9 mg/L. There are no objective criteria by which one can say that a fit is good enough, but we have found in our clinical practice that if most predictions are within 30% of the measured concentrations, that the subsequently calculated optimal doses both make sense and do not result in surprising, unintended follow-up concentrations in stable patients.

(A)

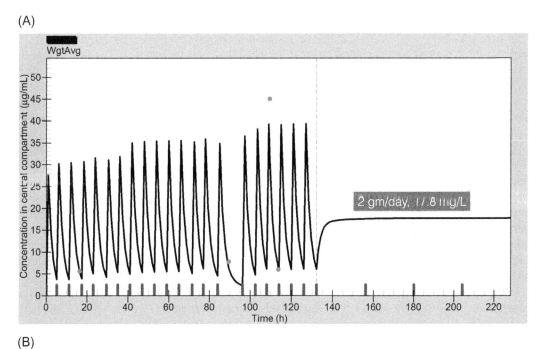

(B)

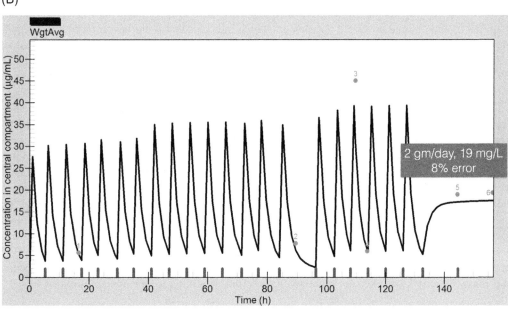

FIGURE 12.4

(A) First fit of vancomycin in BestDose for 7-year-old patient. (B) Second fit showing measured concentrations were close to predicted.

12.9 ISSUES IN FITTING DATA

There are three reasons for concentrations that are not fitted well by a model. The first is that the model is a poor model for the patient. This is a difficult subject to tackle and beyond the scope of this book. Suffice it to say that if a model does a poor job of predicting most concentrations in most patients, then it is not a very useful model for the purposes of clinical therapeutic drug management. One must also be aware of the population used to create the model and determine how relevant such a population is for the current patient.

The second reason for poorly fitted concentrations is that the patient is not stable and that one set of model parameter values cannot adequately describe all concentrations observed over time in a patient. In other words, there is sufficient intra- (within-)patient variability to prevent adequate fitting of all data. If there is an a priori reason to suspect that the patient is unstable, such as a critically ill patient, or a defined reason for a change in pharmacokinetic behavior like initiation of an interacting medication, then it can be helpful to try the interacting multiple model (IMM) approach outlined in Chapter 9. The third reason is simply that the data are incorrect. In particular, timing of samples collected under routine clinical circumstances within hospital settings can be inaccurate and result in poor predictions [45].

In this case, we attempted to use both the hybrid and IMM approaches described in other chapters, in case Reasons #1 or #2, respectively, were responsible for the poorly predicted Concentration #3. Although both improved the fit (not shown), the dose recommendations were either unrealistically low or high. This suggested to us that Reason #3 was at work and that Concentration #3 was perhaps falsely elevated. In fact, when we excluded that concentration, the calculated fit and optimal doses did not change, which indicates that it did not contribute any significant information that influenced the calculation of the patient's Bayesian posterior parameter values.

The estimated daily AUC for the patient was 415 mg × h/L. Based on the measured MIC of 0.5 mg/L, the ratio was 830, more than the target of 400. Nevertheless, one must always regard the patient and recognize that these AUC/MIC efficacy or trough safety targets themselves are averages in a population, and do not represent truly individualized therapy. A single patient presents a unique therapeutic milieu in which the antibiotic must act, and which can change the likelihood of response even when these average targets are achieved. For example, profound immunocompromise may demand a higher AUC/MIC ratio, and an underlying hematologic disorder may require a lower trough to avoid toxicity. Additionally, concentration targets may not be uniformly applicable across all infections. The AUC/MIC target of 400 is derived from patients with pneumonia or blood-stream infections with MRSA, and not central nervous system infections. Unfortunately, this concept of not only individualizing doses and exposures, but individualizing targets, is very much dependent on the existence of readily measured biomarkers for response to therapy (both for efficacy and for toxicity). Efficacy biomarkers, analogous to viral load for HIV, Hepatitis B or Hepatitis C, or galactomannan for aspergillosis, are as yet absent for bacterial infections. Of course, the primary toxicity biomarker for vancomycin is serum creatinine to monitor renal injury.

12.10 THE APPROACH TO THE PATIENT

In this patient's case, we decided to change the shape of the time-concentration profile rather than increase the dose further. It has been our experience that children who receive more than

80 mg/kg/day of vancomycin will frequently and rapidly develop nephrotoxicity, even if such high doses were initially justified by modest exposures. Therefore, we used BestDose to target a continuous infusion with a constant concentration of 18 mg/L, which is a daily AUC of $24 \times 18 = 432$ mg $\times$ h/L, approximately the same AUC as he was getting with 500 mg every 6 h. A priori, then, we expected the dose recommended by BestDose to be approximately $500 \times 4 = 2000$ mg infused continuously over a 24-h period.

Indeed, the optimal calculated continuous infusion to achieve 18 mg/L as a constant concentration was 2028 mg/day, only 1.4% over what we were expecting. We simplified this to 2000 mg/day. We also started rifampin as adjunctive therapy. The predicted vancomycin concentration was 17.5 mg/L (Fig. 12.4A) by the second day of this infusion and the measured was 18.9 mg/L (Fig. 12.4B), an error of -7%, which was acceptable to us. Note that we did not have to wait until some new steady state was achieved. Remarkably, within 24 h of this new regimen, after a week of high fevers and positive cultures, his fevers permanently abated and his cerebrospinal fluid sterilized. It is possible that this was due to rifampin, although as it turns out, adding rifampin to vancomycin may have limited clinical benefit or even be harmful [46].

We have been more systematically evaluating multiple model adaptive control for vancomycin with BestDose at a large public hospital in Los Angeles, CA. During the first year, we enrolled 83 adults who received standard of care vancomycin therapeutic drug monitoring (TDM). The standard dosing for adults with normal renal function was 1 gm intravenously every 12 h. Goal trough concentrations 1 h before the fourth dose were according to the guidelines [15] and dose adjustment to achieve target trough concentrations was intuitive. In the second year, we enrolled 90 further adults, but this time we used BestDose and routinely obtained concentrations to target the estimated daily AUC/MIC to be 400. In the absence of isolated MRSA, we used an AUC target of 400 mg $\times$ h/L (ie, equivalent to a ratio of 400 with an MIC of 1 mg/L). We chose an AUC of 800 mg $\times$ h/L as our upper target, corresponding to the goal ratio for an organism with an MIC of 2 mg/L.

As of the writing of this book, the study is still in progress, and the full results will be published in the peer-reviewed press, but several preliminary results are informative about the use of TDM with and without a pharmacometric tool such as BestDose. Firstly, just as we had found previously [45], there was a great deal of error in the timing of samples in routine clinical practice, with only 40% of troughs actually drawn within 1 h of the next planned or actual dose. Furthermore, 20% were drawn before Doses 1, 2, or 3, which may have been before steady state was achieved. These deviations in sample timing make simple comparison to a predefined steady-state trough range questionable. The second interesting finding was that by trough concentration, about 1/3 of patients were considered therapeutic, whereas 2/3 of those same patients were therapeutic by AUC. Of the nontherapeutic trough concentrations, about 85% were low, which could result in subsequent dose increases, even if the AUC were already therapeutic. In Year Two, because we were managing the patients with BestDose, the average final dose at the end of adjustments was 14.7 mg/kg versus 16.5 mg/kg in year 1 ($P = 0.01$), where the perceived need to increase the trough resulted in higher doses. As one would expect, the number of patients with associated nephrotoxicity in Year One was seven versus none in Year Two ($P = 0.04$). Only 11 (6%) of the 173 patients had a documented MRSA infection, but for up to 72 h after stopping vancomycin in all patients, there was one patient in the first year and none in the second year who experienced a relapse in signs/symptoms of infection ($P = 0.5$). Together, these findings suggest to us that targeting vancomycin AUCs can result in lower doses and less nephrotoxicity, without compromising clinical efficacy. Using a pharmacometric tool like BestDose can accomplish this even with one blood sample for vancomycin concentration measurement in a dosing interval as is currently practiced.

12.11 VORICONAZOLE

Let us now turn our attention to the antifungal drug voriconazole. Voriconazole is the major antifungal drug currently in use that is routinely monitored by serum drug concentration measurement and dose adjustment [47,48]. Neither fluconazole nor amphotericin B in any of its formulations is routinely monitored. Itraconazole and 5-flucytosine are more commonly monitored, but they are less often used. Posaconazole is recommended to be monitored, and the current target concentrations are >0.7 mg/L for prophylaxis and >1.0 mg/L for treatment [48]. Isavuconazole is newly on the market as of the writing of this book, and concentration targets have not yet been established. Finally, echinocandins have also not been routinely monitored in clinical practice due to rare toxicities and uncertain target concentrations.

Voriconazole is a challenging drug to dose precisely and accurately. Numerous reports in adults [49−55], including a prospective randomized trial [56], and in children [34,57,58] have documented improved outcomes when trough concentrations are maintained above 1 mg/L, which is a readily measured clinical surrogate for the full area under the time-concentration curve (AUC) that drives efficacy [59−62].

However, the pharmacokinetic behavior of voriconazole is complex and nonlinear. In many patients, small dose changes are associated with disproportionately large changes in the plasma concentrations of the drug. While more common in adults, nonlinear, saturated pharmacokinetic behavior is readily observed in children who receive higher doses than those that have been approved by regulatory agencies [63]. This nonlinearity also makes half-life and time to steady-state dependent on dose and concentration, complicating the ability to compare steady-state trough concentrations to the accepted therapeutic range of 1−6 mg/L [64], with either unnecessary delays in sampling, or premature sampling and misinterpreted concentrations. It is very difficult to know if a patient is at steady state from a single measured concentration. Furthermore, intuitive or empiric voriconazole dose adjustments result in prolonged patient exposure to the drug outside the therapeutic range in up to half or more children and adults [54,57].

12.12 AN ILLUSTRATIVE PATIENT

The first patient to consider was a 2-year-old, weighing 13.6 kg, whose provider contacted M.N. for assistance with dosing voriconazole as an outpatient. She had autoimmune hepatitis, and she was receiving an immunosuppressive regimen of prednisone. Unfortunately, she developed a positive galactomannan index of 1.63 during routine screening. Her primary provider started her on oral voriconazole 6 mg/kg twice on Day One as a loading dose, followed by 4 mg/kg (55 mg) twice daily thereafter. This is the approved dose for intravenous dosing in adults. The drug is currently not approved in the United States in children under the age of 12 years, although in Europe it is approved for intravenous and oral dosing in children as young as 2 years of age. The approved intravenous pediatric dose from age 2−12 years is 7 mg/kg twice daily, with no loading dose. After age 12, adult dosing is recommended. The approved oral dose for all ages is 200 mg twice daily, regardless of weight.

12.13 **EVALUATION OF DOSAGE GUIDELINES**

Although these doses were based on a parametric population analysis from a large cohort of 82 children enrolled in Phase 1 studies [65], we have always viewed this recommendation as unusual. We can think of no other drug that has the same oral dose from age 2 years through adulthood, regardless of weight. Indeed, our own clinical experience and that of several others suggested that the starting intravenous dose needed to be higher, and the oral dose needed to be weight-based [34,66−69]. In fact, a larger population study that included adolescents and adults subsequently found that children up to 50 kg or 16 years of age should initially be dosed intravenously with 9 mg/kg twice on day one (loading) and 8 mg/kg twice daily thereafter. The oral dosage regimen was revised to 9 mg/kg twice daily.

For this young girl, not surprisingly given the low dose, her provider measured a concentration of <0.1 mg/L 13.75 h after her fourth maintenance dose, according to timing reported by her parents. They also reported that she had not missed any doses. As with the patient whom we discuss in the chapter on HIV therapy, we first decided to use a modeling approach to ascertain whether it was likely that she could have had such a low concentration. We did this to assess the likelihood that her parents had been giving the doses at the times that they had reported.

The following workflow is built into our BestDose software for easy use by clinicians who are unfamiliar with Monte Carlo simulation. Using the patient's age and weight, voriconazole dosing history, and measured voriconazole concentrations, we used BestDose to simulate 1000 versions of the patient by repeatedly sampling from the voriconazole population model parameter value distributions to generate 1000 sets of parameter values. BestDose automatically uses a unique rigorous Monte Carlo simulation technique devised by Dr. Sylvain Goutelle that preserves the nonparametric nature of the models in BestDose [70]. For each set of parameter values, BestDose calculated the concentration of voriconazole at exactly the same time as her sample was reported, after exactly the same doses and times, given her weight and age. From these 1000 possible values for that voriconazole concentration, BestDose computed the percentile of her actual measured concentration, which we set to 0.1 mg/L, relative to the 1000 possible values. This is shown in Fig. 12.5A. Based on the information reported by the family, her measured concentration was at the 49th percentile, placing it squarely in the realm of possibility.

This simulation technique quantifies the probability of adherence, recognizing that it is a stochastic or probabilistic variable, as is much of medicine. There are no absolute thresholds for the determination of adherence, and of course, such a determination only reflects the previous few doses. Nevertheless, it is a helpful technique, and in this case it gave us confidence that this child needed a dose adjustment, and that her parents did not need an in-depth conversation about the importance of taking medicines.

We then set out to design a dosage regimen for her to achieve the desired trough concentration of at least 1 mg/L. Since we were starting from an extremely low voriconazole concentration, which had been censored (see Chapter 4, Optimizing Laboratory Assay Methods for Individualized Therapy), we decided to use the function in BestDose to plan an initial regimen (see Chapter 6, Using the BestDose Clinical Software). We set the target trough concentration to be 2 mg/L. The optimal doses and predicted time-concentration profiles are shown in Fig. 12.5B. Note that because there was no measured concentration, there was no Bayesian posterior. The entire Bayesian prior (ie, the model) was used to calculate the dosages that would optimally achieve the desired target concentration. That is why there

(A)

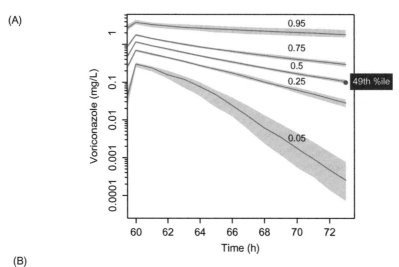

(B)

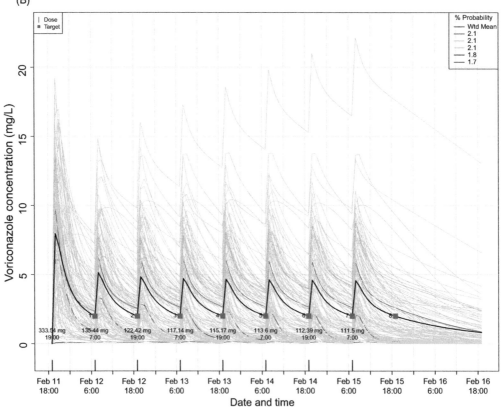

FIGURE 12.5

(Continued on next page)

(C)

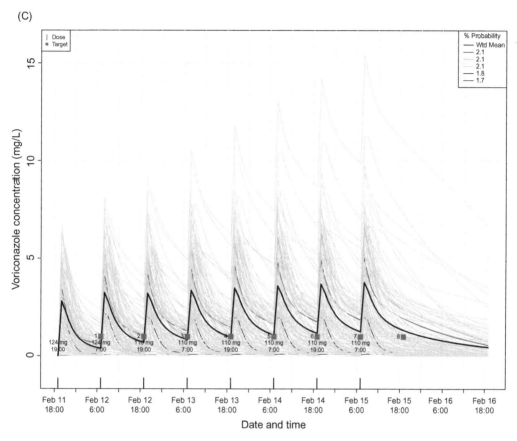

FIGURE 12.5

Managing voriconazole therapy in a 2-year-old outpatient. (A) Simulation to determine if reported outpatient concentration was possible after self-reported dose time. X-axis is time in hours. (B) BestDose plot showing all possible time-concentration profiles as well as the doses most likely to achieve the requested target concentrations. Green squares are the target concentration of 2 mg/L. (C) Projected profile based on dosing that was given, which did not include a loading dose as recommended. Again, green squares are the target concentration, this time 1 mg/L.

are so many possible profiles shown in light gray in Fig. 12.5B, as each profile corresponds to one support point in the population model. As we have stated in Chapter 3, each profile is one of multiple possible models for the patient, and the dark line is the weighted mean profile. Note the tremendous variability in the possible profiles, which reflects the variability in the population for this drug. Even with an initial dose optimized for her weight, she could still possibly have a trough concentration ranging between 0 and 12 mg/L. Nevertheless, based on the optimal dosing, for convenience, we recommended to her provider to load with 9 mg/kg (124 mg) twice on Day One, and to continue with 8 mg/kg (110 mg) twice daily thereafter. The projected profile for this regimen is shown in Fig. 12.5C, and one can easily see that although it is not optimal, by the second day, she would be above the minimum trough concentration of 1 mg/L.

On this regimen, 8.5 h after her ninth maintenance dose, she was still <0.1 mg/L. Before we received the data, the provider gave her two doses of about 11.5 mg/kg (160 mg), followed by maintenance dosing of 9 mg/kg (124 mg). We asked the provider to obtain a concentration earlier in the dose interval to avoid the possibility of a censored value. She had a concentration of 3.4 mg/L measured 2 h after her dose. BestDose predicted that this concentration should have been 3.4 mg/L, so we had a good fit. However, her predicted trough on 124 mg twice daily was 0.04 mg/L. Because we were uncertain about the first measured trough concentration and her overall fit quality, we asked for a repeat measurement, and this time, 10 h and 45 min after the previous dose, it was 1.3 mg/L. Refitting all her data changed the predicted peak of 3.40 mg/L to 3.39 mg/L, which was insignificant, but now the new trough of 1.3 mg/L was predicted to be 1.24 mg/L. Interestingly, her previous unmeasurable trough was now predicted to be 0.45 mg/L, so it is possible that she had parameters that were changing during the time period or that there was some inaccuracy in her modeled dose times, particularly between sampling events. Her galactomannan had increased somewhat, so BestDose predicted that by increasing the dose to 200 mg, she would achieve 1.65 mg/L. The subsequent measured trough was 1.9 mg/L, a prediction error of −13%. She was eventually increased to 220 mg per dose, and BestDose predicted her trough on this dose would be 2.5 mg/L. Indeed, the measured value was exactly that, for a 0% error. Her galactomannan became undetectable and stayed that way.

We chose this patient to illustrate the interplay between adherence, accurate recording of dose and measurement times, and of intra-patient (inter-occasional) variability within a single patient. All of these factors degrade accuracy and precision of predictions, and yet it is still possible to manage such patients. The keys to outpatient management are repeated measurements and patient cooperation and understanding of the process to enable the most accurate data possible.

12.14 ANOTHER ILLUSTRATIVE PATIENT

Inpatients with verified dose and measurement data, particularly if they are receiving intravenous therapy, are of course generally easier to manage. The second patient was a 16-year-old girl, weighing 77 kg, who was severely burned with 35% total body area involved. She developed candidemia with *Candida albicans* from her central venous line, complicated by bilateral candidal chorioretinitis. Her primary team was treating her with voriconazole due to concerns about fluconazole resistance. They wished to minimize nephrotoxicity and to use a drug with good ocular penetration.

Her initial maintenance dose was 200 mg IV twice daily. Trough concentrations ranged between 1.1 and 0.7 mg/L. Her dose was increased to 250 mg IV twice daily, with another trough of 1.1 mg/L. Her primary team wanted a more robust trough concentration that was sustained above 1 mg/L. We input all her data into BestDose, and asked it to calculate a dose that would result in a trough concentration of 1.5 mg/L. Intuitively, one might guess the dose to be 375 mg or 50% higher than her current dose of 250 mg, since the desired trough was 50% higher than her current. However, we must remember that vorioncazole does not have linear pharmacokinetics in many patients, particularly adults. Adolescents are especially unpredictable, as they are physiologically between childhood and full maturity. Indeed, BestDose was able to fit her past concentrations with a weighted mean bias of only 2.35% and imprecision of 2.5%, and calculated that a dose of 300 mg (not 375 mg) would give her a trough concentration of 1.5 mg/L. This is shown in Fig. 12.6. Indeed, her subsequent measured trough

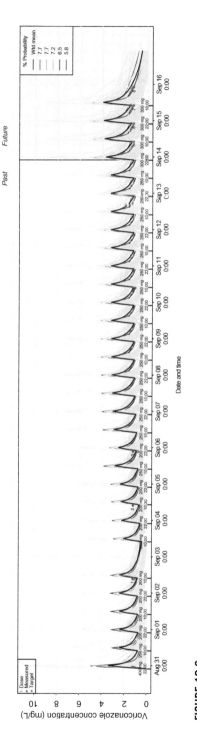

FIGURE 12.6

BestDose plot for voriconazole dosing to achieve a target concentration 12 h after a dose of 1.5 mg/L.

concentration was 1.4 mg/L. Note in the figure that there was a missed dose on Sep. 3. BestDose and any Bayesian method can handle such irregular dosing with ease. She continued on the 300-mg dose with no evidence of active infection.

We have shown that the voriconazole model in BestDose can predict concentrations in adults [71] and children up to age 18 [72]. In both studies, it also calculates the dose to achieve a target concentration (compared to an actual dose resulting in a measured concentration set as the target) with <5% bias with two optimally timed samples at 4 and 12 h after a dose given twice daily. These times were calculated with our MMopt algorithm, discussed in Chapter 8, Monitoring Each Patient Optimally: When to Obtain the Best Samples for Therapeutic Drug Monitoring.

12.15 CONCLUSION

In this chapter, we have provided principles and practices to develop specific concentration targets and to calculate optimal doses to achieve those targets, all for single drug therapy for bacterial or fungal infections. In Chapter 10, Quantitative Modeling of Diffusion into Endocardial Vegetations, the Post-Antibiotic Effect, and Bacterial Growth and Kill we expand upon these ideas with linked pharmacokinetic-pharmacodynamic models, and in Chapter 13, Optimizing Combination Therapy for Bacterial Kill, we extend these ideas to combination drug therapy.

REFERENCES

[1] Craig WA. Basic pharmacodynamics of antibacterials with clinical applications to the use of beta-lactams, glycopeptides, and linezolid. Infect Dis Clin North Am 2003;17:479−501.

[2] Levison ME. Pharmacodynamics of antibacterial drugs. Infect Dis Clin North Am 2000;14:281−91.

[3] Nightingale CH, Ambrose PG, Drusano GL, Murakawa T. Antimicrobial pharmacodynamics in theory and clinical practice. 2nd ed. Informa Healthcare; 2007.

[4] Safdar N, Andes D, Craig WA. In vivo pharmacodynamic activity of daptomycin. Antimicrob Agents Chemother 2004;48:63−8.

[5] Sevillano D, et al. Azithromycin iv pharmacodynamic parameters predicting *Streptococcus pneumoniae* killing in epithelial lining fluid versus serum: an in vitro pharmacodynamic simulation. J Antimicrob Chemother 2006;57:1128−33.

[6] Lodise TP, et al. Pharmacodynamics of an 800-mg dose of telithromycin in patients with community-acquired pneumonia caused by extracellular pathogens. Diagn Microbiol Infect Dis 2005;52:45−52.

[7] Dowell JA, Goldstein BP, Buckwalter M, Stogniew M, Damle B. Pharmacokinetic-pharmacodynamic modeling of dalbavancin, a novel glycopeptide antibiotic. J Clin Pharmacol 2013;48:1063−8.

[8] Pea F, et al. Therapeutic drug monitoring of linezolid: a retrospective monocentric analysis. Antimicrob Agents Chemother 2010;54:4605−10.

[9] Sprandel KA, et al. Population pharmacokinetic modeling and Monte Carlo simulation of varying doses of intravenous metronidazole. Diagn Microbiol Infect Dis 2006;55:303−9.

[10] Noreddin AM, et al. Pharmacodynamic modeling of clarithromycin against macrolide-resistant [PCR-positive mef(A) or erm(B)] *Streptococcus pneumoniae* simulating clinically achievable serum and epithelial lining fluid free-drug concentrations. Antimicrob Agents Chemother 2002;46:4029−34.

[11] Tessier PR, et al. Pharmacodynamic assessment of clarithromycin in a murine model of pneumococcal pneumonia. Antimicrob Agents Chemother 2002;46:1425–34.

[12] Lodise TP, Butterfield JM, Hegde SS, Samara E, Barriere SL. Telavancin pharmacokinetics and pharmacodynamics in patients with complicated skin and skin structure infections and various degrees of renal function. Antimicrob Agents Chemother 2012;56:2062–6.

[13] Meagher AK, et al. Exposure-response analyses of tigecycline efficacy in patients with complicated skin and skin-structure infections. Antimicrob Agents Chemother 2007;51:1939–45.

[14] Passarell JA, et al. Exposure-response analyses of tigecycline efficacy in patients with complicated intra-abdominal infections. Antimicrob Agents Chemother 2008;52:204–10.

[15] Rybak M, et al. Therapeutic monitoring of vancomycin in adult patients: a consensus review of the American Society of Health-System Pharmacists, the Infectious Diseases Society of America, and the Society of Infectious Diseases Pharmacists. Am J Health Syst Pharm 2009;66:82–98.

[16] Barclay ML, Kirkpatrick CM, Begg EJ. Once daily aminoglycoside therapy. Is it less toxic than multiple daily doses and how should it be monitored? Clin Pharmacokinet 1999;36:89–98.

[17] Craig WA, Andes D. Pharmacokinetics and pharmacodynamics of antibiotics in otitis media. Pediatr Infect Dis J 1996;15:255.

[18] Courter JD, Kuti JL, Girotto JE, Nicolau DP. Optimizing bactericidal exposure for β-lactams using prolonged and continuous infusions in the pediatric population. Pediatr Blood Cancer 2009;53:379–85.

[19] Dulhunty JM, et al. Continuous infusion of beta-lactam antibiotics in severe sepsis: a multicenter double-blind, randomized controlled trial. Clin Infect Dis 2013;56:236–44.

[20] Burgess SV, Mabasa VH, Chow I, Ensom MHH. Evaluating outcomes of alternative dosing strategies for cefepime: a qualitative systematic review. Ann Pharmacother 2015;49:311–22.

[21] Lodise TP, et al. Vancomycin exposure in patients with methicillin-resistant *Staphylococcus aureus* bloodstream infections: how much is enough? Clin Infect Dis 2014;59:666–75.

[22] Jung Y, et al. Area under the time-concentration curve to minimum inhibitory concentration ratio as a predictor of vancomycin treatment outcome in methicillin-resistant *Staphylococcus aureus* bacteraemia. Int J Antimicrob Agents 2014;43:179–83.

[23] Holmes NE, et al. Vancomycin AUC/MIC ratio and 30-day mortality in patients with *Staphylococcus aureus* bacteremia. Antimicrob Agents Chemother 2013;57:1654–63.

[24] Brown J, Brown K, Forrest A. Vancomycin AUC24/MIC ratio in patients with complicated bacteremia and infective endocarditis due to methicillin-resistant *Staphylococcus aureus* and its association with attributable mortality during hospitalization. Antimicrob Agents Chemother 2012;56:634–8.

[25] Kullar R, Davis SL, Levine DP, Rybak MJ. Impact of vancomycin exposure on outcomes in patients with methicillin-resistant *Staphylococcus aureus* bacteremia: support for consensus guidelines suggested targets. Clin Infect Dis 2011;52:975–81.

[26] Walsh TJ, et al. Safety, tolerance, and pharmacokinetics of high-dose liposomal amphotericin B (AmBisome) in patients infected with *Aspergillus* species and other filamentous fungi: maximum tolerated dose study. Antimicrob Agents Chemother 2001;45:3487–96.

[27] Hooshmand-Rad R, et al. Retrospective study of the renal effects of amphotericin B lipid complex when used at higher-than-recommended dosages and longer durations compared with lower dosages and shorter durations in patients with systemic fungal infections. Clin Ther 2004;26:1652–62.

[28] Cornely OA, et al. Liposomal amphotericin B as initial therapy for invasive mold infection: a randomized trial comparing a high-loading dose regimen with standard dosing (AmBiLoad trial). Clin Infect Dis 2007;44:1289–97.

[29] Piper L, et al. Fluconazole loading dose pharmacokinetics and safety in infants. Pediatr Infect Dis J 2011;30:375–8.

[30] Clancy CJ, Yu VL, Morris AJ, Snydman DR, Nguyen MH. Fluconazole MIC and the fluconazole dose/MIC ratio correlate with therapeutic response among patients with candidemia. Antimicrob Agents Chemother 2005;49:3171−7.

[31] Goodwin ML, Drew RH. Antifungal serum concentration monitoring: an update. J Antimicrob Chemother 2008;61:17−25.

[32] Walsh TJ, et al. Treatment of invasive aspergillosis with posaconazole in patients who are refractory to or intolerant of conventional therapy: an externally controlled trial. Clin Infect Dis 2007;44:2−12.

[33] Krishna G, Sansone-Parsons A, Martinho M, Kantesaria B, Pedicone L. Posaconazole plasma concentrations in juvenile patients with invasive fungal infection. Antimicrob Agents Chemother 2007;51:812−18.

[34] Neely M, Rushing T, Kovacs A, Jelliffe R, Hoffman J. Voriconazole pharmacokinetics and pharmacodynamics in children. Clin Infect Dis 2010;50:27−36.

[35] Nett JE, Andes DR. Antifungal agents: spectrum of activity, pharmacology, and clinical indications. Infect Dis Clin North Am 2015. Available from: http://dx.doi.org/10.1016/j.idc.2015.10.012.

[36] Andes D, et al. In vivo comparison of the pharmacodynamic targets for echinocandin drugs against *Candida* species. Antimicrob Agents Chemother 2010;54:2497−506.

[37] Andes D, et al. Use of pharmacokinetic-pharmacodynamic analyses to optimize therapy with the systemic antifungal micafungin for invasive candidiasis or candidemia. Antimicrob Agents Chemother 2011;55:2113−21.

[38] Pound MW, Townsend ML, Drew RH. Echinocandin pharmacodynamics: review and clinical implications. J Antimicrob Chemother 2010;65:1108−18.

[39] Gawronski KM, Goff DA, Brown J, Khadem TM, Bauer KA. A stewardship program's retrospective evaluation of vancomycin AUC24/MIC and time to microbiological clearance in patients with methicillin-resistant *Staphylococcus aureus* bacteremia and osteomyelitis. Clin Ther 2013;35:772−9.

[40] Neely MN, et al. Are vancomycin trough concentrations adequate for optimal dosing? Antimicrob Agents Chemother 2014;58:309−16.

[41] Lodise TP, Patel N, Lomaestro BM, Rodvold KA, Drusano GL. Relationship between initial vancomycin concentration-time profile and nephrotoxicity among hospitalized patients. Clin Infect Dis 2009;49:507−14.

[42] Kullar R, Davis SL, Taylor TN, Kaye KS, Rybak MJ. Effects of targeting higher vancomycin trough levels on clinical outcomes and costs in a matched patient cohort. Pharmacother 2012;32:195−201.

[43] Pritchard L, et al. Increasing vancomycin serum trough concentrations and incidence of nephrotoxicity. Am J Med 2010;123:1143−9.

[44] Wong-Beringer A, Joo J, Tse E, Beringer P. Vancomycin-associated nephrotoxicity: a critical appraisal of risk with high-dose therapy. Int J Antimicrob Agents 2011;37:95−101.

[45] Charpiat B, Breant V, Pivot-Dumarest C, Maire P, Jelliffe R. Prediction of future serum concentrations with Bayesian fitted pharmacokinetic models: results with data collected by nurses versus trained pharmacy residents. Ther Drug Monit 1994;16:166−73.

[46] Tremblay S, Lau TTY, Ensom MHH. Addition of rifampin to vancomycin for methicillin-resistant *Staphylococcus aureus* infections: what is the evidence? Ann Pharmacother 2013;47:1045−54.

[47] Smith J, Andes D. Therapeutic drug monitoring of antifungals: pharmacokinetic and pharmacodynamic considerations. Ther Drug Monit 2008;30:167−72.

[48] Ashbee HR, et al. Therapeutic drug monitoring (TDM) of antifungal agents: guidelines from the British Society for Medical Mycology. J Antimicrob Chemother 2014;69:1162−76.

[49] Dolton MJ, et al. Voriconazole pharmacokinetics and therapeutic drug monitoring: a multi-center study. Antimicrob Agents Chemother 2012;56:4793−9.

[50] Troke PF, Hockey HP, Hope WW. Observational study of the clinical efficacy of voriconazole and its relationship to plasma concentrations in patients. Antimicrob Agents Chemother 2011;55:4782−8.

[51] Ueda K, et al. Monitoring trough concentration of voriconazole is important to ensure successful antifungal therapy and to avoid hepatic damage in patients with hematological disorders. Int J Hematol 2009;89:592−9.

[52] Pascual A, et al. Voriconazole therapeutic drug monitoring in patients with invasive mycoses improves efficacy and safety outcomes. Clin Infect Dis 2008;46:201−11.

[53] Smith J, et al. Voriconazole therapeutic drug monitoring. Antimicrob Agents Chemother 2006;50:1570−2.

[54] Mitsani D, et al. Prospective, observational study of voriconazole therapeutic drug monitoring among lung transplant recipients receiving prophylaxis: factors impacting levels of and associations between serum troughs, efficacy, and toxicity. Antimicrob Agents Chemother 2012;56:2371−7.

[55] Miyakis S, van Hal SJ, Ray J, Marriott D. Voriconazole concentrations and outcome of invasive fungal infections. Clin Microbiol Infect 2010;16:927−33.

[56] Park WB, et al. The effect of therapeutic drug monitoring on safety and efficacy of voriconazole in invasive fungal infections: a randomized controlled trial. Clin Infect Dis 2012;55:1080−7

[57] Soler-Palacín P, et al. Voriconazole drug monitoring in the management of invasive fungal infection in immunocompromised children: a prospective study. J Antimicrob Chemother 2012;67:700−6.

[58] Choi S-H, et al. Importance of voriconazole therapeutic drug monitoring in pediatric cancer patients with invasive aspergillosis. Pediatric Blood Cancer 2013;60:82−7.

[59] Siopi M, et al. Susceptibility breakpoints and target values for therapeutic drug monitoring of voriconazole and *Aspergillus fumigatus* in an in vitro pharmacokinetic/pharmacodynamic model. J Antimicrob Chemother 2014;69:1611−19.

[60] Al-Saigh R, Elefanti A, Velegraki A, Zerva L, Meletiadis J. In Vitro pharmacokinetic/pharmacodynamic modeling of voriconazole activity against *Aspergillus* species in a new in vitro dynamic model. Antimicrob Agents Chemother 2012;56:5321−7.

[61] Andes D, Marchillo K, Stamstad T, Conklin R. In vivo pharmacokinetics and pharmacodynamics of a new triazole, voriconazole, in a murine candidiasis model. Antimicrob Agents Chemother 2003;47:3165−9.

[62] Drusano GL. How many steps along the path is too far? Clin Infect Dis 2010;50:37−9.

[63] Neely MN, et al. Voriconazole pharmacokinetics and metabolism to voriconazole-*N*-oxide in children is age independent with more aggressive dosing. Intersci Conf Antimicrob Agents Chemother 2014.

[64] Bruggemann RJM, et al. Therapeutic drug monitoring of voriconazole. Ther Drug Monit 2008; 30:403−11.

[65] Karlsson MO, Lutsar I, Milligan PA. Population pharmacokinetic analysis of voriconazole plasma concentration data from pediatric studies. Antimicrob Agents Chemother 2009;53:935−44.

[66] Spriet I, et al. Voriconazole plasma levels in children are highly variable. Eur J Clin Microbiol Infect Dis 2011;30:283−7.

[67] Walsh TJ, et al. Pharmacokinetics, safety, and tolerability of voriconazole in immunocompromised children. Antimicrob Agents Chemother 2010;54:4116−23.

[68] Michael C, et al. Voriconazole pharmacokinetics and safety in immunocompromised children compared to adult patients. Antimicrob Agents Chemother 2010;54:3225−32.

[69] Shima H, Miharu M, Osumi T, Takahashi T, Shimada H. Differences in voriconazole trough plasma concentrations per oral dosages between children younger and older than 3 years of age. Pediatr Blood Cancer 2010;54:1050−2.

[70] Goutelle S, et al. Population modeling and Monte Carlo simulation study of the pharmacokinetics and antituberculosis pharmacodynamics of rifampin in lungs. Antimicrob Agents Chemother 2009;53:2974−81.

[71] Hope WW, et al. Software for dosage individualization of voriconazole for immunocompromised patients. Antimicrob Agents Chemother 2013;57:1888−94.

[72] Neely M, et al. Achieving target voriconazole concentrations more accurately in children and adolescents. Antimicrob Agents Chemother 2015;59:3090−7.

COMBINATION CHEMOTHERAPY WITH ANTI-INFECTIVE AGENTS

13

G.L. Drusano

CHAPTER OUTLINE

13.1 WHY EMPLOY COMBINATION THERAPY?

There are multiple reasons to employ combination therapy and multiple reasons to avoid it. First, let us examine the reasons to employ it.

13.2 INCREASED SPECTRUM OF EMPIRICAL COVERAGE

It has been well demonstrated [1] that in Hospital-Acquired Bacterial Pneumonia (HABP)/ Ventilator-Acquired Bacterial Pneumonia (VABP), having initial inappropriate therapy results in significantly worse outcomes, such as significantly higher attributable mortality, a higher incidence of septic shock, and a greater number of complications per patient (Table 13.1). Given this, the empirical use of combination therapy in the intensive care unit (ICU) environment, particularly for patients with HABP/VABP, would seem to be a prudent course of action, as this will provide broader empirical coverage for the patient. It is also important to recognize that different ICUs have different organisms prevalent and differing susceptibility profiles. Consequently, empirical choices need to consider the organisms most prevalent in that particular ICU and must take into account the susceptibility profile. It is also important to recognize that hospital-wide antibiograms are **not** adequate for the empirical choice of agent(s) for therapy of ICU-based infections, as the

Individualized Drug Therapy for Patients. DOI: http://dx.doi.org/10.1016/B978-0-12-803348-7.00013-7

Table 13.1 Impact of Appropriate Versus Inappropriate Antimicrobial Chemotherapy on Outcome in ICU Patients With Pneumonia

	Appropriate Rx ($n = 284$)	Inappropriate Rx ($n = 146$)	p-Value
Attributable mortality	16.2%	24.7%	0.04
Complications/patient	1.73 ± 1.82	2.25 ± 1.98	<0.001
Shock	17.1%	28.8%	<0.001

Source: *After Alvarez-Lerma F. Modification of empiric antibiotic treatment in patients with pneumonia acquired in the intensive care unit. ICU-Acquired Pneumonia Study. Intensive Care Med 1996;22:387–94.*

organisms resident in the ICU are, in the main, much more resistant. The intensity of use of antimicrobials in the ICU guarantees that organisms recovered in this setting will be different in kind from organisms rooted in the community and will have a much different susceptibility profile. Furthermore, different ICUs will have different resistance profiles (eg, medical vs surgical vs neurosurgical).

13.3 INCREASED BACTERIAL KILL WITH ADDITIVE OR SYNERGISTIC INTERACTION

Another positive aspect to the use of combination therapy is the possibility of achieving additivity or (hopefully) synergy between the agents in the combination. This gives the possibility of improving the rate of kill of bacteria at the primary infection site. This has a number of positive attributes attached to it.

The first positive attribute is that more rapid bacterial cell kill can help the host immune system in its function of clearing bacteria. Granulocytes are the central mechanism by which the immune system clears most (but not all) bacterial infections. Recently, it was demonstrated that granulocytes are saturable in their killing of bacterial pathogens [2,3], reaching a maximum rate of kill.

In a granulocyte-replete murine thigh infection model [2], *Pseudomonas aeruginosa* and *Staphylococcus aureus* were employed as challenge organisms. There were no interventions with antibacterials. The animals were sacrificed at various times to determine the number of organisms at the infection site over time. These are displayed in Figs. 13.1A and B (*P. aeruginosa*) and Figs. 13.1C and D (*S. aureus*).

It is clear by inspection that both organisms can be killed by the granulocytes up to an inoculum size of about 3×10^6 CFU/g. A smaller inoculum is successfully killed by them. However, above that inoculum size, the organisms are able to grow beyond the maximal ability of the granulocytes to kill them. Below that threshold, the immune system (predominantly the granulocytes) mediates substantial bacterial kill over 24 h (Figs. 13.1A and C). This suggested a Michaelis-Menten-type saturation model, which was then fitted to the data. The model gave a quite acceptable fit to the data (Table 13.2 and Figs. 13.1B and D). This implies that intervention with effective antimicrobial therapy was able to drive the bacterial burden at the infection site to below the half-saturation point

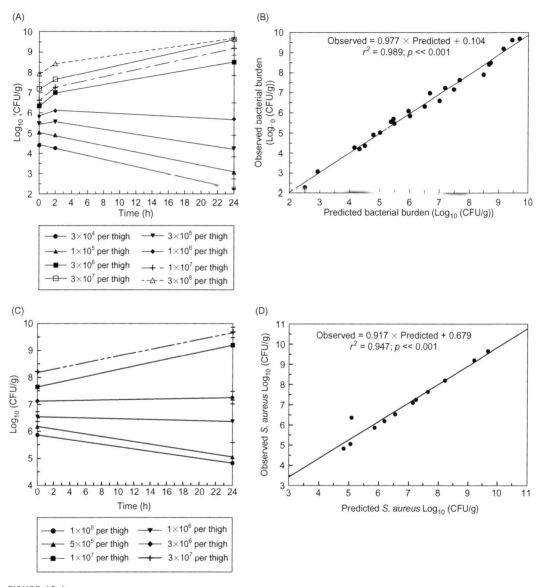

FIGURE 13.1

Effect of initial bacterial burden over time in granulocyte-replete mice with a thigh infection. (A) *Staphylococcus aureus*. (B) Fit of a Michaelis-Menten model to all the data simultaneously (population model). (C) *Pseudomonas aeruginosa* challenge. (D) Fit of a Michaelis-Menten model to all the data simultaneously (population model).

After Drusano GL, Fregeau C, Liu W, Brown DL, Louie A. Impact of burden on granulocyte clearance of bacteria in a mouse thigh infection model. Antimicrob Agents Chemother 2010;54:4368– 72.

Table 13.2 Point Estimates of Model Parameters of a Michaelis-Menten Model for Granulocyte Saturation for *Pseudomonas aeruginosa* and *Staphylococcus aureus* in a Murine Thigh Infection Model

Parameter (units)	$K_{\text{max-growth}}$ (h^{-1})	POPMAX (CFU/g)	$K_{\text{max-kill}}$[a] (h^{-1})	K_m (CFU/g)
Pseudomonas aeruginosa				
Mean	4.299	1.07×10^{10}	1.295	4.30×10^6
SD	3.115	1.02×10^{10}	2.070	3.75×10^6
Staphylococcus aureus				
Mean	5.678	4.24×10^{10}	0.115	5.55×10^6
SD	2.490	3.20×10^9	0.124	2.56×10^6

$K_{max\text{-}growth}$ *is the maximal growth rate of the organism in the mouse thigh; POPMAX is the maximal number of organisms per g of tissue at stationary phase; $K_{max\text{-}kill}$ is the maximal kill rate induced by granulocytes; K_m is the number of organisms per g of tissue at which granulocyte kill is half saturated.*
[a]*Multiplied by the granulocyte number.*
Source: *After Drusano GL, Fregeau C, Liu W, Brown DL, Louie A. Impact of burden on granulocyte clearance of bacteria in a mouse thigh infection model. Antimicrob Agents Chemother 2010;54:4368−72.*

where the granulocytes can kill the infecting pathogen. These experiments are most appropriate to provide insight for skin and skin structure infections.

However, some of the sickest patients with the most serious infections are patients with HABP/VABP. To determine whether this phenomenon was generalizable to pneumonia, we employed a murine pneumonia model in which the pathogen was *P. aeruginosa*. We reached similar findings in this investigation (Figs. 13.2A and B). Of great interest, we also found that the K_m (half-saturation point) and the V_{max} were virtually identical to that seen in the murine thigh infection model. This suggests (but does not prove) that granulocyte saturation may be a generalizable phenomenon across multiple infection sites. Again, this implies that additive or (hopefully) synergistic combination chemotherapy can rapidly decrease bacterial burden to a point where the granulocytes can kill the remaining organisms.

Before examining combination therapy for returning net bacterial burden to a point where net granulocyte bacterial killing can be positive once again, our laboratory used monotherapy to document the ability to return granulocyte kill with treatment of a bacterial burden which had already saturated (ie, markedly exceeded the K_m) the white cells [4]. There were 18 cohorts of mice infected with *P. aeruginosa* in the lung that were treated with the aminoglycoside plazomicin. There were two no-treatment controls. Nine of the treated cohorts were sacrificed at 24 h after therapy initiation (2 h after bacterial challenge). The remaining nine treated were followed for another 24 h without further therapy and sacrificed at Hour 48 after therapy initiation (Hour 50 overall).

Fig. 13.3 demonstrates that the higher plazomicin doses brought the bacterial burden to a point where the granulocytes could then generate another 1−1.5 Log$_{10}$ (CFU/g) bacterial kill in the follow up 24 h without further plazomicin therapy (see Fig. 13.3; after a plazomicin dose of 200mg/kg per day in the first day, the bacterial burden declines between Hour 26 and Hour 50). At the end of the first 24 h, plazomicin concentrations in the epithelial lining fluid were less than 30% of the

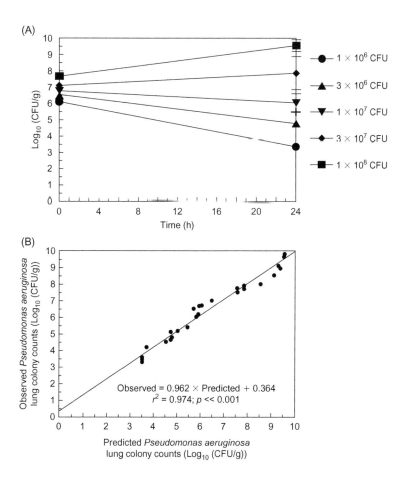

FIGURE 13.2

Effect of initial bacterial burden over time in granulocyte-replete mice with *Pseudomonas aeruginosa* pneumonia thigh infection. (A) *P. aeruginosa* challenge. (B) Fit of a Michaelis-Menten model to the data.

After Drusano GL, Vanscoy B, Liu W, Fikes S, Brown D, Louie A. Saturability of granulocyte kill of Pseudomonas aeruginosa *in a Murine model of pneumonia. Antimicrob Agents Chemother 2011;55:2693–5.*

minimal inhibitory concentration (MIC) and no further drug was administered. We fitted a model to the data. In this instance, we had a kill function, part of which was driven by drug concentrations and part of which was driven by the immune system (the granulocytes). The overall r^2 for the kill function was 0.896 ($p \ll 0.001$). Importantly, the K_m (half-saturation burden) was $2.68 \times 10^6 \pm 6.84 \times 10^5$ CFU/g, which was in excellent agreement with the values from the previous experiments, indicating it is likely that granulocyte saturation is a generalized phenomenon, not specific to the infection site (Table 13.3).

In clinical HABP/VABP, Zaccard et al. [5] performed bronchoalveolar lavage (BAL) in patients with Gram-negative pneumonia and obtained 134 BAL samples (bilateral sampling was performed).

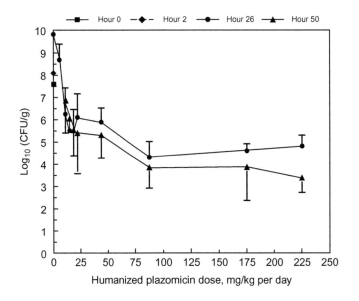

FIGURE 13.3

Plazomicin dose-ranging study and effect on granulocyte unsaturation in a *Pseudomonas aeruginosa* murine pneumonia model.

After Drusano GL, Liu W, Fikes S, Cirz R, Robbins N, Kurhanewicz S, et al. Interaction of drug- and granulocyte-mediated killing of Pseudomonas aeruginosa *in a murine pneumonia model. J Infect Dis 2014;210:1319–24.*

Table 13.3 Point Estimates of Model Parameters of a Michaelis-Menten Model for Granulocyte Saturation for *Pseudomonas aeruginosa* in a Murine Pneumonia Model

Parameter (units)	$K_{max-growth}$ (h^{-1})	POPMAX (CFU/g)	$K_{max-kill}$ (h^{-1})	K_m (CFU/g)
Pseudomonas aeruginosa				
Mean	0.745	8.48×10^{11}	1.97	2.15×10^6
SD	1.01	1.65×10^{11}	3.03	2.66×10^6

Definitions are as in Table 13.2.
Source: *After Drusano GL, Vanscoy B, Liu W, Fikes S, Brown D, Louie A. Saturability of granulocyte kill of* Pseudomonas aeruginosa *in a Murine model of pneumonia. Antimicrob Agents Chemother 2011;55:2693–5.*

The average dilution engendered by the BAL procedure is 30–100 fold (1.5–2.0 Log). Correcting the colony counts for the dilution [6] allowed calculation of the distribution of bacterial burden in patients with VABP. This is displayed in Table 13.4. More than 60% of patients have a bacterial burden that meets or exceeds the granulocyte half-saturation burden. Consequently, in such serious infections, early and adequate antibiotic therapy may supplement granulocyte function, providing more bacterial kill quickly. This may explain the results seen in Table 13.1 by Alvarez-Lerma [1] and others [7,8].

Table 13.4 Dilution Corrected Colony Counts for Patients With Gram-Negative Pneumonia Documented by BAL

Count[a]	Patients # (% of Total)
$\geq 3 \times 10^5$	49 (36.6)
$\geq 3 \times 10^6$	50 (37.3)
$\geq 3 \times 10^7$	35 (26.1)
Total	134 (100)

[a]*CFU/mL BAL fluid.*
Source: *After Zaccard CR, Schell RF, Spiegel CA. Efficacy of bilateral bronchoalveolar lavage for diagnosis of ventilator-associated pneumonia. J Clin Microbiol 2009;47:2918 24; Drusano GL, Lodise TP, Melnick D, Liu W, Oliver A, Mena A. et al. Meropenem penetration into epithelial lining fluid in mice and men and delineation of exposure targets, Antimicrob Agents Chemother 2011;55:3406−12.*

This raises the question whether combination therapy can generate reliable bacterial cell kill enough to reduce the bacterial burden down to that which the granulocytes can then kill. Generally, we refer to the interaction of agents as being additive, synergistic, or antagonistic.

13.4 **WHAT ARE SYNERGY, ADDITIVITY, AND ANTAGONISM?**

Let us first define additivity. The concepts of synergy and antagonism then follow as being significant departures from additivity. Greco and colleagues extensively reviewed this topic [9]. Interested readers are advised to review this paper. There are many competing definitions of additivity. The most common are Loewe Additivity and Bliss Independence.

Loewe Additivity can be understood as additivity giving the same response as a drug being added to itself. Bliss Independence can be thought of as having $Drug_1$ in an exposure that by itself will produce 60% of maximal effect and $Drug_2$ having an exposure producing 40% of maximal effect. The combination for additivity will give a response whereby the final outcome will be the response from $Drug_1$ plus 40% of the remaining possible response from $Drug_2$ (ie, 60% + 16% = 76%). Each definition of additivity has its adherents and detractors. In this chapter, I will set forth data using the Loewe Additivity definition. The choice was driven first because it is easily grasped and intuitive. Second, the choice was made because Greco derived a fully parametric form in which departures from additivity could be straightforwardly detected and tested for statistical significance.

The Greco Equation is shown here:

$$1 = \frac{[drug1]}{IC_{50D1} \times (E/E_{con} - E)^{1/HD1}} + \frac{[drug2]}{IC_{50D2} \times (E_{con} - E)^{1/HD2}} + \frac{\alpha \times [drug1 \times drug2]}{IC_{50D1} \times IC_{50D2} \times (E_{con} - E)^{(1/2HD1 + 1/2HD2)}} \tag{13.1}$$

The top line includes two sigmoid-E_{max} models describing the effects of the two agents. The second line provides the ability to describe departures from strict Loewe Additivity. The interaction parameter is α. If α is zero, the second line drops out and the interaction is additive. If α is positive, we get to "1" sooner than expected, which is defined as synergy. If α is negative, we get to "1" later than expected, which is defined as antagonism. We can calculate a 95% confidence interval around α. If α is positive and the lower 95% bound does not cross zero, then the interaction is statistically significantly synergistic. Likewise, if α is negative and the upper 95% confidence bound does not cross zero, then the interaction is statistically significantly antagonistic. All other interactions are accorded a definition of additivity. Our laboratory expanded this model to allow changing concentration-time profiles and to allow measurements taken over a time course to be analyzed simultaneously [10].

To test whether it is possible to get a truly synergistic interaction with regard to bacterial cell kill, we examined the drug combination of meropenem (a carbapenem) and levofloxacin (a fluoroquinolone). We had previously demonstrated [11] that these agents were synergistic in an in vitro hollow fiber infection model. In this evaluation, we employed our murine pneumonia model using *P. aeruginosa* as the challenge organism. Here, we used a neutropenic animal, as we wished to evaluate the drug interaction by itself without the immune system (granulocytes) [12]. The results are shown in Fig. 13.4. Levofloxacin was administered in a humanized fashion to the mice (ie, the drug was administered in a fractionated fashion with most of the drug administered at therapy

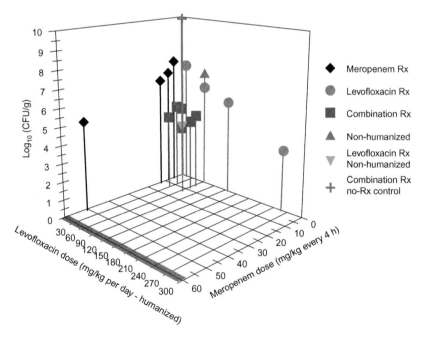

FIGURE 13.4

Effect of a synergistic regimen of meropenem plus levofloxacin on the burden of *Pseudomonas aeruginosa* in a granulocytopenic murine pneumonia model.

See Louie A, Grasso C, Bahniuk N, Van Scoy B, Brown DL, Kulawy R, et al. The combination of meropenem and levofloxacin is synergistic with respect to both Pseudomonas aeruginosa kill rate and resistancesuppression. Antimicrob Agents Chemother 2010;54:2646– 54.

initiation and smaller fractions administered later to make the murine profile more closely resemble the human profile, whereas meropenem was administered on an every 4 h basis). The α value was 2.475 ± 0.120. The 95% confidence interval did not cross zero, indicating that the interaction was synergistic and was statistically significant. Examination of Fig. 13.4 (black diamonds represent meropenem; blue (gray circles in print versions) circles, levofloxacin; red (gray squares in print versions) squares, combination therapy) demonstrates that the effect seen with low doses of the agents in combination achieved the same effect as much larger doses of each drug alone. When one looks at the size of the bacterial kill, the combination therapy at modest doses of each agent produce a 3.5–4.5 Log_{10} (CFU/g) bacterial load reduction. Reference to Table 13.4 indicates that this amount of effect will bring the vast majority of patients down over 1 Log below the half-saturation point, indicating that the combination will add substantial bacterial clearance by way of unsaturating the granulocytes and aiding their function. It should be noted that this combination is very synergistic while many other combinations are less synergistic or are merely additive. We would like to avoid antagonistic regimens if possible. The message is that combination chemotherapy needs to be chosen wisely.

Another example is the combination of fosfomycin plus meropenem [13]. Fosfomycin is an old drug being repurposed for therapy of multiresistant infections. This evaluation was performed in a hollow fiber infection model. In order to make this a substantial challenge, a 10 Log_{10} (CFU/mL) initial bacterial burden was employed. In Fig. 13.5, the meropenem-alone arm produces a 6 Log_{10} (CFU/mL) bacterial kill, but all killing ceases completely after Hour 48. Fosfomycin-alone mediates a 3.5 Log_{10} (CFU/mL) reduction in burden with resistance emergence after Hour 48. The combination reaches an extinction endpoint at Hour 48, mediating a kill of the organisms that meropenem alone could not eradicate, and suppresses all resistance emergence (no less-susceptible subpopulation amplification). One hypothesis that needs evaluation is that the combination is able to kill nonreplicative persister (NRP) phenotype organisms. Given the initial burden, it is likely that all the organisms were in late stationary phase of growth and that there were a substantial number of NRP-phenotype bacteria present as well. The kill of the 10 Log_{10} (CFU/mL) burden in just 48 h is impressive and again leads to the hypothesis that such a combination regimen could shorten therapy duration in serious high-burden infections. The α interaction parameter for these data was 4.78 with a 95% confidence interval of 0.878–8.56, indicating statistically significant synergy. This underlines the importance of choosing combinations that are likely to interact in a positive manner.

13.5 SUPPRESSION OF AMPLIFICATION OF LESS-SUSCEPTIBLE SUBPOPULATIONS

A major use of combination chemotherapy is for suppressing the amplification of a resistant subpopulation. When streptomycin was introduced for treatment of *Mycobacterium tuberculosis* (Mtb), it was clear quickly that resistance emergence was limiting for the use of monotherapy [14]. This story was recapitulated with the introduction of isoniazid. Selkon et al. demonstrated the power of combination therapy [15]. Since this time, combination therapy has been de rigueur for the therapy of tuberculosis.

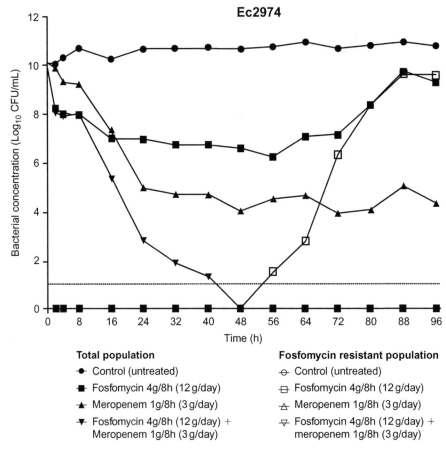

FIGURE 13.5

Effect of a synergistic regimen of fosfomycin plus meropenem on an ESBL-bearing *Escherichia coli* in a hollow fiber infection model. Resistant isolates were only recovered in the fosfomycin-alone arm (hollow squares). No meropenem-resistant isolates were found, but complete cell kill was not achieved. The fosfomycin-meropenem combination completely suppressed all resistance and generated a 10 Log_{10} (CFU/mL) kill (extinction event). Both hollow triangles are at the very bottom of the plot and are therefore not seen.

See Docobo-Pérez F, Drusano GL, Johnson A, Goodwin J, Whalley S, Ramos-Martín V, et al. Pharmacodynamics of fosfomycin: insights into clinical use for antimicrobial resistance. Antimicrob Agents Chemother 2015 e-pub ahead of print.

Recently [10] our laboratory has extended the work of Greco et al. [9] into the realm of resistance suppression. The Greco equation, Eq. (13.1) was embedded into a pharmacokinetic framework that allowed fluctuating drug exposures over time. Furthermore, multiple differential equations were employed to simultaneously model data from organism populations sensitive to both drugs, sensitive to $Drug_1$ but resistant to $Drug_2$, and sensitive to $Drug_2$ but resistant to

$Drug_1$. Given the burdens, the subpopulation resistant to both has a very low probability of existence *a priori*, but the model system is easy to extend to this circumstance, if required. The enabling equations are set forth here:

$$dX_1/dT = R_1 - (CL_1/V_1) \times X_1 \tag{13.2}$$

where R_1 is the piecewise input function for $Drug_1$ and X_1 is the $Drug_1$ amount in the central compartment.

$$dX_2/dT = R_2 - (CL_2/V_2) \times X_2 \tag{13.3}$$

where R_2 is the piecewise input function for $Drug_2$ and X_2 is the $Drug_2$ amount in the central compartment.

$$dN_S/dT = K_{gmax-S} \times N_S \times G - K_{kmax-S} \times M_S \times N_S \tag{13.4}$$

where N_S is the number of organisms susceptible to $Drug_1$ and $Drug_2$; K_{gmax-S} is the maximal growth rate constant for the population sensitive to both $Drug_1$ and $Drug_2$; G is a logistic carrying function, which allows the population to achieve stationary phase; and K_{kmax-S} is the maximal kill rate.

$$dN_{R_1}/dT = K_{gmax-R_1} \times N_{R_1} \times G - K_{kmax-R_1} \times M_{R_1} \times N_{R_1} \tag{13.5}$$

where N_{R_1} is the number of organisms resistant to $Drug_1$ but sensitive to $Drug_2$; K_{gmax-R_1} is the maximal growth rate constant for the $Drug_1$-resistant organisms; G is a logistic carrying function, which allows the population to achieve stationary phase; K_{kmax-R_1} is the maximal kill rate constant for $Drug_1$ and $Drug_2$ in combination for the $Drug_1$-resistant population; and M_{R_1} incorporates Eq. (13.1) for the $Drug_1$-resistant, $Drug_2$-sensitive population.

$$dN_{R_2}/dT = K_{gmax-R_2} \times N_{R_2} \times G - K_{kmax-R_2} \times M_{R_2} \times N_{R_2} \tag{13.6}$$

where N_{R_2} is the number of organisms resistant to $Drug_2$ but sensitive to $Drug_1$; K_{gmax-R_2} is the maximal growth rate constant for the $Drug_2$-resistant organisms; G is a logistic carrying function, which allows the population to achieve stationary phase; K_{kmax-R_2} is the maximal kill rate constant for $Drug_1$ and $Drug_2$ in combination for the $Drug_2$-resistant population; and M_{R_2} incorporates the URSA equation of Greco for the $Drug_2$-resistant, $Drug_1$-sensitive population.

$$G = (1 - (N_S + N_{R_1} + N_{R_2})/POPMAX) \tag{13.7}$$

where POPMAX is the maximal number of organisms per g of tissue at stationary phase.

$$M = (1 - \text{Fractional Effect}) \quad \text{[see above]} \tag{13.8}$$

as derived from the Greco URSA model (see the previous discussion); in this circumstance, E_{con} is set to 1.0.

The use of a multiple bacterial subpopulation model allows independent identification of interaction parameters (α_1 through α_3) that identify the interaction of the drugs for the fully-susceptible population (α_1), as well as subpopulations resistant to $Drug_1$ or $Drug_2$ (α_2 and α_3). This will allow identification of regimens optimal for overall bacterial cell kill as well as resistance suppression for both agents.

This model system has five different system outputs:

System Outputs:
System Outputs 1 and 2: associated with differential Eqs. (13.1) and (13.2) are the measured $Drug_1$ and $Drug_2$ concentrations in the central compartment

$$Output\ 1 = X_1/V_1; \tag{13.9}$$

$$Output\ 2 = X_2/V_2. \tag{13.10}$$

System Output 3 = Total Organism Number = Population sensitive to $Drug_1$ and $Drug_2$ + population resistant to $Drug_1$, sensitive to $Drug_2$ + population resistant to $Drug_2$, and sensitive to $Drug_1$ (as mentioned previously, a population resistant to both $Drug_1$ and $Drug_2$ has not yet been observed). This output is measured by plating on antibiotic-free plates.
System Output 4 = Population resistant to $Drug_1$ and sensitive to $Drug_2$. This output is measured by plating on agar into which $Drug_1$ has been incorporated. The actual concentration employed will differ, depending upon the step size of the resistance mechanism that we are attempting to capture in any experiment with different drugs.
System Output 5 = Population resistant to $Drug_2$ but sensitive to $Drug_1$. This output is measured by plating on agar into which $Drug_2$ has been incorporated. The actual concentration employed will differ, depending upon the step size of the resistance mechanism that we are attempting to capture in any experiment with different drugs.

This approach to modeling combination chemotherapy with a multiple subpopulation model and the URSA equation will allow the "inverted U" mountain type of response to be modeled as was demonstrated in our previous publication [16]. Because of the fully parametric nature of this approach, it allows Monte Carlo simulation to be conducted and allows powerful bridging to humans. This approach allows us to explore combination chemotherapy for cell kill as well as resistance suppression for Mtb, but also for any other circumstance requiring combination chemotherapy.

This approach [10] was applied to a 28-day experiment for Mtb with a treatment of linezolid plus rifampin. The result of the experiment for susceptible and resistant bacterial burdens is shown in Fig. 13.6. The parameter estimates are displayed in Table 13.5. It is clear by inspection that only the highest exposures to linezolid and rifampin (equivalent to the mean exposures from linezolid 600 mg daily plus rifampin either 600 mg or 900 mg daily) were able to provide good cell kill and also to suppress resistance for the duration of the study (see Fig. 13.6, Panels B [cell kill], E, and F [resistance suppression]).

Application of the model to all the data simultaneously was done, and the point estimates of the model parameters and their dispersions are displayed in Table 13.5. Inspection of α_s, α_{r-1}, and α_{r-2} demonstrates that all are negative. However, the 95% confidence intervals for all of these parameters overlap zero, indicating they would be accorded a definition of additive interaction, but with a tendency to antagonism. These values are estimated from all the data simultaneously.

When individual Bayesian posterior parameter estimates are calculated, it becomes possible to examine how the individual combination regimens interact. This is shown in Fig. 13.7. The squares have negative values and the diamonds have positive values (tending toward antagonism and synergy, respectively). In Panel A (susceptible population), 6/9 combination regimens have positive Bayesian estimates for α, whereas in Panels B and C (resistant subpopulations), 8/9 and 7/9 regimens have negative values for α. This clearly indicates that it is much more difficult to prevent

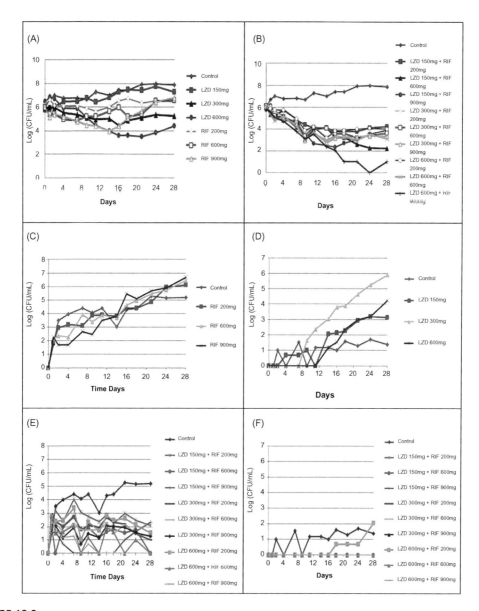

FIGURE 13.6

Impact of multiple monotherapy and combination therapy regimens of linezolid and rifampin on the total and resistant populations of *Mycobacterium tuberculosis*. (A) Effect of LZD and RIF as monotherapies on the total populations of Mtb. (B) Effect of LZD + RIF in combination on the total population of Mtb. (C) RIF-resistant Mtb subpopulation in arms treated with RIF alone. (D) LZD-resistant Mtb subpopulations in arms treated with LZD alone. (E) RIF-resistant Mtb subpopulation in arms treated with RIF in combination with LZD. (F) LZD-resistant *Mtb* subpopulations in arms treated with LZD in combination with RIF.

After Drusano GL, Neely M, Van Guilder M, Schumitzky A, Brown D, Fikes S, et al. Analysis of combination drug therapy to develop regimens with shortened duration of treatment for tuberculosis. PLoS One 2014;9(7):e101311.

Table 13.5 Parameter Estimates for the Fully Susceptible and Resistant Populations of *Mycobacterium tuberculosis* as Determined in a Mathematical Model

Parameter	Units	Mean	Median	Standard deviation
V_1	L	83.5	81.9	22.4
CL_1	L/h	6.20	6.19	0.748
V_2	L	139	141	10.9
CL_2	L/h	30.8	31.5	1.77
POPMAX	CFU/mL	7.85×10^9	7.24×10^8	1.75×10^{10}
K_{gs}	h^{-1}	0.100	0.107	0.0464
K_{ks}	h^{-1}	0.235	0.170	0.130
E_{501s}	mg/L	0.527	0.358	0.389
E_{502s}	mg/L	2.72	2.33	2.38
α_s	—	−0.954	−0.232	4.73
$K_{f13\text{-}01\text{-}9780128033487}}$	h^{-1}	0.0232	0.0198	0.0116
K_{kr1}	h^{-1}	0.274	0.318	0.113
E_{50_1r1}	mg/L	13.5	13.8	2.49
α_{r1}	—	−4.55	−6.11	3.39
$K_{f13\text{-}02\text{-}9780128033487}}$	h^{-1}	0.127	0.133	0.0757
K_{kr2}	h^{-1}	0.251	0.190	0.112
E_{50_2r2}	mg/L	5.92	6.01	0.829
α_{r2}	—	−0.431	−0.950	2.48
H_{1s}	—	4.60	4.64	1.85
H_{2s}	—	2.26	2.35	1.07
H_{1r1}	—	18.4	20.3	6.73
H_{2r2}	—	15.3	15.8	3.23
$INIT_4$	CFU/mL	1.88	2.72	1.87
$INIT_5$	CFU/mL	1.50	1.98	1.14

V_1 and V_2 are volumes of the central compartment for Drugs 1 and 2; CL_1 and CL_2 are clearances for Drugs 1 and 2; K_{gs} and $K_{f13\text{-}01\text{-}9780128033487}$ and $K_{f13\text{-}02\text{-}9780128033487}$ are first-order growth rate constants for the respective sensitive and resistant populations; K_{ks} and K_{kr1} and K_{kr2} are first-order kill rate constants for the respective sensitive and resistant populations; E_{501s}, E_{502s}, E_{50_1r1}, and E_{50_2r2} are the concentrations of the respective drugs at which the kill rate constants are half maximal; α_s, α_{r1}, and α_{r2} are drug interaction constants for the respective populations; H_{1s}, H_{2s}, H_{1r1}, and H_{2r2} are Hill's constants for the respective populations; $INIT_4$ and $INIT_5$ are initial conditions for the population burdens resistant to Drug$_1$, sensitive to Drug$_2$ and sensitive to Drug$_1$, resistant to Drug$_2$, respectively.
Source: After Drusano GL, Neely M, Van Guilder M, Schumitzky A, Brown D, Fikes S, et al. Analysis of combination drug therapy to develop regimens with shortened duration of treatment for tuberculosis. PLoS One 2014;9(7):e101311.

amplification of resistant subpopulations than it is to kill the fully-susceptible population, even with combination agent therapy, mostly because the large MIC change for the resistant clones makes the cell kill rely much more on the partner drug alone.

Another reason for the difficulty in achieving resistant subpopulation suppression is the agents in this combination. Certainly, linezolid is becoming a mainstay of therapy for multidrug-resistant Mtb. Rifampin is arguably our best agent for susceptible Mtb. The problem arises with the step size of resistance for rifampin (ie, the difference in MIC mediated by a mutation in rpoB, the bacterial

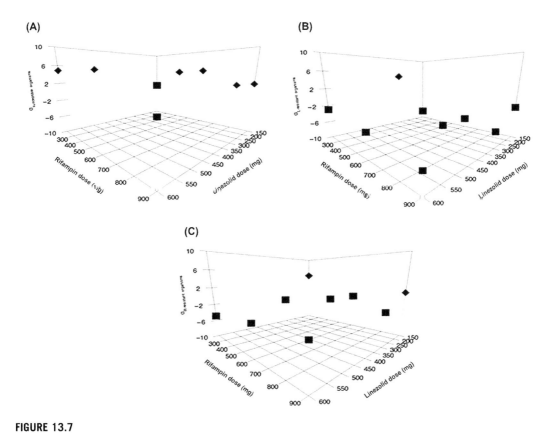

FIGURE 13.7

Bayesian estimates of the drug interaction parameter α for the fully-susceptible population (A), the linezolid-resistant population (B), and rifampin-resistant population (C).

After Drusano GL, Neely M, Van Guilder M, Schumitzky A, Brown D, Fikes S, et al. Analysis of combination drug therapy to develop regimens with shortened duration of treatment for tuberculosis. PLoS One 2014;9(7):e101311.

target site for rifampin). Many point mutations with rpoB will result in a $32-128$ fold increase in the baseline MIC. These single-step mutants virtually nullify all the microbiological activity of rifampin, bringing us into a situation approximating that of monotherapy. Consequently, one of the issues that must be addressed when designing combination therapy is the step size of the MIC change in the mutant subpopulations.

When we administer fixed-dose combinations to large populations of patients, there is a wide range of exposures for each of the agents because of substantial between-patient variability in pharmacokinetic parameter values. This has important implications for therapeutic outcome and for resistance suppression. Because the model is fully parametric, it is possible to perform Monte Carlo simulation for a specific regimen.

In Fig. 13.8, we show the effect of between-patient variability on bacterial burden. In Panel A, the total population burden declines by about 1.5 Log_{10} (CFU/mL) over the course of the

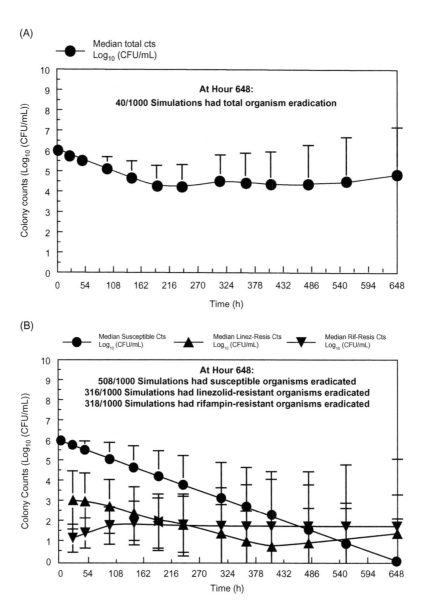

FIGURE 13.8

(A) Monte Carlo simulation (1000 subjects) for the effect of a 600/600 mg regimen of linezolid/rifampin on the total bacterial burden of *Mycobacterium tuberculosis* (B) as well as the fully-susceptible population, linezolid-resistant population, and rifampin-resistant population.

After Drusano GL, Neely M, Van Guilder M, Schumitzky A, Brown D, Fikes S, et al. Analysis of combination drug therapy to develop regimens with shortened duration of treatment for tuberculosis. PLoS One 2014;9(7):e101311.

experiment, with the standard deviations increasing with time. By the end of the experiment only 40/1000 simulated patients (4%) achieve complete population eradication. Examination of Panel B gives insight into this phenomenon. When we explore the effect of the regimen on the different susceptible/resistant subpopulations, the reason becomes clear. Slightly more than 50% of the total 1000 simulated patients had the fully-susceptible population eradicated. For the drug-resistant subpopulations, just shy of 32% of simulated subjects had one or the other resistant population eradicated. As before, only 4% of simulated patients had complete eradication. Consequently, our inability to suppress resistant subpopulation amplification results in trading off (for the most part) susceptible for resistant subpopulations. Because of this, when designing combination regimens, it is imperative to examine the effect of between-patient variability on the ability to kill all the populations or organisms present.

Other examples of resistance suppression have been discussed previously. In Fig. 13.4, the meropenem-levofloxacin combination was able to completely shut off all resistant subpopulation amplification [12]. Likewise, the combination of fosfomycin plus meropenem was able to suppress amplification of all resistant subpopulations of an ESBL-bearing *Escherichia coli* [13]. This is especially impressive as the baseline bacterial burden was 10 Log_{10} (CFU/mL). Clearly, well-chosen combination therapies can deliver both excellent bacterial cell kill as well as suppress amplification of resistant subpopulations.

13.6 SUPPRESSION OF PROTEIN EXPRESSION (IF ONE AGENT IS A PROTEIN SYNTHESIS INHIBITOR)

Cell kill and resistance suppressions are two important issues driving combination chemotherapy. However, there is another reason why combination chemotherapy, where one of the agents is a protein synthesis inhibitor, is advantageous. In certain instances, the protein synthesis inhibitor shuts off expression of a deleterious factor such as a toxin. The laboratory of Rose examined this for *S. aureus* in the monotherapy realm [17]. Our laboratory demonstrated this in the monotherapy realm with the protein synthesis inhibitor linezolid when compared to the fluoroquinolone ciprofloxacin in an in vitro hollow fiber infection model where *Bacillus anthracis* (Table 13.6) was the pathogen [18]. Here, linezolid shut off toxin production by the first sampled time point (3 h), while it took to Hour 24 for ciprofloxacin to shut off toxin production. This demonstration of toxin shut-off resulted in a recommendation from the Centers for Disease Control and Prevention for combination therapy for the therapy of anthrax partially to suppress elaboration of protective antigen, lethal toxin, and edema toxin [19].

Other proteins can be expressed that alter resistance emergence. The best known is the expression of β-lactamase in therapy with β-lactam antibiotics. Our lab examined the agent cefepime against *P. aeruginosa* [20] in the hollow fiber infection model. We employed two isogenic isolates of *Pseudomonas*, the PA01 wild-type isolate and a strain with a very high output of ampC β-lactamase. In Fig. 13.9, we demonstrate the effect of combination therapy on the wild-type isolate. In all instances, therapy with cefepime alone or tobramycin-alone rapidly results in amplification of resistant subpopulations, even at doses/exposures above the largest licensed doses for these

Table 13.6 Effect of Ciprofloxacin and Linezolid Therapies on Protective Antigen (PA) Production by *Bacillus anthracis* Using a Qualitative Immunomagnetic Electro-Chemiluminescence Assay

Therapy	Result[a]										
	0 h	3 h	5 h	8 h	Day 1	Day 2	Day 3	Day 4	Day 6	Day 8	Day 10
Control	−	+	+	+	+	+	+	+	+	+	+
Ciprofloxacin (500 mg every 12 h)	−	+	+	+	−	−	−	−	−	−	−
Linezolid (600 mg every 12 h)	−	−	−	−	−	−	−	−	−	−	−

[a] +, detectable protective antigen; −, below the assay limit of detection of 0.01 ng/mL.
Source: *After Louie A, Vanscoy BD, Heine III HS, Liu W, Abshire T, Holman K, et al. Differential effect of linezolid and ciprofloxacin on toxin production by Bacillus anthracis in an in vitro pharmacodynamic system. Antimicrob Agents Chemother 2012;56:513–17.*

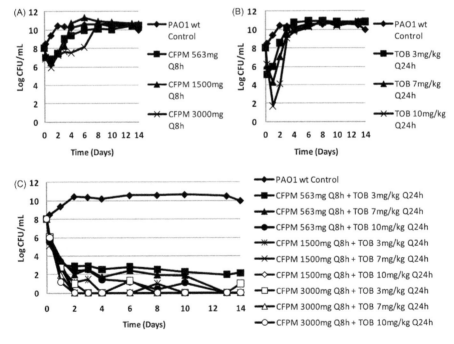

FIGURE 13.9

Effect of cefepime alone, tobramycin alone, and the agents in combination on wild-type *Pseudomonas aeruginosa* PA01 in a hollow fiber infection model. (A) PA01 WT vs cefepime and alone and in combination (cefepime monotherapy arms). (B) PA01 WT vs cefepime and tobra alone and in combination (Tobramycin monotherapy arms). (C) PA01 WT (JNJ) vs cefepime and Tobra Alone and in combination (combination arms).

After Drusano GL, Bonomo RA, Bahniuk N, Bulitta JB, van Scoy B, Defiglio H, et al. Resistance emergence mechanism and mechanism of resistance suppression by tobramycin for cefepime for Pseudomonas aeruginosa. *Antimicrob Agents Chemother 2012;56:231–42.*

drugs. The use of combination therapy with cefepime plus tobramycin caused excellent cell kill and suppression of resistance across a range of doses/exposures for these agents.

This caused us to hypothesize that the aminoglycoside, as a protein synthesis inhibitor, was markedly reducing expression of the β-lactamase. In the next experiment, we chose to identify that the β-lactamase expression was the cause of the resistance emergence. In Fig. 13.10, we generated cefepime exposures equivalent to 32 g/day (8 g every 6 h). In all instances, failure of the regimen with resistance emergence was demonstrated. In one arm of the evaluation, we added the β-lactamase inhibitor NXL-104 (now called *avibactam*) to a submaximal exposure equivalent to 1 g every 6 h. The β-lactamase inhibitor allowed good bacterial cell kill without resistance emergence for a clinically relevant 10−14 days.

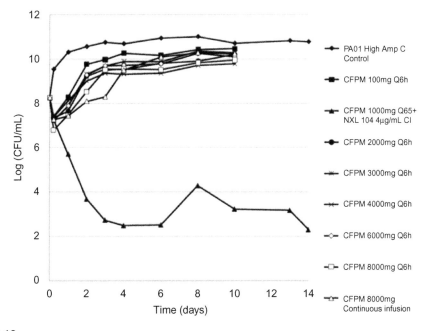

FIGURE 13.10

Effect of escalating regimens of cefepime on *Pseudomonas aeruginosa* PA01 isogenic stable derepressed isolate of *P. aeruginosa*. In one regimen, the β-lactamase inhibitor NXL-104 (now avibactam) is added to a cefepime regimen.

After Drusano GL, Bonomo RA, Bahniuk N, Bulitta JB, van Scoy B, Defiglio H, et al. Resistance emergence mechanism and mechanism of resistance suppression by tobramycin for cefepime for Pseudomonas aeruginosa. *Antimicrob Agents Chemother 2012;56:231−42.*

As part of the evaluation, we also hypothesized that the cefepime exposures in the hollow fiber system would demonstrate a time-dependent decrease. Fig. 13.11 shows that this did indeed occur. All cefepime-alone arms show a time-dependent decrease in cefepime concentration-time profile with the continuous infusion evaluation arm showing the clearest result. Only the arm with the

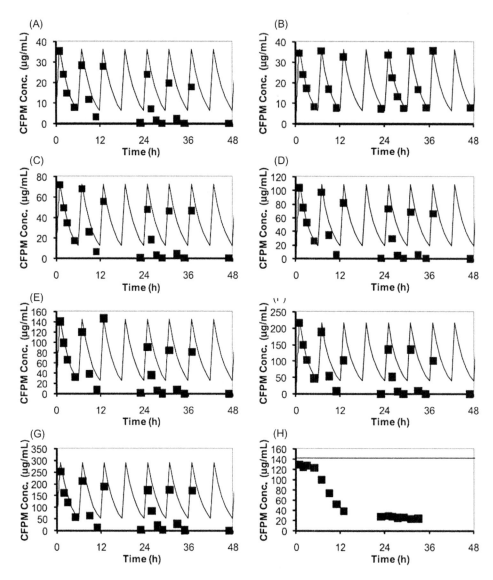

FIGURE 13.11

Impact of ampC β-lactamase production over time on the concentration-time profile of cefepime. Solid lines are the target profile. Squares are the measured (LC/MS/MS) cefepime concentrations. Only panel B, the regimen with the β-lactamase inhibitor NXL-104, attains the desired targets. (A) PA01 High Amp C vs cefepime 1000 mg Q6h. (B) PA01 High Amp C vs cefepime 1000 mg Q6h + NXL-104 4 μg/mL Cl. (C) PA01 High Amp C vs cefepime 2000 mg Q6h. (D) PA01 High Amp C vs cefepime 3000 mg Q6h. (E) PA01 High Amp C vs cefepime 4000 mg Q6h. (F) PA01 High Amp C vs cefepime 6000 mg Q6h. (G) PA01 High Amp C vs cefepime 8000 mg Q6h. (H) PA01 High Amp C vs cefepime 8000 mg continuous infusion.

After Drusano GL, Bonomo RA, Bahniuk N, Bulitta JB, van Scoy B, Defiglio H, et al. Resistance emergence mechanism and mechanism of resistance suppression by tobramycin for cefepime for Pseudomonas aeruginosa. Antimicrob Agents Chemother 2012;56:231–42.

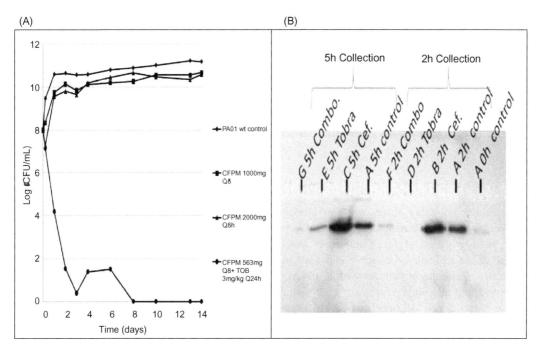

FIGURE 13.12

(A) Effect of combination therapy on *Pseudomonas aeruginosa* PA01. (B) Western blot for the production of ampC β-lactamase for a control flask, a cefepime-alone flask, a tobramycin-alone flask, and a flask with the combination.

After Drusano GL, Bonomo RA, Bahniuk N, Bulitta JB, van Scoy B, Defiglio H, et al. Resistance emergence mechanism and mechanism of resistance suppression by tobramycin for cefepime for Pseudomonas aeruginosa. *Antimicrob Agents Chemother 2012;56:231–42.*

addition of the β-lactamase inhibitor (Panel B) demonstrated that the cefepime concentrations could be maintained unchanged for the full course of therapy. This provides another thread of evidence that the β-lactamase expression was directly linked to the emergence of resistance.

Finally, we demonstrated that the addition of the aminoglycoside (tobramycin in this instance) did directly decrement the expression of the ampC β-lactamase. In Fig. 13.12A, only the combination therapy arm suppressed resistance and achieved a major bacterial cell kill. In Fig. 13.12B, we show a Western blot for ampC β-lactamase. The no-treatment control demonstrates a time-dependent increase in ampC β-lactamase expression, as one might expect with cell growth. The cefepime-only-exposed arm shows an even greater expression. This is somewhat surprising because cefepime is often thought of as a "weak inducer," relative to type II carbapenems like imipenem or meropenem. However, large concentrations of cefepime, such as would be seen for some time after the end of an intravenous infusion, can cause an increase in expression such as that seen here. The tobramycin-alone virtually shuts off all expression while the combination of cefepime plus tobramycin markedly reduces the β-lactamase expression relative to cefepime alone or the no-treatment control. It should be noted that an independent evaluation employing PCR demonstrated the same findings (see [20]).

We also evaluated the drug interaction employing the Greco model. The interaction for cell kill was additive (α value was positive, but the 95% confidence interval overlapped zero). This demonstrates that drug interaction for bacterial cell kill and for resistance suppression are two distinctly separate things, as there was absolute suppression of resistance, yet the interaction for cell kill was only additive and not synergistic. Indeed, even pairs fully antagonistic for bacterial cell kill can still successfully suppress resistance, as demonstrated for Mtb [21,22].

13.6.1 WHY NOT USE COMBINATION THERAPY?

There are also a number of reasons to avoid combination therapy. First, it is difficult to demonstrate convincingly that combination therapy results in better outcomes for all pathogens [23]. Organisms like *P. aeruginosa* and *Acinetobacter* spp. and other nonfermentors may represent a separate group because of their likelihood of multiresistance in the empiric therapy setting. However, one analysis did identify a stratum of patients with a survivorship benefit for combination therapy [24].

Second, not all combinations are synergistic or additive but may be antagonistic. They may not provide bacterial cell kill benefits over that seen with monotherapy, depending on the pathogen.

Third, not all regimens suppress amplification of resistant mutant subpopulations across the broad range of exposures achieved in infected patients (see Figs. 13.6 and 13.8).

Fourth, there is a monetary cost, sometimes substantial, to be paid for combination therapy.

Finally, there is the issue of a drug concentration-driven toxicity occurring from one of the agents in the combination, and there is the possibility of the agents interacting to make the likelihood of toxicity even higher than with monotherapy employing only the toxic agent [25].

Examples include monotherapy-driven toxicities with drugs like aminoglycosides and vancomycin as well as interaction between them. Aminoglycosides are well known to cause an increased probability of nephrotoxicity, indexed to exposure [26]. In Fig. 13.13, the relationship between the probability of nephrotoxicity and aminoglycoside exposure indexed to nephrotoxicity is displayed. It is also important to note that administering the drug on a daily basis ameliorates the likelihood of toxicity when compared to multiple exposures per day of the same total dose (ie, smaller doses more frequently).

Another example is seen with vancomycin administration as a single agent resulting in a higher likelihood of nephrotoxicity [27]. In this evaluation, the probability of vancomycin-driven nephrotoxicity is linked to trough concentrations. There is a significant effect on the probability of nephrotoxicity if the patient is sick enough to be in an ICU (ie, two different logistic regression functions for patients within the ICU and those treated elsewhere). The current recommendation to obtain vancomycin trough concentrations of 15–20 mg/L will drive probabilities of seeing a nephrotoxic event to the 20–30% range.

Furthermore, administering vancomycin and an aminoglycoside together do interact to raise the likelihood of a nephrotoxic episode (see [25] and Fig. 13.13).

Consequently, combinations should be chosen carefully, especially when one or the other of the agents in the combination is known to have clear exposure-related toxicity (Fig. 13.14).

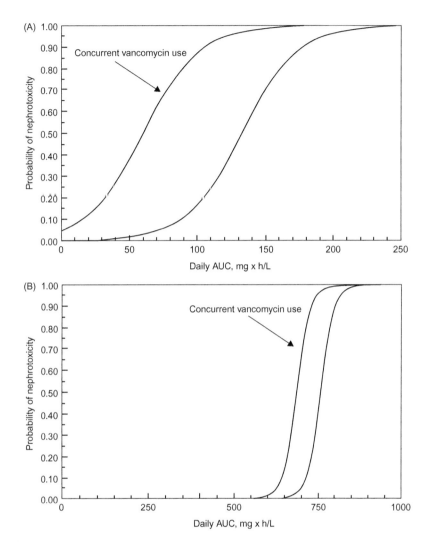

FIGURE 13.13

(A) Logistic regression function for the probability of aminoglycoside nephrotoxicity in patients receiving the drug as half dose every 12 h, either with or without vancomycin. (B) Logistic regression function for the probability of aminoglycoside nephrotoxicity in patients receiving the drug as a single daily dose, either with or without concurrent vancomycin use.

After Rybak MJ, Abate BJ, Kang SL, Ruffing MJ, Lerner SA, Drusano GL. Prospective evaluation of the effect of an aminoglycoside dosing regimen on rates of observed nephrotoxicity and ototoxicity. Antimicrob Agents Chemother 1999;43:1549–55.

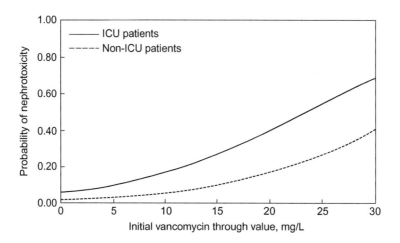

FIGURE 13.14

Logistic regression function for probability of occurrence of nephrotoxicity of patients receiving vancomycin either in the ICU or in non-ICU patients as a function of measured trough concentration.

See Lodise TP, Patel N, Lomaestro B, Rodvold KA, Drusano GL. Relationship between initial vancomycinconcentration-time profile and nephrotoxicity among hospitalized patients. Clin Infect Dis2009;49:507–14

13.7 SUMMARY

Combination chemotherapy for serious infections can provide significant benefits, both for empirical therapy as well as when therapy is definitive. The drawbacks to combination therapy are clear. It is necessary to stress that not all combinations of agents for therapy of serious infections are equally likely to provide benefits that make the drawbacks acceptable (risk/benefit ratio). It is best to use combinations in seriously infected patients and to use combinations that are likely to result in synergistic or additive interaction with regard to bacterial cell kill. Resistance suppression is a major plus for combination therapy (see therapy for tuberculosis). Finally, the ability to decrease protein toxin elaboration or resistance mechanisms such as β-lactamases provides a clear benefit when one of the agents is a protein synthesis inhibitor. Clinicians need to exercise appropriate judgment about starting combination therapy to obtain maximal benefits and to pull back as information about the infection becomes available. In this way, optimal benefit will accrue to the seriously infected patient.

REFERENCES

[1] Alvarez-Lerma F. Modification of empiric antibiotic treatment in patients with pneumonia acquired in the intensive care unit. ICU-Acquired Pneumonia Study. Intensive Care Med 1996;22:387–94.
[2] Drusano GL, Fregeau C, Liu W, Brown DL, Louie A. Impact of burden on granulocyte clearance of bacteria in a mouse thigh infection model. Antimicrob Agents Chemother 2010;54:4368–72.

[3] Drusano GL, Vanscoy B, Liu W, Fikes S, Brown D, Louie A. Saturability of granulocyte kill of *Pseudomonas aeruginosa* in a Murine model of pneumonia. Antimicrob Agents Chemother 2011;55: 2693—5.

[4] Drusano GL, Liu W, Fikes S, Cirz R, Robbins N, Kurhanewicz S, et al. Interaction of drug- and granulocyte-mediated killing of *Pseudomonas aeruginosa* in a murine pneumonia model. J Infect Dis 2014;210:1319—24.

[5] Zaccard CR, Schell RF, Spiegel CA. Efficacy of bilateral bronchoalveolar lavage for diagnosis of ventilator-associated pneumonia. J Clin Microbiol 2009;47:2918—24.

[6] Drusano GL, Lodise TP, Melnick D, Liu W, Oliver A, Mena A, et al. Meropenem penetration into epithelial lining fluid in mice and men and delineation of exposure targets. Antimicrob Agents Chemother 2011;55:3406—12.

[7] Luna CM, Aruj P, Niederman MS, Garzón J, Violi D, Prignoni A, Grupo Argentino de Estudio de la Neumonía Asociada al Respirador group, et al. Appropriateness and delay to initiate therapy in ventilator-associated pneumonia. Eur Respir J 2006;27:158—64.

[8] Kollef KE, Schramm GE, Wills AR, Reichley RM, Micek ST, Kollef MH. Predictors of 30-day mortality and hospital costs in patients with ventilator-associated pneumonia attributed to potentially antibiotic-resistant gram-negative bacteria. Chest 2008;134:281—7.

[9] Greco WR, Bravo G, Parsons JC. The search for synergy: a critical review from a response surface perspective. Pharmacol Rev 1995;47:331—85.

[10] Drusano GL, Neely M, Van Guilder M, Schumitzky A, Brown D, Fikes S, et al. Analysis of combination drug therapy to develop regimens with shortened duration of treatment for tuberculosis. PLoS One 2014;9(7):e101311.

[11] Louie A, Grasso C, Bahniuk N, Van Scoy B, Brown DL, Kulawy R, et al. The combination of meropenem and levofloxacin is synergistic with respect to both *Pseudomonas aeruginosa* kill rate and resistance suppression. Antimicrob Agents Chemother 2010;54:2646—54.

[12] Louie A, Liu W, VanGuilder M, Neely MN, Schumitzky A, Jelliffe R, et al. Meropenem plus levofloxacin is synergistic for the therapy of *Pseudomonas aeruginosa* as tested in a murine model of pneumonia. J Infect Dis 2015;211:1326—33.

[13] Docobo-Pérez F, Drusano GL, Johnson A, Goodwin J, Whalley S, Ramos-Martín V, et al. Pharmacodynamics of fosfomycin: insights into clinical use for antimicrobial resistance. Antimicrob Agents Chemother 2015 e-pub ahead of print.

[14] Medical Research Council. Streptomycin treatment of pulmonary tuberculosis. BMJ 1948;2:769—82.

[15] Selkon JB, Devadatta S, Kullarna KG, Mitchison DA, Narayana AS, et al. The emergence of isoniazid-resistant cultures in patients with pulmonary tuberculosis during treatment with isoniazid alone or isoniazid plus PAS. Bull World Health Organ 1964;31:273—94.

[16] Drusano GL, Liu W, Fregeau C, Kulawy R, Louie A. Differing effect of combination chemotherapy with meropenem and tobramycin on cell kill and suppression of resistance on wild-type *Pseudomonas aeruginosa* PA01 and its isogenic MexAB efflux pump over-expressed mutant. Antimicrob Agents Chemother 2009;53:2266—73.

[17] Pichereau S, Pantrangi M, Couet W, Badiou C, Lina G, Shukla SK, et al. Simulated antibiotic exposures in an in vitro hollow-fiber infection model influence toxin gene expression and production in community-associated methicillin-resistant *Staphylococcus aureus* strain MW2. Antimicrob Agents Chemother 2012;56:140—7.

[18] Louie A, Vanscoy BD, Heine III HS, Liu W, Abshire T, Holman K, et al. Differential effect of linezolid and ciprofloxacin on toxin production by *Bacillus anthracis* in an in vitro pharmacodynamic system. Antimicrob Agents Chemother 2012;56:513—17.

[19] Hendricks KA, Wright ME, Shadomy SV, The Workgroup on Anthrax Clinical Guidelines. Centers for disease control and prevention expert panel meetings on prevention and treatment of anthrax in adults. Emerg Infect Dis 2014;20(2):e130687.

[20] Drusano GL, Bonomo RA, Bahniuk N, Bulitta JB, van Scoy B, Defiglio H, et al. Resistance emergence mechanism and mechanism of resistance suppression by tobramycin for cefepime for *Pseudomonas aeruginosa*. Antimicrob Agents Chemother 2012;56:231−42.

[21] Drusano GL, Sgambati N, Eichas A, Brown DL, Kulawy R, Louie A. The combination of rifampin plus moxifloxacin is synergistic for resistance suppression, but is antagonistic for cell kill for *Mycobacterium tuberculosis* as determined in a hollow fiber infection model. mBio 2010;1(3):e00139−10.

[22] Balasubramanian V, Solapure S, Gaonkar S, Mahesh Kumar KN, Shandil RK, Deshpande A, et al. Effect of co-administration of moxifloxacin and rifampin on *Mycobacterium tuberculosis* in a murine aerosol infection model. Antimicrob Agents Chemother 2012;56:3054−7.

[23] Paul M, Lador A, Grozinsky-Glasberg S, Leibovici L. Beta lactam antibiotic monotherapy versus beta lactam-aminoglycoside antibiotic combination therapy for sepsis. Cochrane Database Syst Rev 2014;1: CD003344. Available from: http://dx.doi.org/10.1002/14651858.CD003344.pub3.

[24] Kumar A, Safdar N, Kethireddy S, Chateau D. A survival benefit of combination antibiotic therapy for serious infections associated with sepsis and septic shock is contingent only on the risk of death: a meta-analytic/meta-regression study. Crit Care Med 2010;38(8):1651−64.

[25] Rybak MJ, Abate BJ, Kang SL, Ruffing MJ, Lerner SA, Drusano GL. Prospective evaluation of the effect of an aminoglycoside dosing regimen on rates of observed nephrotoxicity and ototoxicity. Antimicrob Agents Chemother 1999;43:1549−55.

[26] Drusano GL, Ambrose PG, Bhavnani SM, Bertino JS, Nafziger AN, Louie A. Back to the future: using aminoglycosides again and how to dose them optimally. Clin Infect Dis 2007;45:753−60.

[27] Lodise TP, Patel N, Lomaestro B, Rodvold KA, Drusano GL. Relationship between initial vancomycin concentration-time profile and nephrotoxicity among hospitalized patients. Clin Infect Dis 2009;49:507−14.

CONTROLLING ANTIRETROVIRAL THERAPY IN CHILDREN AND ADOLESCENTS WITH HIV INFECTION

14

M. Neely and N.Y. Rakhmanina

CHAPTER OUTLINE

14.1 INTRODUCTION

Global efforts in the prevention of mother-to-child transmission of HIV have paid off with significant (60%) reduction of new infections among children in 2013, from a peak of 580,000 new pediatric HIV cases recorded in 2001, according to the Joint United Nations Programme on HIV/AIDS (UNAIDS) 2013 Report on the Global AIDS Epidemic (http://www.unaids.org/en/resources/campaigns/globalreport2013/). Despite this progress, according to the World Health Organization (WHO), as of the end of 2014, there were 2.6 million children under 15 years of age living with

Individualized Drug Therapy for Patients. DOI: http://dx.doi.org/10.1016/B978-0-12-803348-7.00014-9

HIV worldwide. There were approximately 220,000 new pediatric infections that year, and 150,000 deaths from AIDS among children (http://www.who.int/hiv/data/en). Adolescents (10−19 years of age) are disproportionally affected by the epidemic, and they are the single age cohort that is increasingly infected. Among 2.1 million adolescents living with HIV worldwide, young girls of Sub-Saharan Africa have the highest incidence of new infections. Most dramatically, AIDS-related deaths among adolescents increased by 50% between 2005 and 2012, while overall AIDS-related deaths decreased by 30%. As of 2013, AIDS has become the second leading cause of death for adolescents globally and the leading cause of death among adolescents aged 10−19 years in Africa.

In countries that have the resources and infrastructure to ensure consistent access to antiretroviral therapy (ART), the trajectory of the perinatally acquired epidemic has been dramatically altered. In the United States, the Centers for Disease Control and Prevention estimated just 162 new perinatal infections in 2010 among children under 15 years of age (http://www.cdc.gov/hiv/pdf/risk_WIC.pdf). However, similar to the worldwide trend, the epidemic continues to disproportionally affect adolescents and youth aged 13 to 24 years, who accounted for an estimated 26% of all new HIV infections in the United States in 2010 (http://www.cdc.gov/hiv/group/age/youth/index.html).

Despite the low burden of HIV infection in developed countries relative to the developing world, the most treatment-experienced children and adolescents presently reside and obtain care in regions of the world such as the United States and Europe [1,2]. Although the number of infected patients receiving ART worldwide has skyrocketed from 1% in 2000 to 40% in 2014, the proportion of children <15 years of age receiving ART worldwide has been static around one-third [3]. In 16 high-burden countries in sub-Saharan Africa most hit by the HIV epidemic, fewer than 10% of children living with HIV received ART in 2013, according to the United Nations. However, with the increasing availability of ART worldwide and following a renewed global call for increased ART coverage in children, the number of treatment-experienced children is expected to sharply rise globally. For these young patients, there is and will be a chronic and pressing need to dose antiretroviral drugs (ARVs) optimally.

There are seven therapeutic classes of 39 unique or combination ARV medications currently marketed as therapy for HIV infection (Table 14.1), and 25 (76%) are licensed in the United States for use in children under 16 years of age. Table 14.1 also includes common abbreviation(s) for each drug, used throughout this review. The US Department of Health and Human Services (DHHS) HIV treatment guidelines from the United States [4] and guidelines from Europe [5] on the use of these ARVs in children and adolescents endorse the role for dose optimization through therapeutic drug monitoring (TDM) or therapeutic drug management in selected patients, as we prefer to define it. Both guidelines cite a lack of evidence to clearly define in whom and when TDM should be considered, how to practice it, and what benefit might be expected. Nonetheless, these and other barriers notwithstanding, the guidelines present the justification for TDM in children and adolescents, including limited published pediatric ARV PK data relative to adults, multiple drug-drug and drug-food interactions, a narrow margin between therapeutic and toxic concentrations, severe consequences for underdosing (ie, development of ARV resistance), a high degree of interindividual PK variability, and limited knowledge about long-term consequences of pediatric ART. Most importantly, there are extensive pathophysiologic changes with pharmacologic impact that occur as a HIV-infected child matures from infancy to adulthood, and this process does not occur with precisely predictable timing or magnitude on an individual scale [6−8]. Dosing of ARVs in pediatric patients depends on chronological age and/or body parameters (eg, height, weight) and requires frequent reassessment particularly during

Table 14.1 Currently Available ARVs With Generic, Trade, and Abbreviated Names, and the Lower Age of FDA Licensure Obtained From Package Inserts

Drug	Lower Age Limit for Licensed Prescribing in the United States
Nucleoside reverse transcriptase inhibitors (NRTIs)	
Abacavir (Ziagen, ABC)	3 months
Didanosine (Videx, Videx EC, ddI)	2 weeks
Emtricitabine (Emtriva, FTC)	Birth
Lamivudine (Epivir, 3TC)	Birth
Stavudine (Zerit, d4T)	Birth
Tenofovir (TFV) disoproxil fumarate (Viread, TDF)	2 years
Zidovudine (Retrovir, ZDV)	Birth
Nonnucleoside reverse transcriptase inhibitors (NNRTIs)	
Efavirenz (Sustiva, EFV)	3 years
Etravirine (Intelence, ETV)	6 years
Nevirapine (Viramune, NVP)	1 month
Rilpivirine (Edurant, RPV)	12 years
Protease inhibitors (PIs)	
Atazanavir (Reyataz, ATV)	3 months
Darunavir (Prezista, DRV)	3 years
Fosamprenavir (Lexiva, FPV)	6 months
Indinavir (Crixivan, IDV)	18 years
Lopinavir/ritonavir (Kaletra, LPV/RTV)	14 days
Nelfinavir (Viracept, NFV)	2 years
Saquinavir (Invirase, SQV)	18 years
Tipranavir (Aptivus, TPV)	2 years
Entry and fusion inhibitors	
Enfuvirtide (Fuzeon, T-20)	6 years
Maraviroc (Selzentry, MVC)	16 years
Integrase inhibitors	
Dolutegravir (Tivicay, DTG)	12 years and $\geq 40\,kg$
Elvitegravir (Vitekta, EVG)	18 years
Raltegravir (Isentress, RAL)	4 weeks
Pharmacokinetic enhancers	
Cobicistat (Tybost, COBI)	18 years
Ritonavir (Norvir, RTV)	Only as an enhancer, starting at 2 weeks of age as LPV/RTV

(Continued)

Table 14.1 Currently Available ARVs With Generic, Trade, and Abbreviated Names, and the Lower Age of FDA Licensure Obtained From Package Inserts *Continued*

Drug	Lower Age Limit for Licensed Prescribing in the United States
Fixed-dose combinations	
Abacavir + Lamivudine (Epzicom)	16 years
Abacavir + Lamivudine + Zidovudine (Trizivir)	variable (>40 kg)
Atazanavir + Cobicistat (Evotaz)	18 years
Darunavir + Cobicistat (Prezcobix)	18 years
Tenfovir TF + Emtricitabine (Truvada)	12 years and weight ≥35 kg
Tenofovir TF + Emtricitabine + Efavirenz (Atripla)	12 years and weight ≥40 kg
Tenofovir DF + Emtricitabine + Rilpivirine (Complera)	18 years
Tenofovir + Emtricitabine + Elvitegravir + Cobicistat (Stribild)	18 years
Tenofovir AF + Emtricitabine + Elvitegravir + Cobicistat (Genvoya)	12 years
Zidovudine + Lamivudine (Combivir)	12 years

Clinical trials are ongoing for the use of elvitegravir, dolutegravir, rilpivirine, and the related FDCs in children <12 years and of darunavir/cobicistat + atazanavir/cobicistat in adolescents <18 years of age.

fast growth at a younger age. Developmental differences in drug absorption, distribution, metabolism, and elimination contribute to high variability and increased risk for suboptimal exposure. The developmental changes occur also in the immunologic system of the child, while the virus evolves, relocates within the reservoirs, and adapts to the new ART exposures. All of these factors mandate rational consideration of ART in every child with strong consideration for using pharmacokinetic (PK) and pharmacodynamic (PD) evaluation for optimal dosing.

In 2011, we published a comprehensive review of ART PK, PD, and pharmacogenomics with respect to both efficacy and toxicity in children [9]. In the present chapter we update this work and focus on a more detailed explanation of illustrative cases where we have used pharmacometric principles to individualize therapy.

14.2 PHARMACOKINETICS (PK)

The study of PK is an attempt to describe the relationship between dose, drug concentration, and time. Concentration is typically measured in the blood, plasma or serum, but may include any other bodily fluid. DHHS guidelines [4] summarize currently available ARV formulations, pharmacokinetics, dosing adjustments for renal and hepatic failure, drug-drug interactions, and major toxicities. In the absence of a defined limited sampling strategy based on rigorously estimated optimal times calculated from pharmacokinetic data, our general approach to sampling, which we have employed in the clinical care of our patients, is the following. A predose sample establishes the baseline, and comparison of this to a predicted postdose sample at the same reported time interval after a dose establishes the likelihood of steady state and provides some estimate of patient adherence. The second sample is around the time of the expected peak concentration. The third sample is generally 2−3 h after the expected peak, to establish some estimate of the elimination or clearance of the drug, enabling predictions of subsequent concentrations at any time point, including a trough. Since many ARVs are adequately described by single-compartment models (see Table 14.2), this sampling scheme will provide rough approximations of key exposure indices (trough or AUC) linked to efficacy or toxicity. Later in this chapter, in the section on TDM, we discuss how a population approach and multiple model (MM) Bayesian adaptive control can be used as a more powerful approach.

Although package inserts and the PK studies included in the DHHS tables describe variability in ARV concentrations or PK parameters such as clearance, typically derived from noncompartmental analytic techniques, variability within and between individuals is not distinguished. This overestimates the true magnitude of between-individual PK parameter variability and can obscure the influence of factors such as age on individual parameter values. In contrast, population PK techniques estimate distributions of PK parameter values globally across the entire study population as well as for the individual subjects within the population, and more accurately partition sources of variability. There are several other advantages to population analyses that are relevant to children. Strict adherence to a sampling schedule is not required. Population and individual parameter values may be estimated with sparse data, even single samples, although accuracy, precision, and predictive power of population PK models will suffer with increasingly sparse data. Perhaps most importantly, population analysis offers a formal method to incorporate what is known about the PK of a drug, eg, in adults, so that estimation of pediatric PK does not begin from a zero-knowledge state. Lastly, because population models are distributions of parameter estimates, they may be used to predict PK parameter values, with measures of statistical regression, and thus ARV concentrations in children who were not part of the study population. This is discussed further in the section on TDM. To our knowledge, other than our older reference [9], there is no published summary of population ARV PK analyses in children. In Table 14.2, we update our summary of pediatric ARV population PK studies.

All population PK models in children include some influence of maturation, because it is well known that significant physiologic changes associated with growth from infancy to adulthood affect the PK behavior of drugs [6,40−43]. Drug clearance, which relates dose to average steady-state concentration, when adjusted for body weight or surface area, appears to increase rapidly through early childhood, reaching values that are higher than those of adults, and which do not subside until late adolescence [44]. Drug clearance can be somewhat normalized for body size across all ages by allometric scaling (eg, $(weight/70)^{0.75}$ where weight is in kilograms) [45], but since drug doses are nonetheless commonly dispensed in milligrams per kilogram, pediatric doses in general are higher than adult doses when adjusted for weight. The maturation process does not proceed at a regular and predictable pace in all individuals, which contributes to PK variability in a manner that is unique to children.

Comparisons between studies in Table 14.2 can be difficult as each model is slightly different. The table includes our own interpretation of the major findings in many studies. Several important trends can be distinguished from Table 14.2 about the PK of ARV in children. First, the disposition of many of the ARV can be described by single-compartment models with first-order elimination or clearance. This implies that in general, concentrations in the blood will be proportional to the dose, eg, doubling the dose doubles the blood concentration. This is not strictly true, since

Table 14.2 Summary of ARV Population PK Studies in Children

Drug	Patients	Dose	Model Summary	Intersubject Variability	Covariates	Notes
NRTI						
Abacavir [10]	$N = 25$ Mean 13.2 years (SD 3.1)	8 mg/kg orally × 1 dose	One compartment with zero-order absorption and first-order clearance	Clearance 63% Volume 52%	None	
Abacavir [11]	$N = 105$ Mean 8.8 years (SD 3.9)	Mean 8.2 mg/ kg twice daily	One compartment with first-order absorption and clearance	Clearance 6% Volume 8% *Exponential model, values are at population means	None	
Abacavir [12]	$N = 69$ Median 5.6 years (0.4–12.8)	16 mg/kg daily (divided once or twice)	Two compartments with first-order absorption and clearance	Clearance 22% Volume 48%	None	
Didanosine [13]	$N = 49$ Median 6.5 years (range 2.5–14.0)	240 mg/m² once daily	One compartment with first-order absorption and clearance	Clearance 127% Volume 83%	None	
Lamivudine [14]	$N = 99$ Median 56 days (range 3–757)	2–4 mg/kg twice daily	One compartment with first-order absorption and clearance	Clearance 34% Volume 31%	⬆︎⬆︎ Age = Clearance	An increased dose in mg/kg is required in older infants
Lamivudine [15]	$N = 580$ Median 7.4 years (range 2 days–18 years)	Mean 7.5 mg/kg/day	Two compartments with first-order absorption and clearance	Clearance 6% Volume 9%	⬆︎⬆︎ Age = Clearance in the first year of life	
Lamivudine [16]	$N = 77$ Median 5.7 years (range 0.4–12.8)	Various	One compartment with first-order, delayed absorption and clearance	Clearance 26% Volume 19% Absorption 66%		
Stavudine [17]	$N = 272$ Median 8.2 years (range 3 days–16 years)	1 mg/kg twice daily	One compartment with zero-order absorption and first-order clearance	Clearance 38% Volume 32%	⬆︎⬆︎ Age = Clearance ⬆︎⬆︎ Age = Volume *In this model, volume and clearance were not adjusted for weight	Adult values for clearance and volume were reached by about 15 years of age
Tenofovir [18]	$N = 93$ Median 14 years (range 5–18)	150–300 mg once daily	Two compartments with first-order absorption and first-order clearance	Clearance 7% Volume 14%	Lopinavir = ⬇︎ Clearance	

Drug [ref]	N / Age	Dosing	Model	Variability	Covariate relationships	Comments
Zidovudine [19]	N = 38 Mean 29.7 weeks (SD 3.0)	<2 weeks: 1.5 mg/kg q12 hours intravenously or orally >2 weeks: 2 mg/kg q8 hours intravenously or orally	One compartment with first-order absorption and clearance	Clearance 33% Clearance maturation 83% Volume 13% Bioavailability 22%	↑Postnatal Age = ↑Clearance Gestational Age >30 weeks = ↑Clearance Furosemide = ↑Clearance ↑Serum Creatinine = ↓Clearance	Increasing dose with postnatal age Preterm infants at greater risk for higher concentrations and potential toxicity Reduced dose with severe renal failure (50% of standard dose)
Zidovudine [20]	N = 83 Mean 19.3 days (SD 27.9)	Various (numerous studies)	Two compartments with first-order absorption, elimination and intercompartmental transfer	Volume 23% Elimination 25%	↑Postnatal Age = ↑Elimination Gestational Age >35 weeks = ↑Elimination	Increasing dose with postnatal age. Preterm infants at greater risk for higher concentrations and potential toxicity
Zidovudine [21]	N = 394 Mean 45.2 months (SD 45)	180 mg/m^2 q6 hours	One compartment with first-order absorption and clearance	Clearance 31% Volume 28% Bioavailability 35%	↑AST = ↓Clearance +ddI = ↓Clearance >2 years = ↑Clearance	May need dose reductions for hepatotoxicity but no definitive recommendation. Coadministration with ddI may lower concentrations, but not significantly, and is not contraindicated
Zidovudine [22]	N = 247 Median 10.8 years (0.15–18)	36–600 mg/day	One compartment with first-order absorption and clearance	Clearance 18% Volume 23%		
Zidovudine-triphosphate [23]	N = 27 Median 19.7 years (range 17–24)	600 mg (zidovudine) once daily	One compartment with first-order elimination	40-fold in predose Zidovudine-Triphosphate	None	Plasma zidovudine is not a good predictor of intracellular zidovudine-triphosphate
NNRTI						
Efavirenz [24]	N = 48 Median 6.4 years (range 2.8–14.7)	Weight band dosing (See Table 14.3)	One compartment with first-order absorption and clearance	Clearance 61%	↑Age = ↓Clearance	Dose in mg/kg decreases with age
Efavirenz [25]	N = 36 Median 6.5 years (range 0.9–19)	Weight band dosing (See Table 14.3)	One compartment with two-phase transitional absorption and first-order clearance	Mean absorption time 54% Clearance 52% Volume 40%	CYP2B6 516 G>T = ↓Clearance Liquid (vs capsule) = ↓Bioavailability	In simulation studies, children with CYP2B6 GG genotype had 50–70% chance of subtherapeutic EFV trough with standard dosing

(Continued)

Table 14.2 Summary of ARV Population PK Studies in Children *Continued*

Drug	Patients	Dose	Model Summary	Intersubject Variability	Covariates	Notes
Nevirapine (Benaboud: 2011 kg)	$N = 30$ Gestational age median 39 weeks (range 33–42)	200 mg to mother	One compartment with first-order absorption and clearance	Clearance 28% Volume 17%		
Nevirapine [26]	$N = 639$ Median 6.5 years (range 0.1–19.5)	150–200 mg/m² twice daily	One compartment with first-order absorption and clearance	Clearance 48% Volume 28%		
Nevirapine [27]	$N = 94$ Median 12.5 months (range 0–93)	100 (21–200 mg) twice daily	One compartment with first-order absorption and clearance	Clearance 10%		
PI						
Atazanavir [28]	$N = 51$ Median 14 years (range 3–18)	300 (100–400) with RTV or 400 (150–600) without RTV	One compartment with first-order absorption and clearance	Clearance 34%	+ RTV = → Clearance	
Fosamprenavir [29]	$N = 137$ Median 10 years (range 0.7–18)	Various	Two compartments with first-order absorption and clearance	Clearance 30% Volume 66%	+RTV = → Clearance Age = ↗ Clearance	Dose in mg/kg decreases with age or with RTV
Fosamprenavir [30]	$N = 212$ Median 6 years (range 0.17–18)	Various	Two compartments with first-order absorption and clearance	Clearance 45% Volume 50%	+RTV, Black race = → Clearance Age = ↗ Clearance	Dose in mg/kg decreases with age or with RTV
Lopinavir [31]	$N = 18$ Median 3.4 months (range 1.6–5.9)	LPV 300 mg/m² bid plus RTV 75 mg/m² bid	One compartment with first-order absorption and clearance	Absorption 178% Clearance 60% Volume 67%		
Lopinavir [32]	$N = 52$ Median 11 years (range 5.3–17.5)	Median 275 mg/m² twice daily	One compartment with first-order absorption (after a delay) and elimination	Absorption 168% Absorption delay 104% Elimination 87% Volume 39%	Age = ↔ Volume	Dose in mg/kg decreases with age
Lopinavir [33]	$N = 157$ Mean 9.1 years (SD 4.8)	Mean 288 mg/m² twice daily	One compartment with first-order absorption fixed equal to elimination	Clearance 31% Volume 44%	Male = ↖ Clearance if age >12 years +Nevirapine = ↖ Clearance	Dose needs to be increased with concomitant nevirapine (see Table 14.3) and adolescent boys may be at greater risk for subtherapeutic concentrations

Drug [ref]	Population	Dose	PK model	Covariate magnitude	Covariate influence	Notes
Lopinavir [34]	N = 96 Median 2 weeks (1 day–102 weeks)	Mean 39 mg/kg 2–3 times daily	One compartment with first-order absorption fixed equal to elimination	Clearance 46% Volume 45%	↑ Age = ↑ Clearance	
Nelfinavir [35]	N = 38 Median 5.3 years (range 0.1–17.9)	30 mg/kg three times daily, or 45 mg/kg twice daily	One compartment with zero-order absorption and first-order clearance	Clearance 26% Volume 26%		
Nelfinavir [36]	N = 182 Median 8.2 years (range 3 days–17 years)	Dose in mg/kg not reported	One compartment with first-order absorption and clearance	Clearance 39% Volume 109%	← Age = ↓ Clearance ←→ Age = Volume	Dose in mg/kg decreases with age
Tipranavir [37]	N = 52 Median NR (range 2–16)	TPV 290–417 mg/m² bid plus RTV 115–167 mg/m²	One compartment with first-order absorption and clearance	Absorption 54% Clearance 53% Volume 13%	→ Age = Volume ←→ Age = Volume	Dose in mg/kg decreases with age
Entry inhibitors						
Enfuvirtide [38]	N = 43 Median 11 years (range 5–16)	2 mg/kg subcutaneously twice daily (maximum 90 mg)	One compartment with first-order absorption and clearance	Absorption 28% Clearance 36% Volume 30%	None	
Integrase inhibitors						
Raltegravir [39]	N = 65 Median NR (range 4 weeks–18 years)	6 mg/kg (granules) for <2 years and (chewable) for 2–12 years; 400 mg film-coated tablet for >12 years	Two compartments with first-order absorption and clearance	Absorption 32% Clearance 34% Volume 108%		

Notes: Except where noted, clearance and volume increase with body size in all models; thus the absolute dose in mg for all ARVs increases with growth. Reported covariate influences are in addition to those of size. First-order absorption, elimination, or clearance indicates a constant fraction of drug per unit of time; zero-order is a constant amount of drug per unit of time. "Absorption" refers to the rate of appearance of drug within the bloodstream, while bioavailability is the extent of drug that reaches the bloodstream and cannot be estimated from oral-only dosing. Significant covariates are in addition to some measure of size—eg, weight, allometric weight, or body surface area, which are a component of any pediatric population PK model.

absorption characteristics and bioavailability may limit the rate and extent of drug transfer from the intestine to blood; however, clinicians will not run the risk of increased drug concentrations disproportionate to small increases in dose, as can be seen for so-called Michaelis-Menten drugs like the antifungal drug voriconazole [46,47].

Secondly, as seen in Table 14.2, intersubject variability of PK parameters can be more than 100%, but in general is approximately 40%. However, most of these studies were not designed to truly assess day-to-day (interoccasion) variability within the same patient, which increases the range of measured drug concentrations in a population [48,49].

14.3 PHARMACODYNAMICS (PD)

Pharmacodynamics (PD) quantifies the relationship between drug concentration and clinical endpoints or effects, desired and otherwise. Although the ultimate goal of ARV therapy is good health, the primary outcomes are typically surrogate markers that include the HIV RNA measured in copies/mL and/or $\log_{10}$ change in viral load, and $CD4^+$ cell count measured as absolute count and percentage of $CD4^+$ lymphocytes. The proximate goal of ART is to reach and sustain peripheral blood viral load below the detection threshold (usually <20 viral copies/mL blood) and to assure retention or full restoration (in case of baseline immune deficiency) of the $CD4^+$ cell count. Immunologic markers ($CD4^+$ cell count) have been most closely tied to predictions of opportunistic infections and survival [50,51], and virologic surrogates have been tied most closely to defining ART adherence and success [4].

The virologic and immunologic surrogates are measured typically closely at the initiation of ART and are monitored at 12−24 weekly intervals thereafter. Therefore, several strategies have been proposed to predict outcomes of ART before or right at the first dose, including target therapeutic concentrations. Because all ARV drugs except MVC have viral rather than human molecular targets, a major assumption for pediatric ART has been that ARV PK-PD behavior would be the same in children as it is in adults. In other words, assuming the retroviral population were identical in a child and an adult, then the antiviral effect should be the same for a given drug concentration. Indeed, all ARV PK studies in children have been designed to find the dose that is associated with exposures (eg, C_{max}, AUC, and especially C_{min}) similar to those already known to be safe and effective in adults. For the simple reason that there are fewer infected children than adults in need of ART, the vast majority of HIV therapeutic studies in children take advantage of this assumption and therefore are small Phase II or Phase IIb designs, rather than large Phase III trials. The following sections review the literature on the relationships between ARVs concentrations, efficacy, and toxicity in children and adolescents. Table 14.3 summarizes this information in the form of suggested pharmacologic efficacy targets, which are taken from the DHHS guidelines [4].

14.3.1 DRUG EXPOSURE AND EFFICACY

14.3.1.1 Nucleoside Reverse Transcriptase Inhibitors (NRTIs)

Since nucleoside reverse transcriptase inhibitors (NRTIs) are active as intracellular triphosphate metabolites, the relationship between plasma drug concentrations and virologic and immunological

Table 14.3 Suggested Therapeutic Drug Trough Concentration or AUC Targets for Children

Drug	Target C_{min} (ng/mL)	Notes
NNRTI		
Efavirenz	1000	
Etravirine	275 (81−2980)	No efficacy target established; value is median (range) from clinical studies
Nevirapine	3000	
PI		
Atazanavir	150	
Darunavir	3300 (1233−7368)	No efficacy target established; value is median (range) from clinical studies in adults given 600 mg twice daily
Fosamprenavir	400	Measured as amprenavir
Lopinavir	1000	
Nelfinavir	800	Parent plus M8 active metabolite
Tipranavir	20,500	Not suggested for PI-naïve patients
Entry inhibitor		
Maraviroc	50	Not suggested for treatment-naïve patients
Integrase strand inhibitor		
Raltegravir	72 (29−118)	No efficacy target established; value is median (range) from clinical studies in adults given 600 mg twice daily

Concentration targets are from DHHS pediatric treatment guidelines [4].

outcomes is not well correlated, and no new pediatric data are available since our previous summary [9]. There are no currently recommended NRTI target concentrations in the treatment guidelines [4].

14.3.1.2 Nonnucleoside Reverse Transcriptase Inhibitors (NNRTIs)

Measurement of EFV plasma concentrations in combination with pharmacogenetic evaluation for the polymorphism of the main drug-metabolizing enzyme cytochrome P (CYP) 450 2B6 continues to be recommended in the US pediatric HIV treatment guidelines for children aged <3 years to avoid suboptimal drug exposure [4].

For NVP, pediatric PK modeling has suggested that the current WHO-recommended NVP dosing in young children who are <10 kg should be increased from 50 mg bid (3−6 kg) and 75 mg (6−10 kg) to 75 mg and 100 mg, respectively, to achieve steady plasma trough concentrations >3000 ng/mL and prevent the development of viral resistance and treatment failure [27].

Plasma efficacy concentrations have not been established for second generation nonnucleoside reverse transcriptase inhibitors (NNRTIs) ETR and RPV to date, and for those drugs, the available therapeutic targets include trough plasma concentrations from the population average C_{min} from the product labels approved by the Food and Drug Administration (FDA) (http://www.dailymed.com).

14.3.1.3 Protease Inhibitors (PIs)

Pediatric ATV PK and PD data are available from the PACTG 1020 A study, which was a phase I/II trial of ATV with and without RTV in pediatric patients aged 3 months to 19 years of age [52]. The study design employed ATV plasma target concentration (AUC of >45 mcg $\times$ h/mL) monitoring to guide therapy and to establish optimum starting doses in treatment-naïve and -experienced children. To achieve the AUC target, dosing without RTV resulted in a very high C_{max}, particularly in younger children. In the younger age cohort, the median RTV-boosted ATV AUC and C_{min} were 44.7 mcg $\times$ h/mL and 589 ng/mL, and for the older cohort, the median RTV-boosted ATV AUC and C_{min} were 41.4 mcg $\times$ h/L and 885 ng/mL. Overall, at Week 24, 84/139 subjects (60.4%) and at Week 48, 83/142 (58.5%) had HIV RNA ≤ 400 copies/mL. At Week 48, 69.5% of naïve and 43.3% of experienced subjects had HIV RNA ≤ 400 copies/mL. These data suggest that, when given with RTV, an ATV C_{min} of at least 600 ng/mL is adequate in naïve children, while much higher ATV exposure is required for experienced patients.

Plasma efficacy concentrations have not been established for newer PI DRV, and combinations of the novel booster cobicistat with DRV and ATV have not been established to date. For those drugs and combinations, the available therapeutic targets include trough plasma concentrations from the population average C_{min} from the FDA-approved product labels (http://www.dailymed.com).

14.3.1.4 Integrase Strand Inhibitors (INSTIs) and Entry Inhibitors (EI)

There have been several studies of integrase strand inhibitor (INSTI) PK in children published since our last review [9]. RAL PK were studied in the phase I/II International Maternal Child Adolescent AIDS Clinical Trials group (IMPAACT) P1066 study [53]. Dose selection was based on achieving target adult PK parameters similar to geometric mean (GM) area under the curve of $14-25 \mu M \cdot h$ and GM 12-h concentration >33 nM in three age cohorts aged 12 to <19 years, 6 to <12 years, and 2 to <6 years. Additional subjects were enrolled in each age cohort to evaluate long-term efficacy, tolerability, and safety. Ninety-three (97%) subjects completed 24 weeks of treatment with 54% achieving HIV RNA <50 copies/mL with a mean CD4 T lymphocyte (CD4) count (%) increase of 119 cells/mm^3 (3.8%). Ninety-one subjects completed 48 weeks of treatment with 57% achieving HIV RNA <50 copies/mL with a mean CD4 count (%) increase of 156 cells/mm^3 (4.6%).

Interpatient and intrapatient variability for PK of RAL were considerable, especially with the film-coated tablets, dictating different dosing recommendations between the film-coated and chewable tablet formulations. Finally, IMPAACT P1066 also evaluated the PK/PD of RAL suspension in 26 infants and toddlers aged 4 weeks to <2 years who were treatment or prophylaxis experienced. A total of 23 (88%) infants completed 48 weeks of treatment with 44% achieving HIV RNA <50 copies/mL with a mean CD4 count (%) increase of 492 cells/mm^3 (7.8%). PK parameters were similar to those achieved for the older cohorts in IMPAACT P1066.

Dolutegravir (DTG) PK and PD in children are being evaluated in an ongoing IMPAACT P1093 open-label trial of HIV-infected children starting at age 4 weeks. The current FDA approval of dolutegravir dosing starting at 12 years of age is based on data from 23 treatment-experienced, INSTI-naive adolescents and intensive PK evaluations from the first 10 participants [54]. There were 9 patients weighing ≥ 40 kg who received 50 mg, and 1 patient who weighed 37 kg and received a 35 mg dose. Their exposures were comparable to those seen in adults receiving 50 mg once daily. After 9/10 participants achieved HIV RNA concentration <400 copies/mL at Week 4, an additional 13 participants were enrolled, and at 24 weeks and 48 weeks, 70% and 61% of overall cohort had achieved HIV RNA concentration <50 copies/mL, respectively. Currently, children aged ≥6 to <12 years are undergoing PK and longer-term follow-up in P1093. To date, data have demonstrated a favorable safety profile, adequate PK, and virologic efficacy through 48 weeks.

Elvitegravir (EVG) is FDA approved for use in combination with a PI plus ritonavir and as fixed-dose combination with PK enhancer cobicistat (COBI), plus FTC and tenofovir disoproxil fumarate (TDF) for adult use only. An ongoing PK study of the adult dosage formulation of EVG/COBI/FTC/TDF in 14 HIV-infected youth aged 13−17 years (weight 35−80 kg) and 14 pediatric patients aged 6−11 years suggested that EVG PK were similar to those in adults [55,56]. Safety and efficacy data at 48 weeks suggested safety and efficacy similar to that seen in adult trials.

A minimally effective plasma concentration relative to in vitro viral susceptibility has not been established for RAL, DTG, or EVG, and population PK parameters (C_{max}, AUC, and C_{min}) are considered as therapeutic targets for these ARVs.

The PK, safety, and efficacy of the EI maraviroc (MVC) in patients aged <16 years have not been established. A dose-finding and efficacy study is under way in children ages 2 to 17 years [57,58]. In this trial, the MVC dose is based upon body surface area and the presence or absence of a potent CYP3A4 inhibitor in the background regimen. Preliminary PK data are encouraging in those on a potent CYP3A4 inhibitor, but low exposures were seen in those not on a potent CYP3A4 inhibitor. Follow-up with participants in this trial continues. Efficacy trough concentrations for MVC have been derived in adult patients with multiple drug-resistant HIV strains only [4].

14.3.2 DRUG EXPOSURE AND TOXICITY

Very little new information on relationships between ARV PK and toxicity in children is available, and it is summarized by drug class here.

14.3.2.1 NRTIs

Concerns for TDF-associated nephro- and bone toxicity prompted the manufacturer to reformulate tenofovir into a new pro-drug formula, tenofovir alafenamide fumarate (TAF), an investigational NRTI that is undergoing adult and pediatric clinical trials in form of the fixed-dose combination (FDC) of EVG/COBI/FTC/TAF (Genvoya) and has been approved by FDA for adolescents starting age of 12 years in fall of 2016. TAF was designed to circulate systemically as the prodrug and undergo conversion to tenofovir intracellularly, achieving higher active metabolite concentrations in peripheral blood mononuclear cells and lower plasma tenofovir exposures compared to TDF. The 48-week data from studies in adolescents ≥12 and <18 years demonstrate rapid virologic response and high rates of virologic success and good tolerability. The study reported a small observed increase in serum C_r, consistent with known effect of COBI in adults. EVG/COBI/FTC/TAF has demonstrated decreased renal biomarkers of inflammation, similar to that observed in adult phase III adult studies. The adolescent study group had increased median spine bone mineral density at Week 24 (+1.3%) compared with a mean decrease (−0.9%) in EVG/COBI/FTC/TDF group, suggesting reduced bone-associated toxicity of TAF versus TDF [59,60].

14.3.2.2 Other ARVs

There have been no updates on the relationship of the plasma exposure of NRTIs, PIs, EIs, or INSTIs to toxicity in pediatric patients since our prior review [9].

14.4 PHARMACOGENOMICS (PG)

Pharmacogenomics (PG) is the study of the interaction between genetic polymorphisms and drug PK or PD. It is relevant because PG factors may influence initial dose selection in an individual patient. It is important to realize, however, that with good population approaches to optimizing individual therapy, the influence of genotypic polymorphisms diminishes greatly after one starts to measure and use drug concentrations, which are the sum of all genotypic (and other) covariates, measured and unmeasured [61]. There are ranges of phenotypic activity (eg, drug PK disposition) within genotypes such that there can be overlap. For example, a genotypically wild-type individual may nevertheless eliminate a drug at a rate consistent with a "slow" genotype, such as was the case for Patient 2 in the TDM section. There are numerous other nongenetic factors that may influence a drug's disposition, such as clearly demonstrated for ETV [62]. Therefore, knowledge of an altered genotype does not immediately suggest the appropriate dose, which must be determined by TDM, as we describe exactly for Patient 2.

With the exception of screening for HLAB*5701 prior to initiating therapy with ABC and determination of the CYP2B6 genotype in young patients (<3 years of age) initiating EFV therapy, there are no current standard practice recommendations to ascertain patients' PG profiles for other ARVs [4]. Polymorphisms in UGT1A1 have been linked to susceptibility to atazanvir-related increases in bilirubin, but as mentioned these are usually not treatment limiting, and routine screening is not recommended [63].

14.5 ARV THERAPEUTIC DRUG MONITORING/MANAGEMENT (TDM)

TDM is the practice of measuring drug concentrations in a single patient for the purpose of optimizing the dose to maximize the likelihood of achieving desired therapeutic goals and avoiding undesirable concentration-dependent effects. By definition, TDM occurs subsequently to consideration of factors that influence the initial dose selection discussed in the previous Pharmacokinetics section, as a patient must have received one or more doses of the drug. There are several reasons to consider TDM in the setting of ART in children and adults: (1) to confirm appropriate concentrations of drug(s) for the given dose and patient, (2) to ascertain the magnitude of drug-drug interactions, (3) to monitor adherence, and (4) to estimate individual PK/PD parameters for rational dose adjustment if necessary. For this last reason, rather than "therapeutic drug monitoring," we prefer the term "therapeutic drug *management*" to convey a more comprehensive process that includes rational management and adaptive control strategies instead of intuitive reactions to measured drug concentrations.

There are numerous reviews, position papers, and guidelines that endorse TDM of ARVs [4,5,64−66]. All of these suggest children as a target population for ARV TDM, while routine use of ARV TDM in adults is considered of no benefit. Nonetheless, it is recognized that under certain circumstances, such as those listed in the preceding paragraph, TDM can be helpful across both patient cohorts. While studies to describe the relationship between plasma drug concentrations and outcomes in children have been described in the Pharmacodynamics (PD) section, the published ARV TDM experience in children, with active dose management in response to measured drug concentrations, is almost nonexistent. Given the physiologic/maturational differences between children and adults, it is difficult, then, to extrapolate the role of routine TDM in children from studies in adults.

The PK of ARVs are sufficiently variable between patients so that the recommended dose ought to be viewed as approximate, even when adjusted for body weight or surface area. The idea that this dose is optimal for all HIV-infected children in all clinical circumstances is simply false. As discussed in the introduction to the PK section, drug clearance, adjusted for body weight, does not subside to adult levels until adulthood. This means that drug doses, when adjusted for body weight, are also greater in children than in adults. As we have pointed out [67], there is a relative dearth of published ARV PK data in children, and the developmental, physiological, psychological, and social changes during this stage of life argue strongly for TDM.

14.6 **MULTIPLE-MODEL BAYESIAN ADAPTIVE CONTROL: CASE EXAMPLES**

As described in numerous chapters throughout this book, a population PK model is a set of descriptive equations with parameter values (clearance, volume of distribution, etc.). When parameter values are reasonably estimated, concentrations of a drug may be predicted at any time during a dosage regimen in an individual with a set of characteristics (eg, weight or creatinine clearance), the effects of which on drug disposition are accounted for by the model equations. Population PK modeling deals with many of the obstacles associated with therapeutic optimization, even in the outpatient setting. Chiefly, population PK models allow for discrimination between the sources of error between observed (measured) versus predicted drug concentrations; ie, variability between patients, between occasions in a single patient, and "residual" variability due to model misspecifications or environmental factors that also influence drug disposition [68]. Moreover, because models provide information on the PK parameter values in a population of patients, the parameter values of an individual patient who belongs to that population, even if not among the original contributors to the model, can usually be estimated fairly well even with only a single measured drug concentration, although precision and accuracy improve with multiple samples from the individual [69−71].

Once a set of therapeutic drug PK parameter estimates exists for an individual patient, the clinician can predict likely blood concentrations in the patient at any given time after a dose. More importantly, the opportunity arises to *control* the dose in a systematic manner to achieve clinically selected target concentrations with maximum precision, and therefore to better control the patient's expected clinical response [70].

In our clinical practice, a population PK model for each drug to be optimized is first necessary. Because of the costs and difficulties associated with conducting a phase I trial *de novo*, when we do not have such data available, we use simulation to make population PK models from available PK data in the peer-reviewed literature, using different modules within the Pmetrics and BestDose software collection, which were called MM-USCPACK at the time.

Because many ARVs can be described adequately by a one-compartment model (see Table 14.2), our general approach is to obtain or derive mean PK parameter estimates with standard deviations for each drug of interest from published pediatric and adult pharmacokinetic trials for three parameters: absorption rate constant (k_a), volume of distribution (V_d), and clearance (CL). We construct models as needed for patients who are Tanner stage 3 or less (children and adolescents), and one for patients who are Tanner stage 4 or 5 (adults). The Tanner breakpoint is one attempt to differentiate pharmaco-physiologic children from adults, adapted from national guidelines [4]. For each model, we simulate fifty sets of parameter values randomly by Monte Carlo sampling [72]. Each parameter set therefore comprises randomly sampled values for k_a, V_d, and CL, from which we can calculate drug concentrations at standardized times after an age-appropriate dose. This collection of simulated drug concentrations is then used by the nonparametric adaptive grid (NPAG) program in Pmetrics [73] to make the population pharmacokinetic model, comprising a collection of estimated points and associated probability of each point in the population, where a point represents a given set of parameter estimates. In summary, with this method, a population PK model for each antiretroviral drug is generated from published parameter estimates without recapitulating multiple clinical trials.

For interpretation of serum drug concentrations obtained randomly from each of the patients, we use BestDose to fit the appropriate model to all the patient's available data points (including measured drug concentrations) to obtain Bayesian posterior distributions for each parameter. When adjustment of a dosage regimen is necessary, this is accomplished using the software's MM dosage design based on the entire distribution of posterior parameter values, to hit the target goals with maximum precision (minimum predicted weighted squared error).

14.7 PATIENTS

We have selected patients who represent clinical challenges appropriate for use of therapeutic drug management and dosage individualization. Although this is a chapter on pediatric patients, we include one adult for illustrative purposes. These have been published previously [74,75], but we provide far more detail here about the pharmacometric and overall therapeutic approaches that we used.

14.8 PATIENT 1. GENERAL TECHNIQUES AND THE NEED FOR NONSTANDARD DOSAGE SCHEDULES

We begin with *Patient 1*, a 45-year-old woman (Tanner stage 5) with a long history of medication intolerance, regimen switching, and changing clinics/providers. We include this adult in our case examples because she provides an excellent illustration of a number of principles that can be applied to pharmacometric TDM for any drug, and we will spend considerable time detailing the techniques that we applied to her care. We recognize that not all readers will have the resources to implement the methods, but for the motivated and trained clinician, we can confirm that such methods have greatly enhanced our own practice of patient care.

Our patient was started on a fosamprenavir (FPV) containing regimen (without ritonavir), 2×700 mg tablets twice daily (total 2800 mg/day). After starting the new regimen, she began to experience daytime fatigue, which she attributed to the morning dose, and she inquired about taking the entire dose at night.

At this point, we identified four options, three without pharmacometrics and one with pharmacometric management. The first option was to tell her that once-daily dosing of FPV without ritonavir is not approved, and therefore she should not take all her medications at night. The second option was to tell her to try the once-daily dosing, and in a month, her viral load would reveal if the regimen is adequate. The third option was to switch her to a different regimen. All three of these options were suboptimal. The first option would have likely resulted in dissatisfaction and her departure from the clinic. The second option was irresponsible, because if the regimen had been subtherapeutic, her HIV would have rapidly developed resistance, which is an irreversible and permanent outcome. The third option would have likely resulted in yet another adverse effect to manage, and she had already tried this approach many times. The fourth and most evidence-based approach was to use a population model of PK and a measured concentration to estimate her PK parameters so that we could predict what might happen were she to take all her pills at night.

As we indicated in our overview, the first hurdle to overcome was to construct a population model of FPV. At the time, none had been published. We turned to noncompartmental data, which was also included in the package insert, for information [76]. For 1400 mg of FPV twice daily, without ritonavir, the reported C_{max} was 4.82 mg/L, T_{max} was 1.3 h, 24-h AUC was 33.0 mg $\times$ h/L, and C_{min} was 0.35 mg/L. Because noncompartmental PK equations are actually the same as one-compartmental equations, we assumed a one-compartment model with linear absorption and clearance. We also recognized that we were going to be using the model in the outpatient setting, with unverified dose times, and thus we felt that this uncertainty could not support any models more complex than the most basic. We could then make use of several equations, shown in Box 14.1, to derive estimates for the parameters in our model: k_a (absorption rate), V_d (volume of distribution), and CL (clearance). For variability, we assumed that the typical variability in the package insert observed PK characteristics also applied to the parameters.

From our estimated parameter values and standard deviations, we then used our Pmetrics software [73] to simulate 50 "patients," or sets of PK parameter values to whom we "administered" 1400 mg twice daily of FPV and calculated concentrations at 12-minute intervals after the fifth dose. By simulation, we mean randomly drawing parameter values from our constructed normal distributions. We directed Pmetrics to add a random amount of noise to each simulated

---

BOX 14.1 USEFUL PHARMACOKINETIC EQUATIONS FOR A ONE-COMPARTMENT MODEL

$AUC = Dose/CL$

$V_d = t\frac{1}{2} * CL/\ln(2)$

$k_e = CL/V_d$ or $k_e = \ln(2)/t\frac{1}{2}$

$C_{max} = Dose * e^{-k_e * T_{max}}/V_d$

$T_{max} = \ln(k_a) - \ln(k_e)/(k_a - k_e)$

concentration, selecting the amount from a normal distribution with mean of 0 and standard deviation of 10% of the simulated value. This is an assay error polynomial with $C_0 = 0$, $C_1 = 0.1$, and $C_2 = C_3 = 0$ (see chapter: Optimizing Laboratory Assay Methods for Individualized Therapy). Since the noise term had a mean of 0, the randomly selected amount could be either positive or negative; ie, the simulated concentration could be increased or decreased randomly.

The next step was to run these 50 simulated patients through the NPAG algorithm in Pmetrics to generate a population model. Finally, after transferring the model to our BestDose software for individualized dosing, we checked the mean steady-state predicted amprenavir time-concentration curve characteristics after 1400 mg dosing, and compared it to the reported characteristics. We had to make minor adjustments to the mean values for the parameter values and re-do the model building process a few times, but eventually we were able to closely reproduce the reported pharmacokinetics of amprenavir when dosed as the pro-drug FPV. Our predicted T_{max} was 1.0 h (vs 1.3); C_{max} was 4.2 mg/L (vs 4.8); AUC was 39.0 mg $\times$ h/L (vs 33.0); and C_{min} was 0.37 mg/L (vs 0.35). To get these values, our mean k_a was 3.0 per h, V_d was 297 L, and CL was 68 L/h. Interestingly, since our exercise, a population model of FPV has been published, and their values for these parameters were 1.0, 202, and 60.1, respectively [30]. Absorption was somewhat slower than we had used, but volume and clearance were quite similar, and well within the range of possible values from our simulations. They included a peripheral tissue compartment, which we did not, and this may have accounted for the slight differences.

Once we had a model, we were ready to use it for our patient. Prior to making changes, we measured a serum amprenavir concentration of 1.4 mg/L 4.5 h after her previous dose. We could only rely on her self-reported time of dosing, but we had explained the need for accuracy to her, and she was very willing to cooperate because she saw that we were investing in her care.

As we have described in several other chapters, we used BestDose to fit our constructed model to her measured concentration and calculate her Bayesian posterior parameter distributions. That is, BestDose individualized the model for her, based on her data. The weighted mean predicted concentration was 1.54 mg/L. We deemed this 10% error to be reasonable. On this standard regimen, her predicted trough concentration was 0.21 mg/L, which was just about the minimum target of 0.23 mg/L for wild-type virus [77], which we knew she had by genotypic testing. One can certainly understand why this regimen of FPV is not recommended for patients who might have need of a slightly higher concentration; ie, those who have already been exposed to protease inhibitors (PIs). Her initial fit is shown in Fig. 14.1.

We were now in a position to ask BestDose to use her individual model to calculate the once-daily dose required to maintain a trough of >0.23 mg/L. This plot is shown in Fig. 14.2. The calculated once-daily dose was about 37,100 mg! On 2,800 mg once daily (her request for all 4 pills at night), her predicted trough concentration was 0.02 mg/L. Clearly, with as much evidence as we could gather, she would not have been able to maintain adequate trough concentrations with a single daily dose.

However, we did not stop there. We first calculated the daily exposure from 2,100 mg (3 pills) at night and 700 mg (1 pill) in the morning, to try and shift the fatigue effect to the evening. Unfortunately, her evening trough concentration was predicted to be 0.11 mg/L, which we felt was too low. However, a regimen of one tablet at 8 am followed by three tablets at 6 pm (a 10−14 h schedule) would be 97% likely to achieve the target of all trough concentrations >0.23 mg/L. After careful and thorough discussion of her probable dose-dependent toxicity, she was changed to this regimen. Her fatigue resolved, and she achieved an undetectable viral load. BestDose perfectly

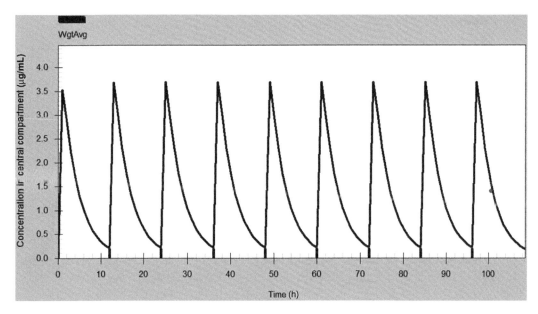

FIGURE 14.1

Time-concentration profile for amprenavir in TDM Patient 1. The red dot is the measured concentration, and the black line is the weighted mean time-concentration curve based on her Bayesian posterior parameter values. Doses are indicated by blue vertical lines at the bottom of the plot.

predicted a follow-up level of 0.9 mg/L obtained 4 h after the morning dose several weeks after beginning the new regimen confirmed that her predicted troughs were likely to be therapeutic, as shown in Fig. 14.3. She maintained an undetectable viral load after starting her new ART regimen.

This patient went beyond the issue not only of changing the dose, but also of changing the dosing schedule as well. While we do not advocate this practice routinely, for some patients it is the only way to achieve a useful "therapeutic alliance" with the physician. If sufficient published data become available to enable construction of a reasonable pharmacokinetic model, and if concentration targets exist, a clinician may at least thoughtfully depart from the usual "standard" dosing regimen in a manner that now can be evidence-based. As always, using therapeutic drug management tools to develop such an individualized regimen does not relieve the clinician of the responsibility to closely monitor her patient, preferably with repeated drug concentrations and Bayesian dosage individualization, to ensure optimal therapeutic efficacy and safety.

Use of repeated measurements is important for another reason. Substantial within-individual variability in orally administered drug concentrations may arise in the outpatient setting, due, eg, to variation in dose times, gastric pH, gastric contents, or drug-drug interactions [48]. Nonetheless, this variability does not preclude therapeutic drug management. However, it must be recognized for appropriate interpretation of results. It is rare in modern medicine to substantially alter any therapy on the basis of a single laboratory result, especially if the information is not immediately life-threatening or corroborated by findings on physical exam. In our practice, repeated measurements are an important component of successful therapeutic drug management. We do not react to a

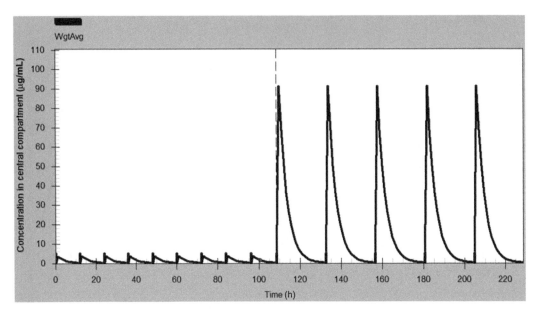

FIGURE 14.2

Predicted profile for TDM Patient 1, were she to take all her fosamprenavir once daily and maintain therapeutic concentrations.

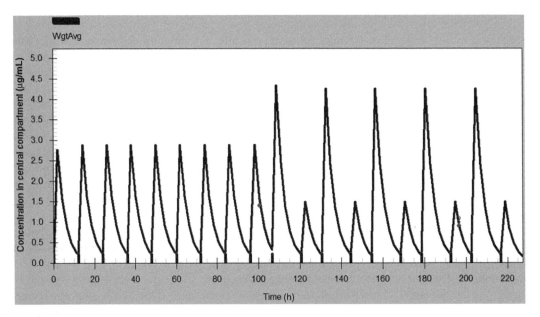

FIGURE 14.3

Confirmatory predicted and measured amprenavir concentrations for TDM Patient 1. The time scale has been compressed for clarity.

single high or low measurement by immediately changing the dose. Rather, we use that information as a guided opportunity to carefully screen for toxicity if necessary, and review the patient's medication-taking behavior, such as appropriate separation from food, concomitant medications like proton-pump inhibitors, missed doses, and regularity of dosing. Repeat testing may demonstrate that therapeutic exposure is possible on the given dose. On the rare occasions that we are unable to reconcile a patient's self-reported behavior with measured drug concentrations, or if we have been unable to document a single concentration within our targeted exposure despite two or three samples, we usually ask the patient to bring her medications with her to the clinic so that we can measure a drug concentration after a witnessed dose.

14.9 **PATIENT 2. UNSUSPECTED IMPAIRED CLEARANCE: PATIENTS NEEDING SMALLER DOSES THAN USUAL**

Patient 2 was a 13-year-old, 26-kg, antiretroviral-naïve African boy (Tanner stage 2), whom we started on his first ART regimen including efavirenz 350 mg once daily in the evening, which was the recommended dose for his age and weight. After two weeks, his mother reported that he had become much too somnolent to attend school since starting the medication, which was a significantly more severe manifestation than the transient drowsiness that may occur after starting EFV [78]. Suspecting that he had impaired drug clearance, possibly due to a polymorphism in his cytochrome P450 2B6 gene [79], we empirically reduced his dose to 200 mg once daily, and by a week after this reduction, his mother reported that he was much more alert and able to attend school again. We measured a serum concentration of 1.37 mg/L 21.5 h after his previous reported dose.

As shown in Table 14.2, the target concentration for EFV is a trough >1 mg/L [4]. It is certainly likely that within 2 h, his concentration would have been still above 1 mg/L, but we wanted to be as certain as possible, since we were using a dose that was just over half of the typical, and a single point mutation (K103N) that can arise from underdosing is sufficient to permanently destroy the antiviral activity of both EFV and NVP [4].

We used the identical approach as we have just described for Patient 1 to construct a model of EFV in children. Using BestDose, his predicted concentration was 1.42 mg/L, an error of only 4%, and his trough was 99.7% likely to be >1 mg/L. Confident in the appropriateness of his dose, we continued, and a follow-up sample obtained several months later on the same low dose, confirmed his therapeutic concentrations. He maintained an undetectable HIV viral load with no further somnolence. In Fig. 14.4, we show the predictions for both concentrations when only the first was used to calculate his Bayesian posterior, and when both were used to calculate the Bayesian posterior. The second concentration, measured 21 h after the preceding dose, was predicted to be 1.40 mg/L, an error of -19%, but still 98.8% likely to have a trough concentration >1 mg/L. When both concentrations were used to generate the posterior, the predictions were 1.49 mg/L (9% error) and 1.48 mg/L (-14% error), and a 99.9% probability to have a trough >1 mg/L. This is one way to get a sense of intraoccasion variability in drug concentrations in the same patient. The prediction of the second concentration changed by only 5% when it was included in the calculation of the Bayesian posterior versus when it was not. In other words, this patient's EFV PK and drug dosing behavior was quite stable, since the estimated PK parameters based only on the first concentration predicted the second very well, and the second concentration did not change the estimation of those

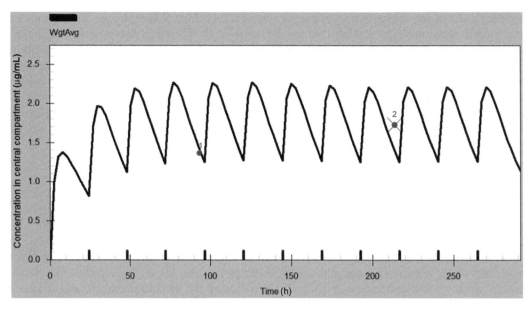

FIGURE 14.4

EFV time-concentration profile for TDM Patient 2. The measured concentration with the red "X" through it was not used to calculate the Bayesian posterior parameter distribution for the patient, so the weighted mean time-concentration profile (black line) is based only on the first measured concentration.

PK parameters much. In an outpatient setting, interoccasion variability is likely due to errors in reported times of doses, but could also be due to unmeasured fluctuation in physiologic states, such as gastric pH, that might affect drug PK and consequently alter time-concentration profiles between occasions. As we discussed for the previous patient, we usually handle this with repeated, confirmatory concentrations, or observed dosing. Lastly, our IMM technique (discussed in chapters: Monitoring the Patient: Four Different Bayesian Methods to Make Individual Patient Drug Models and Optimizing Single-Drug Antibacterial and Antifungal Therapy) is a method to track changing PK parameter values within an individual over time.

This patient illustrates the situation when drug clearance differs substantially from clearance reported in the package literature. In this case, we suspected that it was due to a polymorphism in cytochrome P450 2B6, a key drug-metabolizing enzyme with clinical significance for both EFV and NVP [79,80]. However, there has not been universal agreement in the clinical significance of polymorphisms in this gene with regard to EFV PK [81], and for many drugs, compensatory or alternative pathways exist that mitigate effects of mutations in the gene product primarily responsible for metabolism. In fact, we later proved that he was wild-type with respect to P450 2B6, showing that genotype is not a perfect predictor of dose, as we discussed in the Pharmacogenomics section, and as recognized by the national guidelines, which recommend both genotyping and TDM when managing EFV in children [4]. Again, genomic profiling must always be linked to a pharmacokinetic model of drug behavior.

14.10 **PATIENT 3. LOW CONCENTRATIONS: UNDERDOSING OR POOR ADHERENCE?**

Patient 3 was an 18-year-old woman (Tanner stage 5) who was congenitally infected with HIV. She had been treated with multiple ART regimens over the years, with consistently poor adherence based on a very poor virologic response and chronically low CD4$^+$T lymphocyte count. In an effort to devise a simple regimen, we started her on ARV combination therapy based on unboosted atazanavir 400 mg once daily. While unboosted atazanavir is not recommended for PI-experienced patients, she was not able to tolerate ritonavir, even in low doses for PK boosting.

Unfortunately, her viral load and CD4$^+$ cell count did not improve. Moreover, her total bilirubin did not increase, which is an effect of atazanavir as we discussed earlier. Together, this information strongly suggested that she was not taking her ATV (or other ARVs), however, she continued to insist that she was indeed taking the medicines.

After telling her that we wanted to check her blood to see how appropriate her dose was, we measured an ATV concentration of <10 ng/mL, 18 h after her self-reported previous dose. Could she have taken it? Was she underdosed, or could we conclude nonadherence? Using the same techniques as we have described, we constructed a model of unboosted ATV and used BestDose to fit her concentration to the model. We fitted it with the concentration set at 10 ng/mL and 5 ng/mL as a sensitivity analysis. The plot of all possible time-concentration curves is shown in Fig. 14.5.

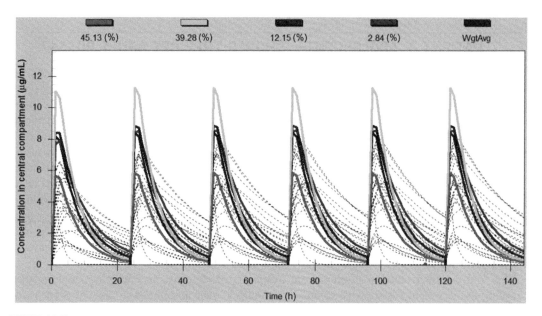

FIGURE 14.5

Possible atazanavir time-concentration profiles for TDM Patient 3, with her measured concentration shown in red at the bottom of the plot. Colors for profiles correspond to the probability of the profile as labeled at the top of the plot. Profiles with dashed lines are very low probability.

Based on our analysis, there was a $10^{-10}\%$ chance of having taken the dose when she said she did, 18 h prior to the measured concentration. When we presented this information to her, she became tearful and admitted that she could not tolerate taking her medicines. She saw that we did not condemn her or chastise her, and this was the beginning of a real therapeutic breakthrough for her, which had not been possible prior to the PK intervention. We were later able to devise a regimen that did work for her, enlist the help of her family, and achieve an undetectable viral load and robust CD4$^+$ cell count for the first time in her life.

A major lesson we learned from this experience was that even though patients often could be confronted with the objective effects of poor adherence on a paper laboratory report; ie, high viral load and low CD4$^+$ count, their admissions of nonadherence became more consistent when confronted with improbably low drug concentrations, which is a direct consequence of not taking the medication. In fact, we altered our practice for nonadherent patients. When nonadherence appears to be entrenched for a patient, we will typically say something like, "We need to check how much drug is in your blood to make sure your dose is right. If you didn't take your medicines in the last 24 h, we will not be able to measure anything and we will have stuck you with a needle for no reason. Should we go ahead?" Countless times, even when the patient had said earlier in the same visit that there were no missed doses, he let us know that we should not bother with the test that day. Again, it is the response to such an admission that determines the next steps, and often we were able to forge a therapeutic alliance to make progress when we responded with compassion and support.

14.11 PATIENT 4. ADOLESCENTS: SHOULD THEY GET ADULT DOSES?

Patient 4 was a 10-year-old girl (Tanner stage 2) who weighed 30.7 kg. Based on the standard pediatric NFV dose of 55 mg/kg, and within formulation limitations, she was prescribed 1875 mg twice daily. Since the recommended "maximum" NFV dose is the smaller adult dose of only 1250 mg twice daily, a random serum concentration of 4.9 mg/L was measured 4 h after her most recent dose to ensure that she was not in a toxic range. From this concentration, her predicted peak concentration on the 1875 mg dose was 5.5 mg/L and her 12-h trough was 2.1 mg/L. By using BestDose to simulate the results on the lower dose of 1250 mg, given her estimated PK parameter distributions, her predicted trough concentration would have been 1.4 mg/L. Because she was tolerating the higher dose, and because her predicted most likely NFV profile was more solidly within a suggested therapeutic range of 1−6 mg/L at the time [77], we elected to continue that larger dose to give her a greater margin above the minimum trough target of 1 mg/L. She did not develop either gastrointestinal or any other toxicity, despite the larger dose, and she continued to have an undetectable viral load.

This is a common problem in adolescent medicine. Adolescents may weigh enough so that, according to the weight-based pediatric dosing guidelines, their absolute dose amount exceeds the typical maximum recommended adult dose. Clinicians are left in a quandary about whether the published dosing cap should be respected, or whether their individual adolescent patient is still pharmaco-physiologically a child. Children typically have higher weight-adjusted volumes of distribution and more rapid clearances than adults [6,41], which reduce drug concentrations after a given dose in these younger patients relative to adults and thus require higher doses when adjusted for body weight. Although guidelines recommend pediatric dosing for those who are Tanner Sexual Maturity Stage 3 and under [4], lack of concentration data and therapeutic drug management increases the risk of improper dosing. Furthermore, the reason for therapeutic failure can be misconstrued to be an adherence problem: on the one hand, patients who are underdosed may be incorrectly labeled as poorly adherent. Alternatively, overdosed patients who are experiencing medication-related adverse effects may be reluctant to admit that they therefore avoid them. The clinician will rightly detect the nonadherence when therapeutic failure is observed, but the true source of the nonadherence—toxicity—may go unrecognized. This example shows clearly that dosage individualization does not simply mean dose reduction to minimize toxicity. It also means giving larger doses than usual when they are warranted in an individual patient, to obtain appropriate benefit.

14.12 **PATIENT 5. EXTRAPOLATING FROM ADULTS TO CHILDREN**

Patient 5 was a 14-year-old male (Tanner stage 4) with poor medication adherence and previous NNRTI resistance. To encourage better adherence, he was changed to a once-daily regimen that included ATV given in combination with low-dose ritonavir. The usual adult dose of ATV is 300 mg when given with ritonavir, so he was started on 200 mg based on his age and small size (height and weight in the 25th percentile). Since there were no published pediatric PK data or dose at the time, we obtained a random ATV concentration of 780 ng/mL 18 h after his previous dose. His predicted trough concentration was 380 ng/mL, above the minimum target of 150 ng/mL [4], so the dose was continued. He initially achieved an undetectable viral load. However, self-disclosed persistently poor adherence allowed his viral load to rebound partially to about 2000 copies/mL, despite a second measured therapeutic concentration (660 ng/mL) of ATV. By having concentration data available, we were able to accurately ascertain that the cause of his virologic failure was indeed due solely to suboptimal adherence, and not because we had underdosed him.

This type of patient is all too familiar to pediatricians, who are commonly faced with the necessity to prescribe medications off label. Although it is preferable to prescribe medications at doses that have already been tested for safety and efficacy, by using therapeutic drug management and Bayesian dosage individualization when necessary, the clinician can ensure that a child's drug exposure is similar to that of safe and effective adult exposures, which is the foundational approach to pediatric phase I/II labeling trials. This is the approach we took to managing a 12-year-old boy on darunavir, who had been accidentally chronically overdosed by three times the adult dose [75]. Through measurement of plasma darunavir concentrations and pharmacometric analysis, we were able to show that the dose that best matched adult exposures was twice the adult dose. Again, we see elements of Patient 4 here; adolescents may need to receive more than adults do, either in mg/kg or in absolute mg doses.

By its very nature, dose optimization is an individual, not a population process. Because of this, illustrative individual case reports such as these provide important supportive evidence in a manner that does not obscure this essentially individual nature of therapy, as may often happen in large clinical trials with limited or no actual individual dose modification [82–84]. Our method for converting reported PK data into population models can be used locally to optimize safety and efficacy in individual patients. Successful and practical TDM using Bayesian adaptive control and individualization of the dosage regimen to achieve desired target goals has been illustrated by the preceding specific clinical examples. In addition to other patients who fit the clinical situations described here, we have used the same techniques to adjust therapy in other settings. We used the same techniques reported here, to establish that the combination of FPV and lopinavir (LPV) resulted in dramatically reduced amprenavir concentrations in a multidrug resistant adolescent. We immediately stopped that combination, prior to published recommendations against using the regimen because of that interaction [85].

Taking advantage of published pharmacologic data and a tool such as the BestDose software, which runs on a server accessed through the web, puts Bayesian adaptive control in the hands of physicians and pharmacists who recognize special patients requiring a more specific and individualized approach to therapy than "one-size-fits-all." It is not possible to know with absolute certainty how patients take their drugs and how to interpret randomly obtained levels. However, in appropriate settings such as those presented here, with a judicious clinician, we argue that therapeutic drug management can be quite practical and is better than blindly trusting the "one-size" dose. Why wait until virologic failure or dose-dependent toxicity to find out, at the patient's medical and financial cost, that such blind trust was misplaced?

14.13 MOVING FORWARD

Despite the recognition of the potential benefits of ART TDM in children, one must recognize the substantial barriers that have limited its use. These barriers exist at all levels of patient care: the individual patient, the therapeutic process, and the scientific-medical culture. At the most individual level, predefined sample times (troughs) generally do not occur when the patient is in clinic with once- or twice-daily ARV regiments, and the exact times of the doses preceding the blood sample are subject to recall bias. Comparisons with target ranges become difficult, and they are even further confounded by between-patient or within-patient (interoccasion) PK variability, in bioavailability, which may obscure reasons for concentrations outside the range.

Barriers related to the therapeutic process include poor availability of ARV concentrations or long turnaround times, lack of expertise to interpret concentration data, especially if obtained outside the "trough window," which is compounded by limited PK data in children, paucity of user-friendly software tools, and reports of poor reimbursement for such services [86].

On the global scale of the entire scientific-medical culture, TDM is hampered by a drug development process geared toward an economically advocated "one-size-fits-all" dose and not target-oriented therapy, limited commitment or mechanisms to update dosing guidelines as postmarket evidence emerges, poor physician training in basic or applied pharmacology, and an insufficient partnership between physicians and clinical pharmacists to dose complex or atypical patients.

All of these factors are intertwined and formidable, yet they may be overcome [87]. When one wishes to estimate a fuller or more accurate exposure than can be obtained from a trough, there have been attempts to define more informative, yet limited sampling strategies. NFV AUC_{0-12}, for example, can be estimated by sampling just prior to and 4 h after a dose [88]. LPV AUC_{0-12} is best predicted by samples 2 and 6 h after a dose [89]. Because of its long half-life, NVP AUC_{0-12} can be estimated by a single blood sample any time between 2 and 4 h after a dose [90]. All of the aforementioned studies were done in adults, and so they should not be considered applicable to children without validation.

While offering some solution, many "limited sampling" approaches suffer from the same problem as traditional TDM of rigid sampling times and an inability to handle patients who are not "typical." On the other hand, population PK techniques, introduced in the section on Basic Techniques, coupled with Bayesian adaptive control allow for prediction of plasma drug concentrations at any time after a dose, given all information known about a patient, such as dose amount, frequency, estimated times of drug administration, and known time(s) of blood sampling (regardless of the elapsed time). Information not specific to the patient, but nonetheless relevant, such as PK behavior in other children or in adults, may also be included in the model to improve the quality of the predictions. The obvious advantage is that one is no longer limited to specific sampling times that may be inconvenient. We have successfully applied these techniques in the care of our own HIV-infected pediatric patients as described previously.

So what is the best approach to optimize ARV therapy in children at present? We believe that the initial dose should be selected on the basis of available dosing recommendations when possible. PG patient profiling is not yet readily accepted and implemented except for HLA typing prior to initiating ABV therapy, or CYP450 2B6 testing prior to initiating EFV therapy in infants and toddlers under 3 years of age. However, as we have stated in the Pharmacogenomics section, individual PG information may be able to identify some (but not all) patients who will need a different starting dose, but it cannot reliably specify the magnitude of departure from standard dosing for a single patient.

In all cases, once therapy is started, virologic, immunologic, and safety parameters should be monitored closely, especially early after treatment initiation. Strongly consider early measurement of drug concentrations within the first one to two weeks to ensure adequate exposure, particularly in treatment-experienced children, or for certain drugs (eg, EFV in young children) regardless of treatment history.

Measurement of drug concentrations may also be helpful when there are clinical responses that are different from what is desired. ARV concentrations can be measured at commercial or research laboratories. Consultation with experts in pediatric HIV pharmacology can be of assistance with the decisions about when to obtain samples for TDM and interpretation of the data. Such experts are available at numerous universities and medical centers, including our own. Good resources for locating them are through large research networks such as the International Maternal Child Adolescent AIDS Clinical Trials group (IMPAACT, http://www.impaactgroup.org) and the Paediatric European Network for Treatment of AIDS (PENTA, http://www.pentatrials.org), or the International Association for TDM and Clinical Toxicology (IATDMCT, http://www.iatdmct.org).

Much progress has been already achieved to optimize ARV therapy in children and adolescents, but much work lies ahead as ART becomes available to more children of diverse ethnic/racial backgrounds worldwide. Reliable and user-friendly software that employs techniques such as Bayesian adaptive control needs to be validated. New pharmacologically relevant genetic polymorphisms will likely be characterized; developmental, physiologic, and psychosocial factors affecting ART adherence and response in children of different continents are not well described; and the role and manner of TDM in different cultural settings needs to be addressed. However, with resources and commitment, the successes of pediatric ART seen thus far in developed countries can be continued, extended, and replicated worldwide.

ACKNOWLEDGMENTS

MN receives support from NIH PHS grants NIGMS R01 GM068968 and NICHD R01 HD070886. NR received support from NICHD K23 1K23HD060452, NIGMS R01 EB005803-01A1, and MO1-RR-020359. The authors have no financial conflicts of interest.

REFERENCES

[1] McConnell MS, et al. Trends in antiretroviral therapy use and survival rates for a large cohort of HIV-infected children and adolescents in the United States, 1989–2001. J Acquir Immune Defic Syndr 2005;38:488–94.

[2] Foster C, et al. Young people in the United Kingdom and Ireland with perinatally acquired HIV: the pediatric legacy for adult services. AIDS Pat Care STDs 2009;23:159–66.

[3] HIV/AIDS, J.U.N.P.O. UNAIDS announces that the goal of 15 million people on life-saving HIV treatment by 2015 has been met nine months ahead of schedule, <unaids.org> at <http://www.unaids.org/>.

[4] Panel on antiretroviral therapy and medical management of HIV-infected children. Guidelines for the use of antiretroviral agents in pediatric HIV infection, <http://www.aidsinfo.nih.gov>; 2015.

[5] Bamford A, et al. Paediatric European Network for Treatment of AIDS (PENTA) guidelines for treatment of paediatric HIV-1 infection 2015: optimizing health in preparation for adult life; 2015.

[6] Kearns GL, Reed MD. Clinical pharmacokinetics in infants and children. A reappraisal. Clin Pharmacokinet 1989;17(Suppl. 1):29–67.

[7] Kearns GL, et al. Developmental pharmacology—drug disposition, action, and therapy in infants and children. New Engl J Med 2003;349:1157–67.

[8] Meibohm B, Laer S, Panetta JC, Barrett JS. Population pharmacokinetic studies in pediatrics: issues in design and analysis. AAPS J 2005;7:E475–87.

[9] Neely MN, Rakhmanina NY. Pharmacokinetic optimization of antiretroviral therapy in children and adolescents. Clin Pharmacokinet 2011;50:143–89.

[10] Cross SJ, et al. Abacavir and metabolite pharmacokinetics in HIV-1-infected children and adolescents. J Acquir Immune Defic Syndr 2009;51:54–9.

[11] Jullien V, et al. Abacavir pharmacokinetics in human immunodeficiency virus-infected children ranging in age from 1 month to 16 years: a population analysis. J Clin Pharmacol 2005;45:257–64.

[12] Zhao W, et al. Population pharmacokinetics of abacavir in infants, toddlers and children. Br J Clin Pharmacol 2012. Available from: http://dx.doi.org/10.1111/bcp.12024.

[13] Hirt D, et al. Didanosine population pharmacokinetics in West African human immunodeficiency virus-infected children administered once-daily tablets in relation to efficacy after one year of treatment. Antimicrob Agents Chemother 2009;53:4399–406.

[14] Acosta E, et al. Population pharmacokinetics of lamivudine in human immunodeficiency virus-exposed and -infected infants. Antimicrob Agents Chemother 2007;51:4297–302.

[15] Bouazza N, et al. Developmental pharmacokinetics of lamivudine in 580 pediatric patients ranging from neonates to adolescents. Antimicrob Agents Chemother 2011;55:3498–504.

[16] Piana C, et al. Covariate effects and population pharmacokinetics of lamivudine in HIV-infected children. Br J Clin Pharmacol 2014;77:861–72.

[17] Jullien V, et al. Age-related differences in the pharmacokinetics of stavudine in 272 children from birth to 16 years: a population analysis. Br J Clin Pharm 2007;64:105–9.

[18] Bouazza N, et al. Population pharmacokinetics of tenofovir in HIV-1-infected pediatric patients. J Acquir Immune Defic Syndr 2011;58:283–8.

[19] Capparelli EV, et al. Pharmacokinetics and tolerance of zidovudine in preterm infants. J Pediatr 2003;142:47−52.

[20] Mirochnick M, Capparelli E, Connor J. Pharmacokinetics of zidovudine in infants: a population analysis across studies. Clin Pharmacol Ther 1999;66:16−24.

[21] Capparelli EV, et al. Population pharmacokinetics and pharmacodynamics of zidovudine in HIV-infected infants and children. J Clin Pharmacol 2003;43:133−40.

[22] Fauchet F, et al. Population pharmacokinetics study of recommended zidovudine doses in HIV-1-infected children. Antimicrob Agents Chemother 2013;57:4801−8.

[23] Flynn PM, et al. Intracellular pharmacokinetics of once versus twice daily zidovudine and lamivudine in adolescents. Antimicrob Agents Chemother 2007;51:3516−22.

[24] Hirt D, et al. Is the recommended dose of efavirenz optimal in young West African human immunodeficiency virus-infected children?. Antimicrob Agents Chemother 2009;53:4407−13.

[25] ter Heine R, et al. A pharmacokinetic and pharmacogenetic study of efavirenz in children: dosing guidelines can result in subtherapeutic concentrations. Antivir Ther 2008;13:779−87.

[26] Nikanjam M, et al. Nevirapine exposure with WHO pediatric weight band dosing: enhanced therapeutic concentrations predicted based on extensive international pharmacokinetic experience. Antimicrob Agents Chemother 2012;56:5374−80.

[27] Foissac F, et al. Evaluation of nevirapine dosing recommendations in HIV-infected children. Br J Clin Pharmacol 2013;76:137−44.

[28] Foissac F, et al. Population pharmacokinetics of atazanavir/ritonavir in HIV-1-infected children and adolescents. Br J Clin Pharmacol 2011;72:940−7.

[29] Fisher J, Gastonguay MR, Knebel W, Gibiansky L, Wire MB. Population pharmacokinetic modeling of fosamprenavir in pediatric HIV-infected patients, American Conference on Pharmacometrics. Tuscon, AZ; 2008.

[30] Barbour AM, Gibiansky L, Wire MB. Population pharmacokinetic modeling and simulation of amprenavir following fosamprenavir/ritonavir administration for dose optimization in HIV infected pediatric patients. J Clin Pharmacol 2014;54:206−14.

[31] Chadwick EG, et al. Pharmacokinetics, safety and efficacy of lopinavir/ritonavir in infants less than 6 months of age: 24 week results. AIDS 2008;22:249−55.

[32] Rakhmanina N, et al. Population pharmacokinetics of lopinavir predict suboptimal therapeutic concentrations in treatment-experienced human immunodeficiency virus-infected children. Antimicrob Agents Chemother 2009;53:2532−8.

[33] Jullien V, et al. Population analysis of weight-, age-, and sex-related differences in the pharmacokinetics of lopinavir in children from birth to 18 years. Antimicrob Agents Chemother 2006;50:3548−55.

[34] Urien S, et al. Lopinavir/ritonavir population pharmacokinetics in neonates and infants. Br J Clin Pharmacol 2011;71:956−60.

[35] Crommentuyn KML, et al. Population pharmacokinetics and pharmacodynamics of nelfinavir and its active metabolite M8 in HIV 1-infected children. Pediatr Infect Dis J 2006;25:538−43.

[36] Hirt DEB, et al. Age-related effects on nelfinavir and M8 pharmacokinetics: a population study with 182 children. Antimicrob Agents Chemother 2006;50:910−16.

[37] Sabo JP, et al. Population pharmacokinetic (PK) assessment of systemic steady-state tipranavir (TPV) concentrations for HIV+ pediatric patients administered tipranavir/ritonavir (TPV/r) 290/115 mg/m^2 and 375/150 mg/m^2 BID, conference on retroviruses and opportunistic infections. Denver, CO; 2005.

[38] Zhang X, et al. Population pharmacokinetics of enfuvirtide in HIV-1-infected pediatric patients over 48 weeks of treatment. J Clin Pharmacol 2007;47:510−17.

[39] Rizk ML, et al. Population pharmacokinetic analysis of raltegravir pediatric formulations in HIV-infected children 4 weeks to 18 years of age. J Clin Pharmacol 2015;55:748−56.

[40] van den Anker JN. Developmental pharmacology. Dev Disabil Res Rev 2010;16:233—8.

[41] Reed MD, Besunder JB. Developmental pharmacology: ontogenic basis of drug disposition. Pediatr Clin North Am 1989;36:1053—74.

[42] Hines RN. Ontogeny of human hepatic cytochromes P450. J Biochem Mol Toxicol 2007;21:169—75.

[43] Hines RN. The ontogeny of drug metabolism enzymes and implications for adverse drug events. Pharmacol Ther 2008;118:250—67.

[44] Anderson BJ, Meakin GH. Scaling for size: some implications for paediatric anaesthesia dosing. Paediatr Anaesth 2002;12:205—19.

[45] Anderson BJ, Holford NHG. Mechanism-based concepts of size and maturity in pharmacokinetics. Annu Rev Pharmacol Toxicol 2008;48:303—32.

[46] Neely M, Rushing T, Kovacs A, Jelliffe R, Hoffman J. Voriconazole pharmacokinetics and pharmacodynamics in children. Clin Infect Dis 2010;50:27—36.

[47] Neely M, et al. Achieving target voriconazole concentrations more accurately in children and adolescents. Antimicrob Agents Chemother 2015;59:3090—7.

[48] Nettles RE, et al. Marked intraindividual variability in antiretroviral concentrations may limit the utility of therapeutic drug monitoring. Clin Infect Dis 2006;42:1189—96.

[49] Fabbiani M, et al. Pharmacokinetic variability of antiretroviral drugs and correlation with virological outcome: 2 years of experience in routine clinical practice. J Antimicrob Chemother 2009;64:109—17.

[50] Dunn D, et al. Current CD4 cell count and the short-term risk of AIDS and death before the availability of effective antiretroviral therapy in HIV-infected children and adults. J Infect Dis 2008;197:398—404.

[51] Dunn D. Short-term risk of disease progression in HIV-1-infected children receiving no antiretroviral therapy or zidovudine monotherapy: a meta-analysis. Lancet 2003;362:1605—11.

[52] Rutstein RM, et al. Long-term safety and efficacy of atazanavir-based therapy in HIV-infected infants, children and adolescents: the pediatric AIDS clinical trials group protocol 1020A. Pediatr Infect Dis J 2015;34:162—7.

[53] Nachman S, et al. Pharmacokinetics, safety, and 48-week efficacy of oral raltegravir in HIV-1-infected children aged 2 through 18 years. Clin Infect Dis 2014;58:413—22.

[54] Viani RM, et al. Safety, pharmacokinetics and efficacy of dolutegravir in treatment-experienced HIV-1 infected adolescents: forty-eight-week results from IMPAACT P1093. Pediatr Infect Dis J 2015;34:1207—13.

[55] Prasitsuebsai W. et al. Pharmacokinetics of elvitegravir in HIV-1 infected pediatric subjects. Conference on retroviruses and opportunistic infections; 2015.

[56] Guar A, et al. Pharmacokinetics, efficacy and safety of an integrase inhibitor STR in HIV-infected adolescents. Conference on retroviruses and opportunistic infections; 2014.

[57] Giaquinto C, et al. Safety and efficacy of maraviroc in CCR5-tropic HIV-1-infected children aged 2 to <18 years. International AIDS society conference on HIV pathogenesis, treatment, and prevention; 2013.

[58] Vourvahis M, et al. Update from study A4001031: maraviroc pharmacokinetics in CCR5-tropic HIV-1-infected children aged 2 to <18 years. International AIDS society conference on HIV pathogenesis, treatment, and prevention; 2013.

[59] Kizito H, et al. Treatment-naïve HIV-1-infected adolescents initiating INSTI-based single-tablet regimens containing tenofovir alafenamide (TAF) or tenofovir disoproxil fumarate (TDF). International AIDS society conference on HIV pathogenesis, treatment, and prevention; 2015.

[60] Kizito H, et al. Week 24 data from a phase 3 clinical trial of E/C/F/TAF in HIV-infected adolescents. Conference on retroviruses and opportunistic infections; 2015.

[61] Åsberg A, et al. Inclusion of CYP3A5 genotyping in a nonparametric population model improves dosing of tacrolimus early after transplantation. Transpl Int 2013;26:1198—207.

[62] Lubomirov R, et al. Pharmacogenetics-based population pharmacokinetic analysis of etravirine in HIV-1 infected individuals. Pharmacogenet Genomics 2013;23:9−18.

[63] Aceti A, Gianserra L, Lambiase L, Pennica A, Teti E. Pharmacogenetics as a tool to tailor antiretroviral therapy: a review. World J Virol 2015;4:198−208.

[64] Acosta E, Gerber JG, Adult Pharmacology Committee of the AIDS Clinical Trials Group. Position paper on therapeutic drug monitoring of antiretroviral agents. AIDS Res Hum Retroviruses 2002;18:825−34.

[65] Fraaij PL A, Rakhmanina N, Burger DM, de Groot R. Therapeutic drug monitoring in children with HIV/AIDS. Ther Drug Monit 2004;26:122−6.

[66] Acosta EP, King JR. Methods for integration of pharmacokinetic and phenotypic information in the treatment of infection with human immunodeficiency virus. Clin Infect Dis 2003;36:373−7.

[67] Rakhmanina NY, Capparelli EV, Van den Anker JN. Personalized therapeutics: HIV treatment in adolescents. Clin Pharmacol Ther 2008;84:734−40.

[68] Ette EI, Williams PJ. Population pharmacokinetics I: background, concepts, and models. Ann Pharmacother 2004;38:1702−6.

[69] Jelliffe RW. The USC*PACK PC programs for population pharmacokinetic modeling, modeling of large kinetic/dynamic systems, and adaptive control of drug dosage regimens. Proc Annu Symp Comput Appl Med Care 1991922−4.

[70] Jelliffe R, Bayard D, Milman M, Van Guilder M, Schumitzky A. Achieving target goals most precisely using nonparametric compartmental models and 'multiple model' design of dosage regimens. Ther Drug Monit 2000;22:346−53.

[71] Jelliffe RW, Maire P. Goal-oriented, model-based drug regimens. Comput Biol Med 2001;31:145−6.

[72] Metropolis N, Ulam S. The monte carlo method. J Am Stat Assoc 1949;44:335−41.

[73] Neely MN, van Guilder MG, Yamada WM, Schumitzky A, Jelliffe RW. Accurate detection of outliers and subpopulations with Pmetrics, a nonparametric and parametric pharmacometric modeling and simulation package for R. Ther Drug Monit 2012;34:467−76.

[74] Neely M, Jelliffe R. Practical therapeutic drug management in HIV-infected patients: use of population pharmacokinetic models supplemented by individualized Bayesian dose optimization. J Clin Pharmacol 2008;48:1081−91.

[75] Rakhmanina NY, Neely MN, Capparelli EV. High dose of darunavir in treatment-experienced HIV-infected adolescent results in virologic suppression and improved CD4 cell count. Ther Drug Monit 2012;34:237−41.

[76] Wire MB, Shelton MJ, Studenberg S. Fosamprenavir: clinical pharmacokinetics and drug interactions of the amprenavir prodrug. Clin Pharmacokinet 2006;45:137−68.

[77] Kappelhoff BS, et al. Practical guidelines to interpret plasma concentrations of antiretroviral drugs. Clin Pharmacokinet 2004;43:845−53.

[78] Starr SE, et al. Efavirenz liquid formulation in human immunodeficiency virus-infected children. Pediatr Infect Dis J 2002;21:659−63.

[79] Saitoh A, et al. Efavirenz pharmacokinetics in HIV-1-infected children are associated with CYP2B6-G516T polymorphism. J Acquir Immune Defic Syndr 2007;45:280−5.

[80] Gatanaga H, et al. Successful efavirenz dose reduction in HIV type 1-infected individuals with cytochrome P450 2B6 *6 and *26. Clin Infect Dis 2007;45:1230−7.

[81] Burger D, et al. Interpatient variability in the pharmacokinetics of the HIV non-nucleoside reverse transcriptase inhibitor efavirenz: the effect of gender, race, and CYP2B6 polymorphism. Br J Clin Pharmacol 2006;61:148−54.

[82] Torti C, et al. A randomized controlled trial to evaluate antiretroviral salvage therapy guided by rules-based or phenotype-driven HIV-1 genotypic drug-resistance interpretation with or without concentration-

controlled intervention: the resistance and dosage adapted regimens (RADAR) study. Clin Infect Dis 2005;40:1828−36.

[83] Bossi P, et al. GENOPHAR: a randomized study of plasma drug measurements in association with genotypic resistance testing and expert advice to optimize therapy in patients failing antiretroviral therapy. HIV Med 2004;5:352−9.

[84] Clevenbergh P, Garraffo R, Durant J, Dellamonica P. PharmAdapt: a randomized prospective study to evaluate the benefit of therapeutic monitoring of protease inhibitors: 12 week results. AIDS 2002;16:2311−15.

[85] Acosta E, et al. Combining fosamprenavir with lopinavir/ritonavir substantially reduces amprenavir and lopinavir exposure: ACTG protocol A5143 results. AIDS 2005;19:145−52.

[86] Reidenberg MM. A new look at the profession of clinical pharmacology. Clin Pharmacol Ther 2008;83:213−17.

[87] Neely M, Jelliffe R. Practical, individualized dosing: 21st century therapeutics and the clinical pharmacometrician. J Clin Pharmacol 2010;50:842−7.

[88] Regazzi MB, et al. Limited sampling strategy for the estimation of systemic exposure to the protease inhibitor nelfinavir. Ther Drug Monit 2005;27:571−5.

[89] Alexander C, et al. Simplification of therapeutic drug monitoring for twice-daily regimens of lopinavir/ritonavir for HIV infection. Ther Drug Monit 2004;26:516−23.

[90] Veldkamp AI, et al. Limited sampling strategies for the estimation of the systemic exposure to the HIV-1 nonnucleoside reverse transcriptase inhibitor nevirapine. Ther Drug Monit 2001;23:606−11.

INDIVIDUALIZING TUBERCULOSIS THERAPY

15

S. Goutelle and P. Maire

CHAPTER OUTLINE

15.1 INTRODUCTION: THE WHO AND PUBLIC HEALTH APPROACH TO ANTI-TB DRUG DOSING: ONE-SIZE-FITS-ALL

About 70 years after the first clinical trial that investigated the use of streptomycin in tuberculosis (TB) and more than 40 years after the introduction of the so-called short-course chemotherapy [1], the global burden of TB is still considerable worldwide. In 2013, the World Health Organization (WHO) estimated that 9 million people developed TB, and 1.5 million died from the disease. Most TB cases occur in Asia (56%) and Africa (29%). HIV-infected patients represent approximately 13% and 25% of new TB cases and deaths in these areas, respectively [2].

The rationale for the treatment of drug-susceptible TB is based on the results of clinical investigations conducted between the mid-1940s and mid-1980s, which have been nicely reviewed by Fox et al. [3]. Those clinical trials have proven the overall efficacy of the so-called short-course combination chemotherapy of TB that is still in use today.

Individualized Drug Therapy for Patients. DOI: http://dx.doi.org/10.1016/B978-0-12-803348-7.00015-0

Table 15.1 Daily Dose of First-Line Antituberculosis Drugs Recommended by the World Health Organization (WHO) in Adult Patients

Drug	Daily Dose (Range) in mg/kg of Body Weight	Maximum Dose (mg)
Isoniazid	5 (4–6)	300
Rifampicin	10 (8–12)	600
Pyrazinamide	25 (20–30)	–
Ethambutol	15 (15–20)	–

The current standard short-course recommended by the WHO for new patients with drug-susceptible pulmonary TB is as follows:

1. A 2-month intensive phase with HRZE: isoniazid (H), rifampicin (or rifampin, R), pyrazinamide (Z), and ethambutol (E).
2. A 4-month continuation phase with HR.

The WHO-recommended doses of HRZE [4] are presented in Table 15.1. The doses are expressed in mg/kg. Body weight is currently the only covariate that is taken into account to individualize anti-tubercular (anti-TB) drug doses. It is noteworthy that doses of isoniazid and rifampicin are capped at 300 and 600 mg/day, respectively, without any justification. That means, though, that a maximum dose of 300 mg of isoniazid is only 4.3 mg/kg for a 70-kg person and that a maximum rifampin dose of 600 mg is only 8.6 mg/kg for a similar patient, as in Table 15.1, all of which sounds somewhat arbitrary.

The drugs should be administered daily. A thrice-weekly regimen (with increased doses) is considered an acceptable alternative provided that the drug intake is directly observed and the patient is unlikely to be coinfected with HIV.

Since 2006 the WHO has carried out a global plan to stop TB [5], notably based on directly observed therapy (DOT). It should be acknowledged that the fight against TB coordinated by the WHO has been fairly successful in reducing TB burden (ie, TB morbidity and mortality), as TB prevalence and mortality rate fell by an estimated 41% and 45% between 1990 and 2013, respectively [2]. However the efficacy of TB treatment still remains suboptimal.

It has long been stated that the effectiveness of the 6-month treatment regimen of TB was excellent, as the seminal clinical trials showed relapse rates as low as 2–5% [1,3]. However, these numbers, obtained from studies performed in the 1970s and 1980s, do not reflect the reality and diversity of what happens in practice today. In 2012 the WHO reported an average success rate of 86%, success being defined as cure or treatment completion. Treatment success substantially varies across regions, with rates as low as 69% and 72% in Russia and Brazil, respectively. However the actual cure rate might be even much lower. Recent randomized controlled trials have reported cure rates of DOT as low as 64% in Pakistan [6] and 76% in Thailand [7].

Drug resistance is also a crucial issue in TB control. In 2013 an estimated of 3.5% of new cases, but fully 20.5% of previously treated cases, were multidrug-resistant TB (MDR-TB). MDR is defined as resistance to both isoniazid and rifampicin, which are the most bactericidal drugs in the reference combination therapy.

Extensively drug-resistant TB (XDR-TB) has also emerged as a major threat in the last decade. It is defined as resistance to isoniazid and rifampicin, plus at least one fluoroquinolone and at least one second-line injectable drug (ie, amikacin, kanamycin, or capreomycin). XDR-TB cases have been reported in more than 100 countries. In 2013, about 9% of MDR-TB cases were actually XDR. Resistance rates are especially high in Eastern Europe and Central Asia where MDR may represent more than 20% of new cases (Belarus, Kazakhstan, and Moldova) and XDR accounts for more than 20% of cases in some countries (Georgia, Lithuania, and Kazakhstan) [2]. Data on drug resistance are unavailable in many countries [2].

Treatment of MDR- or XDR-TB requires the use of at least five agents based on the results of drug susceptibility testing. Such treatment is long (at least 18−24 months), very expensive, and poorly tolerated. Drugs used in MDR and XDR drug regimens include old oral anti-TB drugs (eg, ethionamide, *para*-aminosalicylic acid), injectable drugs (aminoglycosides), fluoroquinolones (eg, moxifloxacin, levofloxacin) and new agents such as bedaquiline, which was approved in the United States in late 2012. Those drugs often cause adverse drug reactions, including nephrotoxicity, hearing loss, neuropathy, and severe cutaneous reactions [8].

As recently pointed out by Alsultan and Peloquin, if the current regimen and dosages of anti-TB drugs were fully adequate, treatment failure and the observed increase of resistance should not be happening [9]. Although the WHO strategy has strongly contributed to the global decrease in TB burden, there is a body of data suggesting that the "one-size-fits-all" approach to drug dosing is not optimal, that patients may be developing resistance on these dosage regimens, and that patients may benefit from dose individualization of anti-TB drugs.

15.2 THE RATIONALE FOR DOSE INDIVIDUALIZATION OF ANTI-TB DRUGS

15.2.1 PHARMACOKINETIC VARIABILITY

Large interindividual pharmacokinetic (PK) variability has been described for most anti-TB drugs. As an example, Fig. 15.1 shows the distribution of isoniazid concentrations in plasma and the lung epithelial lining fluid (ELF) measured in 80 subjects without TB [10].

A 10- to 20-fold variation in isoniazid or isonicotinylhydrazide (INH) levels was observed in those subjects, all of whom received the same INH dose. The variability was even greater in lung than in plasma. Large variability in plasma and pulmonary exposure has been reported for other agents including rifampicin [11,12], pyrazinamide [13,14], ethambutol [15], and fluoroquinolones [16]. Variability in the oral absorption of anti-TB drugs appears to be an important determinant of overall variability [12,14,17]. Some special populations, notably HIV-infected patients and patients with diabetes mellitus, may have poor absorption of anti-TB drugs [18,19].

For rifampicin, intraindividual variability in drug clearance, due to enzymatic autoinduction, is also an important PK characteristic. Rifampin induces its own metabolism, which results in a progressive increase in its clearance and a decrease in drug exposure after the first weeks of therapy. The reduction in rifampin area under curve (AUC) may range from 40% to 80% after 3 weeks of therapy [20]. It is most surprising to note that this significant change in rifampicin drug clearance has never been taken into account to adjust rifampicin dosage during such prolonged treatment.

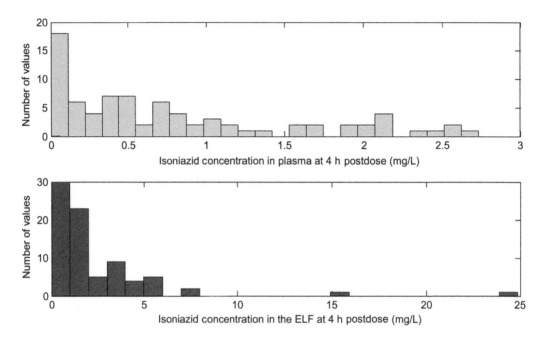

FIGURE 15.1

Histograms of isoniazid concentrations measured in plasma and epithelial lining fluid (ELF) in 80 subjects.
All subjects received 300 mg of oral isoniazid once daily for 5 days. Isoniazid concentration in plasma and ELF
was measured 4 h after the fifth dose.

*Data are from Conte JE, Jr., Golden JA, McQuitty M, Kipps J, Duncan S, McKenna E, et al. Effects of gender, AIDS, and acetylator
status on intrapulmonary concentrations of isoniazid. Antimicrob Agents Chemother 2002;46(8):2358–64.*

Because of PK variability, when patients are given the same dose of anti-TB drugs, even on a
mg/kg basis, great variability in drug exposure is observed [21]. Such variability is generally
ignored in current fixed dosing guidelines, while it clearly affects treatment outcome (see below).

Because of such variability in a significant proportion of patients, the concentrations of anti-TB
drugs associated with the standard doses are often too low; that is, lower than the expected
values [22]. There have been many reports of low anti-TB drug concentrations [18,19,21,23–26], indicating that the standard doses cannot ensure achieving a standard adequate exposure in all individuals.

15.2.2 PHARMACODYNAMIC VARIABILITY

Susceptible strains of *Mycobacterium tuberculosis* do not exhibit much variation in minimum
inhibitory concentrations (MICs). In a study of more than 7900 clinical isolates of *M. tuberculosis*
in the Netherlands, 90–95% of MIC values fell within three $\log_2$ dilutions (ie, an eightfold
range) [27]. However, if the MIC is included in a PK/PD objective such as a target C_{max}/MIC or
AUC/MIC ratio (as discussed next), such variation in susceptibility should be taken into account,
as a twofold increase in drug exposure would be required to compensate for a twofold increase in
MIC, for example [28].

Just as with PK variability, variability in *M. tuberculosis* MIC is currently not taken into account in designing the drug doses. However, it would make good sense. For patients infected with very susceptible strains, smaller doses of drugs would be sufficient and perhaps safer, while more aggressive doses may well be required for patients with poorly susceptible strains in order to eradicate the microorganisms.

15.2.3 PHARMACOKINETIC–PHARMACODYNAMIC RELATIONSHIPS

A major argument supporting the dose individualization of anti-TB drugs is that quantitative PK/PD relationships have now been described for most anti-TB agents. The amount of experimental and clinical data supporting these relationships is considerable. These data will be briefly summarized here. More details can be found in reviews from our group [29] and others [30,31].

For rifampicin, its bactericidal effect has been shown to be exposure-dependent, that is, the effect correlates with the AUC_{24}/MIC ratio, the relationship being described by a nonlinear sigmoidal relationship (Hill equation). This has been shown in cultures of *M. tuberculosis*, inside macrophages, and in mice [32,33]. In humans, rifampicin AUC has also been shown to correlate with early bactericidal activity [30,34], and low exposure has been identified as a significant predictor of poor outcome (microbiologic failure, relapse, or death) of standard combination therapy in a study from Pasipanodya et al. [26]. In addition, in vitro data have shown that rifampicin postantibiotic effect and prevention of resistance were also exposure dependent, but those responses were most closely linked to C_{max}/MIC ratio [33].

Isoniazid microbial kill and prevention of resistance have been shown to correlate with both the AUC_{24}/MIC and C_{max}/MIC ratios [35,36]. In patients, Donald et al. have shown a linear correlation between INH early bactericidal activity and the natural logarithm of the AUC [37]. Low isoniazid AUC was also a predictor of poor outcome in the study from Pasipanodya et al. [26].

For pyrazinamide, in vitro data have shown that the PK/PD relationships were different for the microbial kill (linked to AUC_{24}/MIC) on the one hand and resistance suppression (linked to the percentage of time spent above the MIC, $T >_{MIC}$) on the other [38]. In clinical studies, low pyrazinamide C_{max} [21] and AUC_{24} [26] have been significant predictors of poor outcome of combination therapy.

The bactericidal effect of ethambutol was also linked to AUC_{24}/MIC, while acquisition of resistance appears to correlate with $T >_{MIC}$ in vitro, as a somewhat higher proportion of resistance was observed for once weekly regimens compared with daily regimens, despite similar total AUC [39].

Finally, for quinolone agents, both microbial kill and prevention of resistance were linked to the AUC_{24}/MIC ratio in vitro [40,41]. However the global effect was a double effect, as levels of exposure associated with a good bactericidal effect were also associated with maximum amplification of drug resistance. This is probably due to the amplification of a drug-resistant subpopulation that may preexist in the inoculum.

To summarize, quantitative nonlinear Hill relationships between drug exposure (AUC, C_{max}, or T_{MIC}) and both bactericidal effect and suppression of drug resistance have been described for most anti-TB drugs. Those relationships provide the rationale for setting a target peak serum concentration or a target exposure to be achieved to optimize efficacy and/or minimize the emergence of drug resistance; for example, AUC_{24}, or C_{max} associated with 90% of maximal effect, for a given MIC.

Fewer data are available regarding the relationship between drug PK and toxicity. It has been shown that isoniazid hepatotoxicity, ethambutol-induced visual disturbances, and moxifloxacin-induced QT prolongation are all exposure-dependent effects. However, no specific target of "safe" exposure has been derived. Further research is necessary to better understand this point. A recent study has shown a quantitative relationship between amikacin cumulative AUC and ototoxicity in patients treated for MDR-TB [42]. This is a motivating example.

15.2.4 CONCLUSION: ONE SIZE CANNOT FIT ALL

As a consequence of variability in the PK and MIC of anti-TB drugs, and the existence of quantitative exposure-effect relationships, different individual patients cannot have the same exposure and thus the same effect from a given "one-size-fits-all" dosage regimen. Fig. 15.2 summarizes the concepts presented in this chapter. It shows the exposure—effect relationships of rifampicin presented

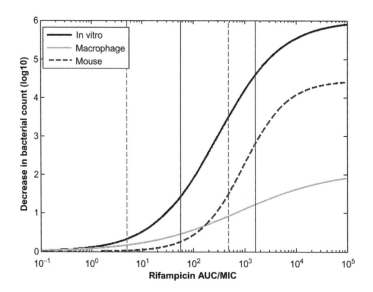

FIGURE 15.2

Rifampicin exposure—effect relationships. The three curves display the decrease in the counts of *Mycobacterium tuberculosis* H37Rv as a function of rifampicin AUC/MIC ratio in vitro, within macrophages and in the mouse model. The exposure—effect curves obtained in vitro and in macrophages are thought to reflect the best possible effect of rifampicin on extracellular bacteria in pulmonary ELF and on intracellular bacteria in alveolar cells, respectively. The curve from the mouse model may be viewed as an "in between," mixed effect, similar to the overall effect on the total bacterial load in humans. The vertical lines show the 5th and 95th percentiles of the distribution of AUC_{24}/MIC in the ELF (dashed red lines) and in alveolar cells (solid blue lines) for the standard 600-mg dose of rifampicin. Data are from a previous simulation study from our group [43]. A fixed MIC of 0.2 mg/L was selected, which is the most frequently observed value in clinical isolates [27]. Original data and curve equations are from Jayaram R, Gaonkar S, Kaur P, Suresh BL, Mahesh BN, Jayashree R, et al. Pharmacokinetics-pharmacodynamics of rifampicin in an aerosol infection model of tuberculosis. Antimicrob Agents Chemother 2003;47(7):2118—24.

above and a simulated distribution of pulmonary rifampicin AUC/MIC values associated with the current recommended dose of 600 mg of rifampicin [43], for a MIC of 0.2 mg/L.

This figure clearly shows that for a significant proportion of subjects, rifampicin exposures in lungs are in the lowest part of the exposure—effect curves and thus are clearly suboptimal.

In addition, there is both experimental and clinical evidence supporting the role of PK variability in acquired drug resistance and treatment failure [44,45]. These are additional arguments for the need to better control targeted drug exposure with individualized dosage regimens.

One might suggest that we could simply use higher doses of anti-TB drugs to optimize efficacy. While this strategy might make sense for some agents (eg, the rifamycins), it may not be clinically appropriate for others at the population level, because of exposure-dependent adverse drug reactions. For example, isoniazid hepatotoxicity, ethambutol induced visual disturbances, and moxifloxacin-induced QT prolongation are all exposure-dependent reactions [29]. For such drugs, the use of higher doses would increase the risk of such severe adverse drug reactions. In our opinion, this is only acceptable at the individual level, if the expected benefit outweighs the expected risk. Also, in some patients infected with very susceptible *M. tuberculosis* (low MIC), such higher doses would be unnecessary.

The only way to deal with both PK/PD variability and the need to hit a desired target exposure is to individualize drug dosing for each patient, according to that patient's PK characteristics and those of the infecting organism.

15.3 HOW TO INDIVIDUALIZE ANTI-TB DRUG REGIMENS

15.3.1 GENOTYPING

Among TB drugs, isoniazid is the main candidate for genotype-based dose individualization. Isoniazid is metabolized mainly by hepatic *N*-acetyltransferase 2 (NAT2) into an acetylated derivative having no anti-TB activity. Fast (F) and slow (S) alleles coding for NAT2 have been described. The elimination phenotype and NAT2 genotype are concordant, and three acetylator types may be distinguished: fast (homozygous FF), intermediate (heterozygous FS), and slow (homozygous SS) [46,47].

A genotype-based dose adjustment has been proposed for isoniazid, which is actually a modern development of phenotype-based dosing approach based on acetylation testing such as the method developed by Vivien et al. [48].

Because most INH activity in combination therapy occurs in the early days [49], Donald et al. have proposed genotype-based dosing of isoniazid to optimize the early bactericidal activity of this drug. At the standard dose of 5 mg/kg, they estimated that the probabilities of achieving an INH exposure associated with 90% of maximal EBA were 100%, in homozygous slow acetylators and 96.3% in heterozygous fast acetylators, but only 25% in homozygous fast acetylators.

In slow acetylators, a 3-mg/kg dose would be sufficient to achieve 100% target attainment (and might be safer than the current recommended dose in this group), while homozygous fast acetylators would need at least 6-mg/kg of INH to ensure the same efficacy [50]. Similarly, Kinzig-Shippers et al. have suggested doses of 2.5, 5, and 7.5 mg/kg to achieve similar INH exposure in homozygous slow, heterozygous fast, and homozygous fast acetylators, respectively [51].

However, because genetics only explain part of INH PK variability, and because there is significant overlap in the distribution of PK parameters such as half-life between fast and slow acetylators, genotype-based dosing is not the most accurate dosing approach available. Indeed, genotyping turns out to be simply another way to classify the drug PK into groups, while it is much more useful clinically to monitor drug concentrations and quantify the PK for optimal individualization of therapy. Genotyping, and other methods that look for covariates rather than observing directly the behavior of the drug, miss the opportunity to track the actual behavior of the drug in each patient, which also takes into account all the effects of all the potential drug interactions and genetic effects we have not discovered yet. Tracking the drug behavior itself lets us study and control the disposition of the drug, and its response to all the known and yet unknown factors responsible for its behavior rather than only considering the effect of only a single covariate [52].

15.3.2 THERAPEUTIC DRUG MONITORING (TDM) OF ANTI-TB DRUGS

Because the antimicrobial effect and, for some agents, resistance suppression are exposure dependent, monitoring concentrations of anti-TB drugs in individual patients appears to be a useful approach to individualize drug regimens and make them more effective.

Peloquin has been an active researcher in this field in the last 20 years. His reviews provide comprehensive data on why and how to perform TDM of anti-TB drugs [9,22]. So far, TDM of anti-TB drugs has not yet been recommended in all patients, but it has been suggested as a useful approach in patients who are slow to respond to treatment (ie, with sputum smear cultures still positive after 2 months); to manage drug–drug interactions, especially with antiretroviral drugs used in patients coinfected with HIV; and in patients who often show poor drug absorption, such as patients infected with HIV or patients with diabetes [9].

Because the half-life of some anti-TB drugs (isoniazid, rifampicin) is short, monitoring trough concentration can be poorly informative, if detectable. It has been recommended to collect a sample at about 2 h postdose to get a reasonable estimate of the peak for most drugs when given orally, and a second sample at about 6–7 h postdose to detect possible delayed absorption and to track information of the drug elimination. Of note, these recommended sampling times are empirical and are not based on optimal sampling theories. Those may be useful in the TDM of anti-TB drugs [53]. Table 15.2 shows the expected values of C_{max} for major anti-TB drugs. More details can be found in the original publications of Peloquin [9,22].

For some drugs, recent studies have identified a threshold of exposure associated with a favorable outcome in combination therapy. In a cohort of 225 patients treated in Botswana, Chideya and colleagues have observed that low pyrazinamide C_{max} (<35 mg/L, median dose, 35 mg/kg) was a significant predictor of poor combination therapy outcome, defined as treatment failure or death during treatment. After adjustment for other factors, patients with pyrazinamide $C_{max}<35$ mg/L were three times more likely to have poor outcomes than patients with $C_{max} \geq 35$ mg/L.

The predictive value of pyrazinamide exposure was confirmed by Pasipanodya and colleagues in a study in 142 patients in South Africa [26]. Pyrazinamide C_{max} was the most important predictor of 2-month sputum culture conversion, with a cutoff estimated at 58 mg/L. Patients with pyrazinamide C_{max} greater than this value had a sevenfold greater probability of treatment success compared to those who had C_{max} below this value.

In addition, low pyrazinamide exposure was the most important predictor of poor long-term outcome (failure, relapse, or death up to 2 years), with a pyrazinamide AUC_{24} breakpoint estimated at 363 mg·h/L. The rate of good outcome was 80% in patients with pyrazinamide AUC_{24} above this threshold, compared to only 55% in patients with pyrazinamide AUC_{24} below this value.

Table 15.2 Usual and Target Exposures for First-Line Anti-TB Drugs and Fluoroquinolones

Drug	Usual Adult Daily Dose	Usual C_{max} (mg/L)[a]	Usual T_{max} (h)[a]	Usual AUC_{24} Range (mg · h/L)[b]	Target Exposure Based on Clinical Evidence[c]
Isoniazid	300 mg 4–5 mg/kg	3–6	0.75–2	4–32	
Rifampicin	600 mg 10 mg/kg	8–24	2–4	5–140	$AUC_{24} > 13$ mg · h/L
Ethambutol	20–25 mg/kg	2–6	2–3	14–86	
Pyrazinamide	1500 mg 25–35 mg/kg	20–60	1–2	270–680	$C_{max} \geq 35$ mg/L $AUC_{24} > 363$ mg · h/L
Levofloxacin	500–1000 mg	8–13	1–2	100–360	
Moxifloxacin	400 mg	3–5	1–2	15–84	

[a]Adapted from Alsultan A, Peloquin CA. Therapeutic drug monitoring in the treatment of tuberculosis: an update. Drugs 2014;74 (8):839–54. Epub 2014/05/23.
[b]Adapted from Peloquin CA, Hadad DJ, Molino LP, Palaci M, Boom WH, Dietze R, et al. Population pharmacokinetics of levofloxacin, gatifloxacin, and moxifloxacin in adults with pulmonary tuberculosis. Antimicrob Agents Chemother 2008;52 (3):852–7; Peloquin CA, Jaresko GS, Yong CL, Keung AC, Bulpitt AE, Jelliffe RW. Population pharmacokinetic modeling of isoniazid, rifampin, and pyrazinamide. Antimicrob Agents Chemother 1997;41(12):2670–9; Magis-Escurra C, Later-Nijland HM, Alffenaar JW, Broeders J, Burger DM, van Crevel R, et al. Population pharmacokinetics and limited sampling strategy for first-line tuberculosis drugs and moxifloxacin. Int J Antimicrob Agents 2014;44(3):229–34. Epub 2014/07/06..
[c]Adapted from Chideya S, Winston CA, Peloquin CA, Bradford WZ, Hopewell PC, Wells CD, et al. Isoniazid, rifampin, ethambutol, and pyrazinamide pharmacokinetics and treatment outcomes among a predominantly HIV-infected cohort of adults with tuberculosis from Botswana. Clin Infect Dis 2009;48(12):1685–94; Pasipanodya JG, McIlleron H, Burger A, Wash PA, Smith P, Gumbo T. Serum drug concentrations predictive of pulmonary tuberculosis outcomes. J Infect Dis 2013;208(9):1464–73. Epub 2013/08/01.

Rifampicin $AUC_{24} \leq 13$ mg/L was identified as an additional predictor of poor clinical outcome in patients with pyrazinamide AUC_{24} over 363 mg/L, as well as isoniazid $AUC_{24} \leq 52$ mg/L in patients with pyrazinamide AUC_{24} over 363 mg/L in combination with rifampicin AUC over 13 mg · h/L. Overall, more than 91% of patients with poor clinical outcome received at least one of these three drugs with a low AUC.

As a result, breakpoint values of AUC_{24} identified in that study [26] may serve as target values to optimize clinical response to TB treatment, at least for pyrazinamide and rifampicin. In our opinion, the breakpoint value identified for isoniazid AUC_{24} may not be relevant because it was the third and least important predictor of outcome in the regression tree analysis performed by this group, and so its value, which is very high [54], may hold true only for a small group of patients. Also, it is noteworthy that individual MIC values were not available in either of the studies from Chideya and Pasipanodya.

Because AUC is emerging as the PK index linked to antimicrobial and clinical effect of several anti-TB drugs, it appears desirable to estimate it in clinical practice. As with other drugs, a noncompartmental estimation of AUC is virtually impossible in routine practice as it requires many concentration measurements within a dose interval. Equations based on limited sampling strategies at fixed sampling times have been proposed to estimate the AUC of first-line anti-TB drugs [55]. It has been suggested that samples taken at 1, 4, and 6 h postdose would provide the best estimation of the AUC of first-line anti-TB drugs simultaneously. Although this approach is interesting, it is not at all flexible, as the proposed equations cannot be used if the predefined sampling times are not closely respected, and they are not directly linked to the subsequent dosage regimens required to hit a desired target most precisely. That is a major weakness of such limited sampling strategies that are designed simply to estimate an AUC.

15.3.3 BAYESIAN DOSE INDIVIDUALIZATION

As with other drug classes presented in this book, it is possible to perform Bayesian individualization of anti-TB drug regimens. The general principles of the approach apply [56]. One can estimate the individual PK parameters of anti-TB drugs based on a population PK model and the observed concentrations in individual patients, derive good individual estimates of PK quantities of interest such as C_{max} or AUC_{24}, and finally calculate an individualized dosage regimen to hit a target drug concentration or exposure.

Parametric and nonparametric population PK models are available for the major anti-TB drugs from the literature [12,17,54,57] and may be implemented in dosing software such as the BestDose clinical software for maximally precise dosage regimens (available at www.lapk.org).

The general advantages of the Bayesian individualized approach hold just as true for anti-TB drugs as they do for any other drug:

1. Bayesian estimation can be performed with only a single measured concentration, although more are better for optimal individualization.
2. There is no need to wait for the steady state to interpret the results correctly and simulate a future regimen.
3. Dose adjustment can be computed precisely based on the model equations, while this can only be done judgmentally by the physician using the raw TDM data alone.
4. The entire individual PK profile of serum concentrations can be calculated, and therefore also the patient's individual AUC, which is the PK quantity linked to the effect for most anti-TB agents; this can be directly compared with the patient's clinical behavior during this time, and a desired target goal can be selected on clinical grounds and a dosage regimen developed to hit it with maximum precision.
5. Samples can be taken at any time and that time can be accurately recorded to the nearest minute using military time. Furthermore, these samples may be obtained over several dosing intervals. AUCs can be easily obtained. This flexibility is desirable in routine clinical practice, and it is also an advantage over the regression equations based on limited sampling strategies discussed earlier in this chapter.

Unfortunately, Bayesian methods of dose adjustment appear to have been little used in optimizing TB therapy. To our knowledge, no study has yet evaluated the potential benefits of this approach in TB patients. Such work may well be expected to yield useful data and improved therapeutic outcomes, as has been the case in many other areas of drug therapy as discussed in the other chapters in this book.

15.4 CONCLUSIONS

Dosage regimens recommended by the WHO and public health agencies for treating both drug-usceptible and drug-resistant TB consist of fixed doses or doses adjusted to body weight. This "one-size-fits-all" dosing approach has had the major advantage of being simple and thus easily applicable worldwide. However the individual patient becomes lost in the masses that are treated this way.

The public health, fixed-dose approach ignores important determinants of the response to treatment, including the large PK variability in the PK of anti-TB drugs, variability in *M. tuberculosis* susceptibility to drugs (MIC), and the existence of quantitative exposure−effect relationships.

However major progress has been made in the knowledge of those determinants in the last 15 years. In particular, quantitative relationships between anti-TB drug exposure (eg, AUC_{24} or C_{max}) and antimicrobial effect, emergence of resistance, and clinical outcome itself have been determined and now can provide rational target values to be selected and achieved for patients. Those advances strongly suggest that individualization of anti-TB drug therapy should be useful to improve patients' response to treatment and to minimize further development of resistance.

Very importantly, PK variability of single anti-TB drugs has been shown to influence the clinical outcome of combination therapy [21,26,45]. Thus, one should not think that combination therapy can necessarily compensate for poor dosing of individual drugs. Because of this, it is important that we should optimize the use of each agent.

The translation of PK/PD concepts into clinical practice requires methods to monitor and control the PK/PD response to anti-TB drugs not just for populations of patients, but especially for each individual patient.

The first thing we suggest is to determine the MIC of each clinical isolate of *M. tuberculosis* from each patient. This is the job of microbiology laboratories that are already aided by the WHO within its Stop TB strategy [5]. If the MIC is not available yet (eg, at the start of therapy) or cannot be determined, one should use the most probable value, based on the local microbial epidemiology (MIC distribution).

Then, one should monitor the patient's therapy using TDM, collect individual PK data, model the drug behavior, and derive the quantities (AUC_{24}, C_{max}) linked to the response. Currently the optimal way to do this is to perform TDM combined with Bayesian estimation of PK parameters. Finally, one has to calculate the optimal dosage of drugs to reach predefined targets (AUC_{24}/MIC, C_{max}/MIC, or anything else). Population PK models, especially nonparametric models, and clinical software are available to implement this Bayesian approach to achieve optimally individualized dosing for each patient.

This integration of MIC values and drug concentration measurements in Bayesian individualization of dosage regimens of anti-TB drugs has been recently advocated by the group led by Gumbo [58]. We totally agree with their views. The individualized approach may also lead to doses of drugs that are significantly lower (in case of infection with a low MIC strain and/or slow drug elimination) or significantly greater (if the MIC of the isolate and/or drug clearance is high) than the current standards. While the use of individualized doses may raise concerns about the tolerance of some anti-TB drugs (for example, pyrazinamide), this approach is actually the most reasonable way to deal with the issue of drug toxicity. It can prevent unnecessary high drug exposure in patients who only need small doses to get the desired response. It may also be most useful to monitor both the disease response and concentration-dependent toxicities when high doses appear necessary in other individuals, by controlling the drug exposure most precisely [59], in combination with careful clinical monitoring.

Ideally, optimal individualized dosage regimens of anti-TB drugs should take into account toxicity in addition to efficacy and prevention of resistance. As pointed out above, available data on anti-TB drug toxicity are not sufficient to derive quantitative relationships between drug PK and adverse drug reactions and define the upper limits for safe exposure. Further research on this point is needed. Today, toxicity of anti-TB drugs remains poorly predictable from drug exposure, and clinical monitoring is always the best way to deal with this issue in individual patients.

As pointed out by Srivastava and Gumbo [58], the main barriers to the development of individual dosing approaches of TB drugs are apparent complexity and cost. Because the world TB burden is mostly born by low-income countries with limited health care systems, our suggestions may sound unrealistic. While individualized therapy may not yet be economically feasible in such low-income countries, it is entirely realistic and certainly can begin in the more developed areas. As the world develops, in future years, it may well be possible for this approach to spread further into these presently underserved areas. In addition, technical progress, such as dried blood spots for measurement of drug concentrations [60] may help. Obviously, the main solution to the problem is money. What is needed to develop this dosing approach is support to develop TDM laboratories, similar to what has been done for microbiology laboratories within the WHO Stop TB program.

Complexity and sophisticated mathematics are not the real issue. The use of PK/PD concepts and easy-to-use Bayesian PK software currently available on laptop computers in clinical practice simply requires proper training of users, like any other technique in medicine. This activity can be centralized, with reference centers performing it for a defined geographical area, just as transplant therapy is now individualized by a central reference service over the web for many areas of France. This very well-used approach is discussed in the chapter on transplantation.

Finally, as pointed out again by Gumbo's group [58], dose individualization and PK/PD-based optimization of TB therapy may well be cost-effective, considering the cost of lost lives, and of retreatment and treatment of secondary resistant TB cases that the individualized approach can help to prevent.

To conclude, dose individualization of anti-TB drugs is a rational approach that should improve the outcome of TB therapy. This approach is similar to what has been proposed and largely applied in practice for many other antimicrobial agents [61], as well as for many other drugs discussed in this book.

However, TB treatment has been rigidly standardized and coordinated at the international level by the WHO, in spite of the increasing scientific evidence supporting individualization of anti-TB dosage drug regimens. We are concerned that the fixed-dose paradigm in TB treatment is unlikely to change unless major clinical evidence shows the superiority of another dosing approach. There is an urgent need for clinical trials comparing individualized, goal-oriented, model-based dosages versus fixed-dose regimens of anti-TB drugs. It would be a great thing for the world when we can change from the fixed-dose approach, where the individual is nothing, to an individualized approach where the individual is everything, as he or she truly should be.

REFERENCES

[1] Mitchison DA. The diagnosis and therapy of tuberculosis during the past 100 years. Am J Respir Crit Care Med 2005;171(7):699−706.

[2] World Health Organization. Global Tuberculosis Report 2014. Geneva: World Health Organization; 2014 WHO/HTM/TB/2014.08.

[3] Fox W, Ellard GA, Mitchison DA. Studies on the treatment of tuberculosis undertaken by the British Medical Research Council tuberculosis units, 1946−1986, with relevant subsequent publications. Int J Tuberc Lung Dis 1999;3(10 Suppl. 2):S231−79.

[4] World Health Organization. Treatment of tuberculosis: guidelines for national programmes. 4th ed. Geneva: World Health Organization; 2009.

[5] World Health Organization. The STOP TB Strategy. Geneva: World Health Organization. 2006 WHO/HTM/TB/2006.368.

[6] Walley JD, Khan MA, Newell JN, Khan MH. Effectiveness of the direct observation component of DOTS for tuberculosis: a randomised controlled trial in Pakistan. Lancet 2001;357(9257):664−9.

[7] Kamolratanakul P, Sawert H, Lertmaharit S, Kasetjaroen Y, Akksilp S, Tulaporn C, et al. Randomized controlled trial of directly observed treatment (DOT) for patients with pulmonary tuberculosis in Thailand. Trans R Soc Trop Med Hyg 1999;93(5):552−7.

[8] Shin SS, Pasechnikov AD, Gelmanova IY, Peremitin GG, Strelis AK, Mishustin S, et al. Adverse reactions among patients being treated for MDR-TB in Tomsk, Russia. Int J Tuberc Lung Dis 2007;11(12):1314−20. Epub 2007/11/24.

[9] Alsultan A, Peloquin CA. Therapeutic drug monitoring in the treatment of tuberculosis: an update. Drugs 2014;74(8):839−54. Epub 2014/05/23.

[10] Conte Jr. JE, Golden JA, McQuitty M, Kipps J, Duncan S, McKenna E, et al. Effects of gender, AIDS, and acetylator status on intrapulmonary concentrations of isoniazid. Antimicrob Agents Chemother 2002;46(8):2358−64.

[11] Conte JE, Golden JA, Kipps JE, Lin ET, Zurlinden E. Effect of sex and AIDS status on the plasma and intrapulmonary pharmacokinetics of rifampicin. Clin Pharmacokinet 2004;43(6):395−404.

[12] Wilkins JJ, Savic RM, Karlsson MO, Langdon G, McIlleron H, Pillai G, et al. Population pharmacokinetics of rifampin in pulmonary tuberculosis patients, including a semimechanistic model to describe variable absorption. Antimicrob Agents Chemother 2008;52(6):2138−48.

[13] Conte Jr. JE, Golden JA, Duncan S, McKenna E, Zurlinden E. Intrapulmonary concentrations of pyrazinamide. Antimicrob Agents Chemother 1999;43(6):1329−33.

[14] Wilkins JJ, Langdon G, McIlleron H, Pillai GC, Smith PJ, Simonsson US. Variability in the population pharmacokinetics of pyrazinamide in South African tuberculosis patients. Eur J Clin Pharmacol 2006;62(9):727−35.

[15] Conte Jr. JE, Golden JA, Kipps J, Lin ET, Zurlinden E. Effects of AIDS and gender on steady-state plasma and intrapulmonary ethambutol concentrations. Antimicrob Agents Chemother 2001;45(10):2891−6.

[16] Peloquin CA, Hadad DJ, Molino LP, Palaci M, Boom WH, Dietze R, et al. Population pharmacokinetics of levofloxacin, gatifloxacin, and moxifloxacin in adults with pulmonary tuberculosis. Antimicrob Agents Chemother 2008;52(3):852−7.

[17] Wilkins JJ, Langdon G, McIlleron H, Pillai G, Smith PJ, Simonsson US. Variability in the population pharmacokinetics of isoniazid in South African tuberculosis patients. Br J Clin Pharmacol 2011;72(1):51−62. Epub 2011/02/16.

[18] Peloquin CA, Nitta AT, Burman WJ, Brudney KF, Miranda-Massari JR, McGuinness ME, et al. Low antituberculosis drug concentrations in patients with AIDS. Ann Pharmacother 1996;30(9):919−25.

[19] Sahai J, Gallicano K, Swick L, Tailor S, Garber G, Seguin I, et al. Reduced plasma concentrations of antituberculosis drugs in patients with HIV infection. Ann Intern Med 1997;127(4):289−93.

[20] Smythe W, Khandelwal A, Merle C, Rustomjee R, Gninafon M, Bocar Lo M, et al. A semimechanistic pharmacokinetic-enzyme turnover model for rifampin autoinduction in adult tuberculosis patients. Antimicrob Agents Chemother 2012;56(4):2091−8. Epub 2012/01/19.

[21] Chideya S, Winston CA, Peloquin CA, Bradford WZ, Hopewell PC, Wells CD, et al. Isoniazid, rifampin, ethambutol, and pyrazinamide pharmacokinetics and treatment outcomes among a predominantly HIV-infected cohort of adults with tuberculosis from Botswana. Clin Infect Dis 2009;48(12):1685−94.

[22] Peloquin CA. Therapeutic drug monitoring in the treatment of tuberculosis. Drugs 2002;62(15):2169−83.

[23] Kimerling ME, Phillips P, Patterson P, Hall M, Robinson CA, Dunlap NE. Low serum antimycobacterial drug levels in non-HIV-infected tuberculosis patients. Chest 1998;113(5):1178−83.

[24] Mehta JB, Shantaveerapa H, Byrd Jr. RP, Morton SE, Fountain F, Roy TM. Utility of rifampin blood levels in the treatment and follow-up of active pulmonary tuberculosis in patients who werè slow to respond to routine directly observed therapy. Chest 2001;120(5):1520−4.

[25] van Crevel R, Alisjahbana B, de Lange WC, Borst F, Danusantoso H, van der Meer JW, et al. Low plasma concentrations of rifampicin in tuberculosis patients in Indonesia. Int J Tuberc Lung Dis 2002;6(6):497−502.

[26] Pasipanodya JG, McIlleron H, Burger A, Wash PA, Smith P, Gumbo T. Serum drug concentrations predictive of pulmonary tuberculosis outcomes. J Infect Dis 2013;208(9):1464−73. Epub 2013/08/01.

[27] van Klingeren B, Dessens-Kroon M, van der Laan T, Kremer K, van Soolingen D. Drug susceptibility testing of *Mycobacterium tuberculosis* complex by use of a high-throughput, reproducible, absolute concentration method. J Clin Microbiol 2007;45(8):2662−8. Epub 2007/06/01.

[28] Gumbo T. New susceptibility breakpoints for first-line antituberculosis drugs based on antimicrobial pharmacokinetic/pharmacodynamic science and population pharmacokinetic variability. Antimicrob Agents Chemother 2010;54(4):1484−91.

[29] Goutelle S, Bourguignon L, Maire P, Jelliffe RW, Neely MN. The case for using higher doses of first line anti-tuberculosis drugs to optimize efficacy. Curr Pharm Des 2014;20(39):6191−206.

[30] Pasipanodya J, Gumbo T. An oracle: antituberculosis pharmacokinetics-pharmacodynamics, clinical correlation, and clinical trial simulations to predict the future. Antimicrob Agents Chemother 2011;55(1):24−34.

[31] Gumbo T, Angulo-Barturen I, Ferrer-Bazaga S. Pharmacokinetic-pharmacodynamic and dose-response relationships of antituberculosis drugs: recommendations and standards for industry and academia. J Infect Dis 2015;211(Suppl. 3):S96−106. Epub 2015/05/27.

[32] Jayaram R, Gaonkar S, Kaur P, Suresh BL, Mahesh BN, Jayashree R, et al. Pharmacokinetics-pharmacodynamics of rifampin in an aerosol infection model of tuberculosis. Antimicrob Agents Chemother 2003;47(7):2118−24.

[33] Gumbo T, Louie A, Deziel MR, Liu W, Parsons LM, Salfinger M, et al. Concentration-dependent *Mycobacterium tuberculosis* killing and prevention of resistance by rifampin. Antimicrob Agents Chemother 2007;51(11):3781−8.

[34] Diacon AH, Patientia RF, Venter A, van Helden PD, Smith PJ, McIlleron H, et al. Early bactericidal activity of high-dose rifampin in patients with pulmonary tuberculosis evidenced by positive sputum smears. Antimicrob Agents Chemother 2007;51(8):2994−6.

[35] Jayaram R, Shandil RK, Gaonkar S, Kaur P, Suresh BL, Mahesh BN, et al. Isoniazid pharmacokinetics-pharmacodynamics in an aerosol infection model of tuberculosis. Antimicrob Agents Chemother 2004;48(8):2951−7.

[36] Gumbo T, Louie A, Liu W, Brown D, Ambrose PG, Bhavnani SM, et al. Isoniazid bactericidal activity and resistance emergence: integrating pharmacodynamics and pharmacogenomics to predict efficacy in different ethnic populations. Antimicrob Agents Chemother 2007;51(7):2329−36.

[37] Donald PR, Sirgel FA, Venter A, Parkin DP, Seifart HI, van de Wal BW, et al. The influence of human *N*-acetyltransferase genotype on the early bactericidal activity of isoniazid. Clin Infect Dis 2004;39(10):1425−30.

[38] Gumbo T, Dona CS, Meek C, Leff R. Pharmacokinetics-pharmacodynamics of pyrazinamide in a novel in vitro model of tuberculosis for sterilizing effect: a paradigm for faster assessment of new antituberculosis drugs. Antimicrob Agents Chemother 2009;53(8):3197−204.

[39] Srivastava S, Musuka S, Sherman C, Meek C, Leff R, Gumbo T. Efflux-pump-derived multiple drug resistance to ethambutol monotherapy in *Mycobacterium tuberculosis* and the pharmacokinetics and pharmacodynamics of ethambutol. J Infect Dis 2010;201(8):1225−31.

[40] Gumbo T, Louie A, Deziel MR, Parsons LM, Salfinger M, Drusano GL. Selection of a moxifloxacin dose that suppresses drug resistance in *Mycobacterium tuberculosis*, by use of an in vitro pharmacodynamic infection model and mathematical modeling. J Infect Dis 2004;190(9):1642−51.

[41] Shandil RK, Jayaram R, Kaur P, Gaonkar S, Suresh BL, Mahesh BN, et al. Moxifloxacin, ofloxacin, sparfloxacin, and ciprofloxacin against *Mycobacterium tuberculosis*: evaluation of in vitro and pharmacodynamic indices that best predict in vivo efficacy. Antimicrob Agents Chemother 2007;51(2):576−82 Epub 2006/12/06.

[42] Modongo C, Pasipanodya J, Zetola NM, Williams S, Sirugo G, Gumbo T. Amikacin concentrations predictive of ototoxicity in multidrug-resistant tuberculosis patients. Antimicrob Agents Chemother 2015;59(10):6337−43.

[43] Goutelle S, Bourguignon L, Maire PH, Van Guilder M, Conte Jr. JE, Jelliffe RW. Population modeling and Monte Carlo simulation study of the pharmacokinetics and antituberculosis pharmacodynamics of rifampin in lungs. Antimicrob Agents Chemother 2009;53(7):2974−81.

[44] Srivastava S, Pasipanodya JG, Meek C, Leff R, Gumbo T. Multidrug-resistant tuberculosis not due to noncompliance but to between-patient pharmacokinetic variability. J Infect Dis 2011;204(12):1951−9 Epub 2011/10/25.

[45] Pasipanodya JG, Srivastava S, Gumbo T. Meta-analysis of clinical studies supports the pharmacokinetic variability hypothesis for acquired drug resistance and failure of antituberculosis therapy. Clin Infect Dis 2012;55(2):169−77 Epub 2012/04/03.

[46] Parkin DP, Vandenplas S, Botha FJ, Vandenplas ML, Seifart HI, van Helden PD, et al. Trimodality of isoniazid elimination: phenotype and genotype in patients with tuberculosis. Am J Respir Crit Care Med 1997;155(5):1717−22.

[47] Hickman D, Sim E. N-acetyltransferase polymorphism. Comparison of phenotype and genotype in humans. Biochem Pharmacol 1991;42(5):1007−14.

[48] Vivien JN, Thibier R, Lepeuple A. La pharmacocinétique de l'isoniazide dans la race blanche. Rev Mal Respir 1973;1(5 − 6):753−72.

[49] Mitchison DA. Role of individual drugs in the chemotherapy of tuberculosis. Int J Tuberc Lung Dis 2000;4(9):796−806.

[50] Donald PR, Parkin DP, Seifart HI, Schaaf HS, van Helden PD, Werely CJ, et al. The influence of dose and N-acetyltransferase-2 (NAT2) genotype and phenotype on the pharmacokinetics and pharmacodynamics of isoniazid. Eur J Clin Pharmacol 2007;63(7):633−9.

[51] Kinzig-Schippers M, Tomalik-Scharte D, Jetter A, Scheidel B, Jakob V, Rodamer M, et al. Should we use N-acetyltransferase type 2 genotyping to personalize isoniazid doses?. Antimicrob Agents Chemother 2005;49(5):1733−8.

[52] Asberg A, Midtvedt K, van Guilder M, Storset E, Bremer S, Bergan S, et al. Inclusion of CYP3A5 genotyping in a nonparametric population model improves dosing of tacrolimus early after transplantation. Transpl Int 2013;26(12):1198−207. Epub 2013/10/15.

[53] Jelliffe R. Optimal methodology is important for optimal pharmacokinetic studies, therapeutic drug monitoring and patient care. Clin Pharmacokinet 2015 Sep;54(9):887−92.

[54] Peloquin CA, Jaresko GS, Yong CL, Keung AC, Bulpitt AE, Jelliffe RW. Population pharmacokinetic modeling of isoniazid, rifampin, and pyrazinamide. Antimicrob Agents Chemother 1997;41(12):2670−9.

[55] Magis-Escurra C, Later-Nijland HM, Alffenaar JW, Broeders J, Burger DM, van Crevel R, et al. Population pharmacokinetics and limited sampling strategy for first-line tuberculosis drugs and moxifloxacin. Int J Antimicrob Agents 2014;44(3):229−34. Epub 2014/07/06.

[56] Jelliffe RW, Schumitzky A, Bayard D, Milman M, Van Guilder M, Wang X, et al. Model-based, goal-oriented, individualised drug therapy. Linkage of population modelling, new 'multiple model' dosage design, Bayesian feedback and individualised target goals. Clin Pharmacokinet 1998;34(1):57−77. Epub 1998/02/25.

[57] Peloquin CA, Bulpitt AE, Jaresko GS, Jelliffe RW, Childs JM, Nix DE. Pharmacokinetics of ethambutol under fasting conditions, with food, and with antacids. Antimicrob Agents Chemother 1999;43(3):568−72.

[58] Srivastava S, Gumbo T. Integrating drug concentrations and minimum inhibitory concentrations with Bayesian-dose optimisation for multidrug-resistant tuberculosis. Eur Respir J 2014;43(1):312−13. Epub 2014/01/02.

[59] Jelliffe R, Bayard D, Milman M, Van Guilder M, Schumitzky A. Achieving target goals most precisely using nonparametric compartmental models and "multiple model" design of dosage regimens. Ther Drug Monit 2000;22(3):346−53.

[60] Vu DH, Alffenaar JW, Edelbroek PM, Brouwers JR, Uges DR. Dried blood spots: a new tool for tuberculosis treatment optimization. Curr Pharm Des 2011;17(27):2931−9. Epub 2011/08/13.

[61] Drusano GL. Antimicrobial pharmacodynamics: critical interactions of 'bug and drug'. Nat Rev Microbiol 2004;2(4):289−300.

INDIVIDUALIZING TRANSPLANT THERAPY

16

P. Marquet and A. Åsberg

CHAPTER OUTLINE

16.1 INTRODUCTION

Calcineurin inhibitors (CNI; cyclosporine A, tacrolimus) are the cornerstones of most immunosuppressive protocols for solid organ transplant (SOT) recipients. Cyclosporine A (CsA) was approved in 1983, and about 10 years later tacrolimus (Tac) was introduced. Nowadays most centers use Tac as their standard CNI.

The CNIs are usually combined with proliferation inhibitors such as mycophenolate and/or steroids. In recent years, the search for less nephrotoxic immunosuppressive therapies has been intense, and in the last 15 years, sirolimus and everolimus, two inhibitors of the protein called "mammalian Target of Rapamycin (mTOR)"—because it was discovered as the target of rapamycin, the first name given to sirolimus—have been approved in different solid organ transplantation settings, depending on countries. mTOR inhibitors (mTORis) have since then gained momentum, used either in combination with low-dose CNIs or in CNI withdrawal/avoidance protocols [1]. Their relative lack of nephrotoxicity is the advantage sought, but widespread use is limited by a high discontinuation rate [2,3].

In the early posttransplantation period, patients may also receive induction therapy with either interleukin 2 receptor alpha-chain (CD25) antibody (IL2-RA)—ie, basiliximab—or a T-cell depleting agent such as thymoglobulin.

Despite many efforts to find specific or universal "immunometers" for individualizing immunosuppressive therapy, transplant physicians still basically rely on pharmacokinetic measures, usually standard therapeutic drug monitoring (TDM), measuring trough concentrations and

Individualized Drug Therapy for Patients. DOI: http://dx.doi.org/10.1016/B978-0-12-803348-7.00016-2

adjusting the doses based on predefined targets, or even using clinical impression or judgment. This applies in particular to CNIs, mTORis, and to a lesser extent (for reasons described later) mycophenolate.

Some centers, however, use the ELISPOT or other assays [4−6] that measure T-cell activation capacity, ie, the residual capacity of T-cells to replicate when stimulated despite the inhibitory effect of immunosuppressive drugs present in the sample. Some data on the use of more straightforward pharmacodynamic biomarkers, such as calcineurin activity to individualize CNI dosing [7−10] and p70S6-kinase activity for mTORi dosing [11] have also been reported. None of these pharmacodynamic biomarkers seemed to predict drug clinical response better than its blood concentration, and none is currently used clinically.

This chapter presents the current dose adjustment strategies for CNIs, mTORis, and mycophenolate, as well as tools based on pharmacokinetic modeling.

16.2 CALCINEURIN INHIBITORS (CNI)

16.2.1 CYCLOSPORINE A

CsA was first commercialized as soft gelatin capsules, an oral solution, and an intravenous formulation under the brand name Sandimmune in the early 1980s, and then in the late 1990s as a microemulsion named Neoral, formulated as soft gelatin capsules and an oral solution with faster absorption, and improved and more consistent bioavailability.

In blood, CsA is extensively distributed in erythrocytes and to a lesser extent in white blood cells, while in plasma, 90% is bound to lipoproteins and albumin. It is extensively metabolized by CYP3A in the liver to many metabolites that are mainly excreted in bile but are also found in blood and urine.

16.2.1.1 Cyclosporine A pharmacokinetics

CsA has high inter-individual pharmacokinetic variability and a narrow therapeutic index. Low exposure leads to acute and chronic graft rejection. High exposure is associated with frequent nephrotoxicity, cardiovascular, and metabolic disorders. It is therefore considered to be a critical dose drug, and individual dosage adjustment based on patient exposure has been recommended by the regulatory agencies since the first years after the drug was released.

16.2.1.2 Therapeutic drug monitoring (TDM) of cyclosporine A

Whole blood trough concentration (C_0) of CsA has been most generally used to adjust dosage for transplant patients, despite a weak correlation with acute rejection (AR) and toxicity in kidney [12] and liver [13] transplantation. After the advent of the improved Neoral formulation with more reproducible pharmacokinetics, efforts were made to find a better exposure biomarker.

Peak drug concentrations (C_{max}) and inter-dose area under the concentration-time curve (AUC) are considered to be better predictors of efficacy and/or toxicity than C_0. Cyclosporine blood concentrations 2, 3, or 4 h postdose were also proposed as alternatives to C_0, as rough estimates of C_{max}. For example, the drug concentration at 2 h postdose (C_2) was found to be a better predictor of immunosuppressive activity than C_0 in heart-transplant recipients [14]. A comparative prospective study in liver transplant recipients showed that C_2 monitoring with predefined target values led to higher Neoral dose and less moderate-to-severe AR episodes than C_0 monitoring [15]. Hence, a global recommendation for C_2 monitoring in kidney and liver transplantation by Novartis, the drug manufacturer, was more adopted by the transplantation centers in the United States than in Europe, owing to the alleged difficulty in programing and carrying out blood sampling at exactly 2 h postdose in a routine consultation setting.

Inter-dose AUC (ie, most generally $AUC_{0-12\,h}$) is more informative than C_0 because it correlates better with rejection in patients with kidney transplants [16−18]. However, $AUC_{0-12\,h}$ estimation based on a complete pharmacokinetic profile requires multiple blood samples over a 12-h period, which is uncomfortable for the patient and costly. For this reason, limited sampling strategies (LSS) coupled with multiple-linear regression equations have been developed for CsA monitoring, since they allow for the estimation of $AUC_{0-12\,h}$ using fewer blood samples. Many authors have proposed such equations (eg, Refs. [19−21]), the typical form of which is: $AUC_{0-12h} = a + b \times C_x + c \times C_y + d \times C_z$ where a, b, c, and d are estimated coefficients and C_x, C_y, and C_z are CsA blood concentrations measured at times x, y, and z. However, this method is not flexible, as it requires drug administration and blood sampling according to a preset strict schedule, and can only estimate the AUC and not C_{max} or any other pharmacokinetic parameter. Moreover, the different equations published all employed different sampling time points, and only a few were validated prospectively in an independent population.

As a better alternative, maximum a posteriori probability (MAP) Bayesian estimation of AUC in individual patients based on CsA population pharmacokinetic models has been employed, as it has the advantage of predicting the main individual pharmacokinetic parameters and may even take into account the patient's pathophysiological characteristics. Such Bayesian estimators are also more flexible as sampling times can be slightly different from the theoretical ones (provided they are accurately recorded using military time, 0000 to 2359 h, for example).

16.2.1.3 Pharmacokinetic modeling of CsA

Many different population pharmacokinetic models were proposed for CsA, from the more classical "first-order absorption with or without lag-time, two-compartment" models to more elaborate ones, in particular with regard to the drug absorption phase. Indeed, CsA exhibits flat and delayed absorption profiles, with a correlation between the delay and the peak width. Such a pattern was proposed to be characteristic of a gamma distribution (of which the exponential—ie, first-order—distribution is a particular case), which was then amply used to develop population pharmacokinetic models in kidney [22], liver, heart, lung, and bone marrow transplantation. As an alternative, an Erlang distribution (a simplification of the gamma distribution that can be described as a chain of transfer compartments between the depot and the central compartment) was employed as it can be more easily implemented in commercial pharmacokinetic modeling software [23−25].

A recent paper reviewed 31 population pharmacokinetic studies of CsA in kidney, liver, heart, lung, and bone marrow transplantation [25,26], of which one-third involved pediatric patients. Twelve concerned the Sandimmune and twenty the Neoral formulation. This review confirmed the variety of models used, partly depending on the type of exposure data available (sometimes only retrospectively collected C_0 values) and the partial or even absent validation of many. Above all, it highlighted that body weight, hematocrit, time after transplantation, cystic fibrosis, and the co-administration of calcium channel blockers (mostly diltiazem but also verapamil) or azole antifungal drugs (itraconazole and ketoconazole) were covariates with a definite effect on CsA pharmacokinetics, while recipient age, liver function, and intake of P-glycoprotein inhibitors had a possible, yet inconclusive, influence. Moreover, it emphasized that the analytical method used had an influence on pharmacokinetic parameter estimation, and that it could be solved by introducing a scaling factor and attributing different residual variability models to each assay [24].

More than 30 published papers reported population pharmacokinetic models of CsA exposure. These models were based either on pharmacokinetic (PK) parameter distributions derived from individual PK modeling [27,28] or on population PK models developed using parametric methods, mostly NONMEM (eg, Refs. [23,24,29−31]) or Abbott PKS [32], or using nonparametric methods such as those implemented in NPEM2 [33] and the Pmetrics software [34]. This last study even compared population models developed using two independent parametric modeling approaches (NONMEM and iterative two stage (ITS) Bayesian modeling) and the nonparametric adaptive grid method (Pmetrics). All predicted CsA $AUC_{0-12 h}$ with minimal bias using only three blood samples (C_0, C_1, C_4) in hematopoietic stem cell transplant patients, and applying all three approaches to the same individual data further increased the reliability of CsA dose adjustment.

Several of these population models have been made accessible to the transplant community since 2005 through a secured website (https://pharmaco.chu-limoges.fr) where all inter-dose AUC results and dose recommendations are validated by trained pharmacologists [35].

16.2.1.4 Clinical validation

Validation of $AUC_{0-12 h}$ monitoring was conducted in a single randomized, multicenter trial studying kidney transplant patients to compare CsA dose adjustment based on C_0 or $AUC_{0-12 h}$ estimates obtained by means of multiple linear regression (MLR) equations based on 3 and then 2 time-points. Different $AUC_{0-12 h}$ and C_0 target ranges were aimed for over the posttransplantation Weeks 2−4 and 5−12. Patients and CsA dose were comparable across the two groups. However, no difference was found in terms of incidence of AR episodes, or incidence and severity of adverse drug effects [36]. It may mean that $AUC_{0-12 h}$ monitoring performed no better than C_0, or maybe that the AUC estimates were not accurate enough.

Bayesian estimation of CsA $AUC_{0-12 h}$ employing blood concentrations measured predose and at 1 and 3 h postdose was used in a comparative, randomized "CNI-sparing" study in renal transplantation [37], where a 50% decrease in CsA exposure relative to usual care was tested using $AUC_{0-12 h}$ as a more robust index of drug exposure than C_0. It showed accurate and almost immediate achievement of the two $AUC_{0-12 h}$ target levels, clear separation of the two study arms in terms of exposure, low inter-individual exposure variability (typical CV = 20%), and better outcome in the dose-sparing arm. Although obviously not a validation of AUC monitoring, this study at least showed the good performance of the individual Bayesian estimation procedure used for dose adjustment.

Finally, although CsA has been largely supplanted by Tac in kidney and liver transplantation, it is still largely used in thoracic and bone marrow transplantation, meaning that, more than 30 years after the drug was first approved, improvements in individualized drug dosing are still to be expected. As for many other critical dose drugs, it is mainly the clinical validation of the sophisticated yet accessible tools that have been developed over the years that is still missing, especially of optimal design in TDM protocols and the use of multiple model dosage design for maximal precision in target achievement.

16.2.2 TACROLIMUS

Tac has a narrow therapeutic window and significant comorbidity if not optimally dosed, including acute and long-term effects limiting optimal outcome in these patients. The obvious risk of rejection if dosing too low must be carefully balanced against the many side effects associated with excessive doses. Such side effects include nephrotoxicity, neurotoxicity, increased blood pressure, dyslipidemia, disrupted glucose metabolism, etc. [38]. Most of these side effects are initially reversible but may cause irreversible damage with time, such as profound fibrosis in the transplanted kidney after long-term CNI use [39]. To obtain a good balance in long-term immunosuppression, there has been a specific focus on minimization/withdrawal strategies based on stratification directed by different biomarkers [40]. In these programs, it will be even more important to be able to perform TDM and Bayesian dosage individualization to avoid under-immunosuppression

16.2.2.1 Tacrolimus pharmacokinetics

Tac has a large pharmacokinetic variability, both intra- and inter-individual. Despite many investigations to find explanations for this variability, much is still not known. For example, the dose requirements change with time after transplantation, and even if many covariates have been investigated, the full description of this change with time is still lacking [41−44].

Tac is a lipophilic drug with rapid absorption, but in many cases it has a significant lag time prior to absorption following oral administration [42]. Its absolute bioavailability is low, typically in the range of $15 - 25\%$, but with a high interindividual variability [45]. Tac binds strongly to plasma proteins and erythrocytes, with an unbound fraction of less than 1% [45−47]. The association with erythrocytes is also temperature dependent. This is why whole blood concentrations are used when investigating Tac pharmacokinetics and for TDM [48].

Tac is a low extraction drug metabolized by CYP3A. Less than 1% is excreted unchanged into urine [45]. Especially *CYP3A5*3* and *CYP3A4*22*, but also other polymorphisms in genes coding Tac metabolic enzymes and membrane transporters, have been shown to influence Tac pharmacokinetics [49−51].

16.2.2.2 Tacrolimus TDM

Due to the temperature-dependent free fraction mentioned previously, most centers measure whole blood concentrations of Tac. In theory, since Tac shows such a low free fraction ($<1\%$), it would be a good candidate for monitoring free concentrations, but owing to the analytical challenges with both the temperature-dependent distribution in blood and the fact that Tac shows high adherence to many types of surfaces, such as walls of Vacutainer tubes and Cryotubes, it is not feasible for high throughput analyses [46].

In most centers, TDM of Tac is performed by trough concentration measurements without using any specific tools to help with dose adjustments. Despite better associations between AUC and other single time-point measurements than C_0, no clinical benefits for measuring Tac concentrations at such time points, like C_2 monitoring for CsA, have been presented [52,53]. The appropriate therapeutic window for trough concentrations of Tac has been lowered since its introduction. The comparative, randomized Symphony clinical trial showed that the low-Tac arm, aiming for Tac trough concentrations between 3 µg/L and 7 µg/L, had better renal function, an approximately twice lower AR rate and a few %-point better one-year graft survival compared to normal- or low-dose

CsA [54]. Still, it is important to note that normal-dose tacrolimus was not investigated in this trial. However, many centers in this study aimed higher than the Tac C_0 target range, and the actual mean Tac trough concentration obtained was more in the range of $5-8$ μg/L [55], at least in the early posttransplant phase with subsequent tapering into the "Symphony range" of below 7 μg/L.

Most of the Tac dose adaptation following transplantation is performed based only on clinical impression, and is obviously dependent on skilled transplant physicians. When the trough concentration is out of range, the treating physician makes a "best guess" on what the appropriate change will be and draws blood after a few days for confirmation. In the early posttransplant phase, blood is drawn more frequently, even before steady-state conditions are fully obtained after a dose adjustment, which makes the interpretation of the results from such trough concentration monitoring even more challenging when not using assisting software tools. Implementation of optimally designed TDM protocols should also help here and also make it possible to dose to achieve a desired AUC target without excessive sampling within a dose interval.

Different tools to assist in dose adaptation of patients have been developed. Most are based on pharmacokinetic calculations, including population pharmacokinetic modeling or neural networks [56,57]. In many cases simplified algorithms, including a few patient characteristics and one or more blood concentration measurements within a dose interval have been used to help with dose individualization. Some of the population pharmacokinetic models have been combined with MAP Bayesian analysis to help individualize Tac doses [58−64]. The ISBA service (ImmunoSuppressants Bayesian dose Adjustment) available on the Internet is based on this approach and has helped clinicians with dose adaptions for Tac for almost 10 years now. In a recent analysis of more than 2000 requests for Tac dose adjustments, the ISBA service has been able to suggest potential AUC targets [41]. Although solid documentation is lacking, drug exposure, both measured as C_{max} and AUC, is linked to Tac therapeutic as well as adverse clinical effects [65−67]. A recent consensus report suggests that interdose AUC best describes systemic exposure of Tac [68]. Utilizing only trough concentrations limits the information on individual pharmacokinetics, even if advanced population pharmacokinetic models are used to analyze the data. Moving toward AUC-based targets and implementing optimally designed TDM protocols should significantly increase the amount of information obtained about each individual patient's pharmacokinetics and hopefully make the targeting and dosage even more precise.

A recent study comparing a generic Tac formulation with the original Prograf formulation in renal transplant recipients illustrates the limitations of only monitoring trough concentrations. In this bioequivalence study, the two formulations showed similar trough concentrations. However, when analyzing AUC and C_{max}, it was clearly shown that the two formulations were not bioequivalent [69].

Applying AUC monitoring will, however, increase the demand for data handling if full 12-/24-h pharmacokinetic profiles are to be obtained, and this is generally not clinically feasible. Combining tools like BestDose, which showed good performance in a clinical setting using trough concentrations [70], and AUC targeting using $2-3$ blood concentrations within a dose interval, will most probably be an even better and clinically applicable tool for individualized dosage.

With regard to the initial dosage regimen, most centers have used a fixed dose, adjusted to the patient's body weight. Recently, some centers have introduced different starting doses based on the patient's *CYP3A5* genotype, giving patients expressing active CYP3A5 (*1/*3 or *1/*1) double dose [64,71,72]. A few centers use more advanced algorithms including *CYP3A5* and *CYP3A4* genotypes, age, days posttransplant, use of calcium channel blocker, and if on a steroid sparing protocol or

Stepwise process of model-based dosing

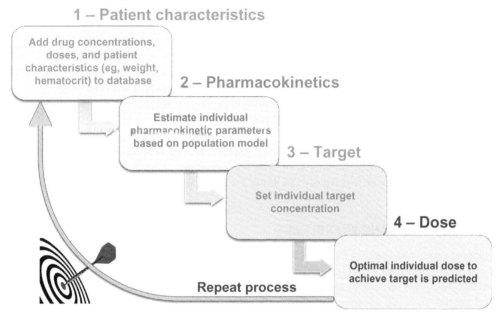

FIGURE 16.1

Steps used to individualize drug doses based on population PK model based computer tools.

Adapted from Elisabet Størset.

not for estimating an individualized starting dose, as nicely reviewed by Andrews et al. [73]. Pretransplant phenotyping of Tac pharmacokinetics has also been tested [74]. Even though many such starting dose algorithms have been described in the literature, their clinical performance has seldom been evaluated. In some instances, when used in other populations than those in which they were developed, such algorithms actually performed poorly [75]. There are also data showing that with information from 3 to 4 consecutive trough concentrations from a patient, proper Bayesian estimators have enough information about Tac pharmacokinetics to overlook *CYP3A5* genotype information, as it is actually redundant for appropriate dose adaption [64]. However, further TDM is still needed to get a proper dose individualization related to time after transplantation [41].

Many Tac population pharmacokinetic models have been reported, using either one or two compartments [26,43,44,59,63,64,76−82]. The more important covariates identified were *CYP3A5* genotype, hematocrit, steroid dose, and time after transplantation. However, clinical validation was generally lacking. We adopted a stepwise process of Tac dosing with a population pharmacokinetic tool (Fig. 16.1). This was shown to be a powerful tool for individualized dose adaptation in renal transplant recipients in the early posttransplant phase [70]. This prospective, randomized controlled trial, comparing the achievement of Tac trough concentration targets by using or not using the population pharmacokinetic model and Bayesian dosage individualization incorporated in the BestDose application of Pmetrics, strongly suggests that such tools should have a future role in the clinic. In addition to better target achievement, this kind of software tool also allows more flexible sampling procedures, as prespecified time-points for concentration measurements are not mandatory. It will also be easy to implement AUC monitoring when using them.

Combining population pharmacokinetic models with optimal sampling times will potentially even further strengthen the precision and capability of these tools when an AUC target is sought. This will in addition make the logistics easier in the outpatient setting as the samples can be drawn at times that suit the patient without having to be within rigidly prespecified time-points.

Another "technique" that would make a big difference when combined with population pharmacokinetic models in dose adaption is dried blood spot analysis of Tac [83−84]. Being able to get several concentrations within a dose interval from the patients without them having to be at the clinic would permit numerous high-information samples in each patient. Another field that potentially may improve TDM of Tac in the future is measurement of drug concentrations closer to the site of the drug effect, such as inside T-lymphocytes for efficacy [85,86] or inside renal tissue for nephrotoxicity [87].

16.2.3 SIROLIMUS AND EVEROLIMUS

Sirolimus (rapamycin) was the first mTORi in clinical use. Everolimus is a derivative of sirolimus with better solubility and improved oral bioavailability [88]. Due to an additive nephrotoxic effect, mTORis should only be combined with CNIs in reduced dosages of both types of drugs [89,90]. Several studies show an advantageous effect on renal function in immunosuppressive protocols in which mTORis are included [91−93]. These patients also tend to have lower rates of viral infections and malignancy compared to standard CNI-based therapies [94−97]. mTORis are usually also the preferred immunosuppressive drugs in case of malignancies in transplanted patients [98].

However, these drugs are not free from side effects. The dominant ones are anemia, thrombocytopenia, elevated triglyceride and cholesterol levels [99−102]. Stomatitis and diarrhea are also common [103], but the most serious, even though less frequent, side effect is noninfectious pneumonitis [104].

16.2.3.1 mTORi pharmacokinetics

Both sirolimus and everolimus are rapidly absorbed and have a low oral bioavailability. Absolute oral bioavailability has not been established in humans but is estimated to be between 15% and 25%, somewhat higher for everolimus than for sirolimus [105−107]. Food strongly delays absorption and decreases C_{max}. It is therefore important that mTORis are consistently administered either with or (preferably) without food [108−111].

Even though cyclosporine is a weak CYP3A inhibitor, it significantly inhibits everolimus metabolism [101,102,109,110,112−114]. In addition to CYP3A, CYP2C8 is involved in the metabolism of mTORis, which are also substrates of P-gp [115,116]. Their elimination is mainly via metabolism and subsequent biliary excretion [117,118]. These drugs are, as are CNIs, highly distributed into erythrocytes in blood. In the plasma compartment, a majority of the drug is bound to plasma proteins and lipoproteins [101,102,119]. Everolimus has a shorter terminal half-life than sirolimus (about 24 h vs about 60 h) [117,120], but both drugs can potentially be dosed once daily. However, only sirolimus is usually given QD, while everolimus is administered BID.

16.2.3.2 mTORi TDM

mTORis have narrow therapeutic windows and high inter- and intra-individual variability [117,121]. TDM is therefore indicated and so far has often been based on whole blood trough concentration measurements. Most centers use C_{trough} as an exposure biomarker, while some use the AUC (estimated using 2- or 3-sample algorithms) [105]. AUC is the preferred systemic exposure measure, but due to clinical applicability, C_{trough} is more commonly used based on the clinical interpretation that the correlation between C_{trough} and AUC appears reasonable [99,100,122].

There are, however, reports that disagree with this assumption [123], but it has at least been shown that intracellular concentrations in leukocytes correlate well with whole blood concentrations [124], which is not the case for CNIs [86,125].

The C_{trough} targets proposed in the literature are different for sirolimus and everolimus. In combination with CNIs, one has usually aimed for a C_{trough} between 5 µg/L and 15 µg/L for sirolimus and $3-8$ µg/L for everolimus. Without concomitant CNI, the respective target ranges are $10-20$ µg/L for sirolimus and $6-10$ µg/L for everolimus [2,99,100,103,126−132].

Unlike for the CNIs, few population pharmacokinetic models have been described for mTORis [105,133], and none have been validated for clinical use for dose adaption in transplanted patients so far. In the study of Moes et al. [105], however, aiming for a maintenance everolimus AUC_{0-12} of 120 µg × h/L resulted in low AR rates, and well-preserved renal function.

As always, the literature is not fully consistent, but currently there are no strong data showing any significant influence on everolimus dosing of polymorphisms in *CYP3A* or *P-gp* genes [105,124,134,135]. For sirolimus, however, patients expressing CYP3A5 should probably have a 1.5-fold to twofold higher starting dose compared to *CYP3A5*3/*3* patients, especially if not in combination with CNIs [133,136−138].

16.2.4 MYCOPHENOLATES

Mycophenolic acid (MPA) is an immunosuppressant indicated in combination with CsA or Tac to prevent rejection following organ transplantation. It is an inhibitor of inosine monophosphate dehydrogenase (IMPDH), a key enzyme in the synthesis of DNA. Activated lymphocytes express the inducible isozyme IMPDH2 in addition to the constitutional isoform IMPDH1 and would be more susceptible to MPA inhibitory activity than other cells. However, MPA also has proliferation inhibition activity on fast-renewal cell lines such as erythrocytes, neutrophils, or enterocytes, which is likely to be the cause of some of its frequent adverse effects, such as neutropenia, anemia, and diarrhea, respectively.

MPA is commercially available in two formulations: the ester prodrug mycophenolate mofetil (MMF) and an enteric-coated sodium salt, mycophenolate sodium (EC-MPS). The role of TDM for MPA is still debated, and the controversy about its utility was recently reviewed [139,140]. However, this controversy only concerns the ester prodrug MMF because TDM is hardly feasible for EC-MPS. Indeed, in some patients, EC-MPS has very unpredictable pharmacokinetics, particularly at nighttime when absorption can be seriously delayed so that morning predose levels are the actual C_{max} of the evening dose, presumably due to the combination of a distal absorption site and slow enteric motility at night.

16.2.4.1 Pharmacokinetics of mycophenolic acid

MMF and EC-MPS are completely hydrolyzed to MPA by esterases in the gut wall, blood, liver, and tissue. Oral bioavailability of MPA is >80% when administered as MMF and approximately 72% for EC-MPS. MPA peak concentration usually occurs $1-2$ h after MMF administration. EC-MPS has a median lag time of $0.25-1.25$ h in MPA absorption after the morning dose, while absorption after the evening dose, as mentioned previously, can be much more delayed.

MPA binds $97-99\%$ to serum albumin. It is metabolized in the gastrointestinal tract, liver, and kidney by the phase II enzymes uridine diphosphate glucuronosyltransferases (UGTs).

7-O-MPA-glucuronide (MPAG) is the major metabolite of MPA. It is present in plasma at 20- to 100-fold higher concentrations than MPA, but is not pharmacologically active. MPAG has an enterohepatic cycle with deconjugation by gut microflora, with secondary MPA absorption peaks about $6-12$ h postdose, which contributes approximately 40% to the total area under the plasma concentration-time curve (AUC). The mean elimination half-life of MPA ranges from 9 h to 17 h [141].

After MMF administration, MPA has large interindividual PK variability as a result of numerous factors such as liver and renal function, serum albumin levels, or associated drugs with which it has pharmacokinetic interactions, such as CsA and corticosteroids. The dose-standardized MPA AUC can vary 10-fold between kidney transplant recipients and 20-fold between liver transplant patients. In patients with severe renal impairment, liver disease, or hypoalbuminemia, MPA plasma protein binding may be altered, increasing its free fraction and the apparent oral clearance (CL/F) of total MPA. This results in a reduction in total MPA AUC while MPA free concentration, the exchangeable and supposedly active concentration, is minimally altered. Therefore, total MPA concentrations should be interpreted with caution in such cases.

CsA inhibits the biliary excretion of MPAG, reducing the enterohepatic recirculation of MPA, so that its $AUC_{0-12\,h}$ is approximately $30-40\%$ lower than when the drug is given alone, or also when given with Tac or sirolimus. Also, high dosages of corticosteroids may induce the expression of UGTs, reducing exposure to MPA by increased metabolism [141]. Finally, there is a time-dependent increase in dose-standardized MPA AUC of about 40% over the first 3 months posttransplantation [142].

16.2.4.2 Exposure-effect relationships: mycophenolate

For MMF, several observational studies over the first year posttransplantation have found that MPA AUC_{0-12h} was better correlated with patient outcome than was any single concentration-time point, and that patients with AR had lower mean MPA $AUC_{0-12\,h}$ than those without AR [143–145]. A recent retrospective analysis of a large group of patients showed a significant association between the longitudinal exposure to MPA (MPA AUC over time) and AR ($p = 0.0081$) [144]. A subanalysis of the same population even showed that it was a predictor of MMF efficacy at large (AR, graft loss or death), while longitudinal exposure to CsA or Tac was not [146]: each 1 mg × h/L increase of MPA $AUC_{0-12\,h}$ was associated with a 4% decreased risk of an event (hazard ratio = 0.96; 95% confidence interval: $0.93-0.99$).

In renal transplant recipients on MMF and CsA, a randomized concentration-controlled trial (RCCT) compared the incidence of AR between patients dose-adjusted to reach low (16.1 mg × h/L), intermediate (32.2 mg × h/L), or high (60.6 mg × h/L) MPA $AUC_{0-12\,h}$ [147]. Although after Day 21, the mean MMF dose was reduced, the mean MPA AUC gradually increased and target MPA

AUC values were exceeded in all three groups. There was a highly statistically significant relationship between biopsy-proven acute rejection (BPAR) and individual median $AUC_{0-12\,h}$ ($p < 0.001$) or C_0 ($p = 0.01$), but not individual mean MMF dose ($p = 0.082$). In contrast, patients who were prematurely withdrawn due to adverse events had a significantly higher mean MMF dose ($p < 0.001$), while there was no difference for median C_0 ($p = 0.512$) or $AUC_{0-12\,h}$ ($p = 0.434$).

Consensus conferences and reports on MMF TDM all preferred drug dosing based on MPA interdose $AUC_{0-12\,h}$ rather than C_0, and recommended a target MPA $AUC_{0-12\,h}$ range 30–60 mg × h/L over the first 6 months post–kidney or heart transplantation, when MMF is used in combination with cyclosporine and steroids [140,148,149]. This target window was mostly based on the exposure achieved in the intermediate group of the RCCT study [147].

However, it is frequently said that AUC monitoring would not be feasible owing to clinical constraints, which is counting without LSS and pharmacokinetic modeling. Indeed, LSS can be used to estimate the $AUC_{0-12\,h}$ with a limited number of time points (typically from 2 to 4), provided MLR equations (see below) or Bayesian estimators have previously been set up in the population.

16.2.4.3 Multiple linear regression (MLR) equations for AUC estimation

Many MLR equations have been published in transplantation for all organs, as well as in populations with autoimmune diseases, both for MMF and EC-MPS [150–153]. As for CsA, the MLRs proposed were very diverse in terms of sampling times and coefficients, even for the same transplanted organ. In 2010, Barraclough et al. identified 78 MLR with LSS for MPA, which they tested in parallel on a rather small group of patients (69 full AUC profiles, from 25 patients cotreated with CsA and 20 with Tac) [154]. Twelve of the 25 MLR for CsA-cotreated recipients and one of the 53 MLR for Tac-cotreated recipients displayed acceptable (less than 15%) bias and imprecision. In the CsA group, the highest predictive power was obtained with one MLR that used four points in the first 6 h postdose (predose, 1, 3, and 6 h postdose; $r^2 = 0.84$, median percentage prediction error (MPPE) 1.6%, median absolute percentage prediction error (MAPE) 7.8%) and one that used 4 time points in the first 4 h postdose (predose, 1, 2, and 4 h postdose; $r^2 = 0.76$, MPPE -0.8%, MAPE 10.2%). In the Tac group, the best MLR used 2 time points in the first 4 h postdose (predose and 4 h postdose; $r^2 = 0.80$, MPPE -3.0%, MAPE 13.6%). The authors concluded that "high variability in performance of MLR with LSS highlights the importance of validating any MLR before applying it to a different population." Attention to comedication use is of particular relevance when choosing an MLR with LSS. As already mentioned for CsA, other obvious limitations of MLR with LSS are that they cannot estimate other exposure indices such as C_{max} or take into account covariates (eg, comedication or transplant type). Contrary to population pharmacokinetic models and Bayesian individualized models, they are not at all flexible with respect to blood sample timing.

16.2.4.4 Pharmacokinetic modeling: mycophenolate

The first efficient parametric population PK models developed for MPA after oral administration of MMF concerned rather simple clinical situations, such as stable kidney transplant recipients on CsA (ie, with reduced enterohepatic recirculation). These models had two compartments and first-order absorption, with or without a lag time [155–157]. The first two studies found that MPA oral clearance was significantly, although loosely, positively correlated with bodyweight while the third found MPA clearance to be significantly influenced by sex, creatinine clearance, plasma albumin, and CsA daily dose following the equation $CL = 32.5 \times (CLCR/48)^{-0.12} \times (Alb/30)^{-1.07} \times (CsA/450)^{0.31} \times 1.11^{sex}$, and MPA distribution volume to be correlated with creatinine clearance and plasma albumin following the equation $V1 = 91 \times (CLCR/48)^{-0.62} \times (Alb/30)^{-1.13}$.

More complex models were rapidly proposed to describe MPA pharmacokinetic profiles in the first weeks posttransplantation, owing to obvious secondary peaks often attributed to enterohepatic recirculation. Using in-house individual PK modeling software, Prémaud et al. [158,159] proposed a one-compartment model with a double gamma distribution to describe the absorption phase in the immediate period after renal transplantation, while single- and double-absorption models performed equally well after 3 months. More recently, Saint-Marcoux et al. [61] found that the same double gamma absorption model adequately described MPA profiles in children with idiopathic nephrotic syndrome not given CNI, which is consistent with the higher enterohepatic circulation of MPAG/MPA in the absence of CsA. Using parametric population modeling, Musuamba et al. [160] developed a two-compartment model with first-order absorption and lagtime for MPA coadministered with CsA, to which a compartment for MPAG and a gastrointestinal compartment were added in the case of sirolimus co-medication to describe enterohepatic cycling of MPAG/MPA (Fig. 16.2). The only significant covariate on MPA concentrations was the glomerular filtration rate as estimated by the Nankivell formula [160].

Sherwin et al. [161] employed a rather complex structural model for MPA in patients with systemic lupus erythematosus, with a gallbladder compartment for enterohepatic recycling and bile release time related to meal times, with first-order absorption and single series of transit compartments, leading to 11 PK parameters to estimate (one was fixed) (Fig. 16.2). However, the correlation between individual predicted and observed MPA concentrations was not optimal, and in any case not as good as that of the metabolite MPAG.

In an effort to describe the influence of combined genetic polymorphisms and renal function on MPA PK, Colom et al. [162] developed an even more complex model with an intestine compartment, two compartments for MPA, two for MPAG, and one for acyl-MPAG (a possibly active, minor MPA metabolite), with linear elimination from the central MPAG compartment and the acyl-MPAG compartment. Enterohepatic circulation was modeled by transport of MPAG to the intestine compartment. Interestingly, this transport was significantly decreased with increasing CsA trough concentrations, while MPAG and AcMPAG plasma clearances were significantly decreased with decreased renal function. As a result, enterohepatic circulation was significantly reduced with high CsA C_0 values and good renal function. No significant influence of the genetic polymorphisms tested was found.

Some of these complex models may be overparameterized, which may compromise the identification of covariates, their performance in an independent population set, or their clinical applicability.

Prémaud et al. [163] compared parametric (NONMEM) and nonparametric (NPAG) modeling of MPA in pediatric renal transplant patients, using what may be an oversimplified two-compartment model with first-order absorption and a lag time. Wider ranges of individual PK parameters and large skewness and kurtosis values (ie, far from normal distributions, which are a prerequisite of parametric methods) were obtained with NPAG, especially for the elimination constant (k_e). Bayesian forecasting of MPA exposure using the NPAG population PK parameters as priors yielded a better predictive performance, with a significantly smaller bias than the NONMEM model. It was concluded that nonparametric analysis is preferable to parametric in case of nonnormal distribution of any one of the PK parameters, and is more suited to clinical applications such as optimal, maximally precise dosage individualization.

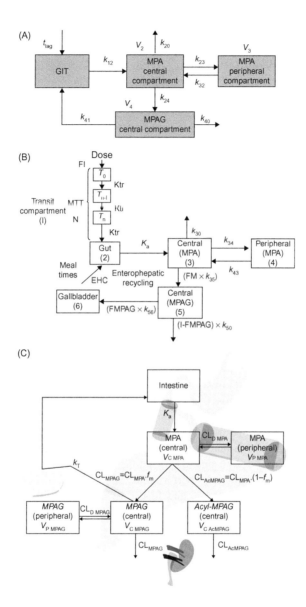

FIGURE 16.2

Examples of complex structural pharmacokinetic models proposed to describe mycophenolic acid concentration-time profiles with secondary peaks, generally attributed to enterohepatic recirculation of MPAG/MPA.

Reproduced with permission from (A) Musuamba FT, Rousseau A, Bosmans JL, Senessael JJ, Cumps J, Marquet P, et al. Limited sampling models and Bayesian estimation for mycophenolic acid area under the curve prediction in stable renal transplant patients co-medicated with ciclosporin or sirolimus. Clin Pharmacokinet 2009;48(11):745–58; (B) Sherwin CM, Fukuda T, Brunner HI, Goebel J, Vinks AA. The evolution of population pharmacokinetic models to describe the enterohepatic recycling of mycophenolic acid in solid organ transplantation and autoimmune disease. Clin Pharmacokinet 2011;50(1):1–24; (C) Colom H, Lloberas N, Andreu F, Caldés A, Torras J, Oppenheimer F, et al. Pharmacokinetic modeling of enterohepatic circulation of mycophenolic acid in renal transplant recipients. Kidney Int 2014;85(6): 1434–43.

Dong et al. [164] developed a PK/PD model for MPA using a two-compartment model with a semi-mechanistic transit compartment absorption and a simplified inhibitory E_{max} model to describe the relationship between MPA plasma concentration and IMPDH activity in mononuclear cells. Similar to previous reports [61,165], they found a nonlinear relationship between dose and MPA exposure. Covariate analysis identified body weight to be significantly correlated with CL/F. For the population PK/PD analysis, individual PK parameter estimates from post hoc Bayesian estimation were used as inputs to the PD model of IMPDH activity [164]. Prémaud et al. [166] also modeled MPA PK/PD using NONMEM, but considering T-cell proliferation, intracytoplasmic IL-2 and TNF-α expression, and membrane CD71 and CD25 expression as more distal pharmacodynamic biomarkers. They found that both CD25 and CD71 expression and T-cell proliferation were clearly reduced with increasing MPA concentrations, in contrast to IL-2 and TNF-α expression. The CD25, CD71 expression, and T-cell proliferation profiles were adequately fitted using a sigmoid inhibitory E_{max} model, showing a transient MPA concentration-dependent decrease in T-cells expressing CD25 and CD71, and a strong reduction of T-cell proliferation in patients given MMF.

16.2.4.5 Bayesian estimation of mycophenolate AUC

Staatz and Tett [167] identified and reviewed 14 studies that used maximum a posteriori Bayesian estimation (MAP-BE) to predict MPA $AUC_{0-12 h}$ based on a few measured MPA plasma concentration-time points. Of them, at least three studies found that the same 3 time-point strategy, at 20 min, 1 h, and 3 h postdose, yielded the best individual $AUC_{0-12 h}$ estimation performance: bias values between -8.2% and 7.7%, and RMSE between 12.0% and 20.5% in renal transplant patients from Day Seven to more than 3 months posttransplantation [155,161], and bias $= -0.8\%$ and RMSE $= 14.2\%$ in pediatric patients with idiopathic nephrotic syndrome [61]. Payen et al. [155] found that two sampling times, at 1 and 4 h postdose, allowed precise and accurate $AUC_{0-12 h}$ estimation (bias: 0.9 mg $\times$ h/mL; precision 6.02 mg $\times$ h/mL). The 1 h-4 h-6 h model was more accurate, but was deemed not to be clinically applicable by the authors. Musuamba et al. [76] compared MLR and MAP-BE and found that the best LSS was predose, 0.66 h and 2 h postdose with MLR, and predose, 1.25 h and 2 h postdose with Bayesian estimation, and that MLR yielded poorer $AUC_{0-12 h}$ estimation performance than MAP-BE ($r^2 = 0.79$, bias $= 0.9\%$, RMSE $= 14\%$ vs $r^2 = 0.93$, bias $= -0.4\%$, and RMSE $= 12.4\%$). In 2013, Musuamba and colleagues compared MLR and Bayesian estimation of MPA $AUC_{0-12 h}$ (in combination with tacrolimus AUC) using the same 1.5 h and 3.5 h two-time-point LSS in 65 renal transplant patients and also found that BE provided better results than MLR ($r^2 = 0.90$ and RMSE $= 13\%$ for BE vs $r^2 = 0.66$, RMSE $= 24\%$ for MLR) [77].

As described in a recent review paper [164], multiple population models for MMF in solid organ transplantation and autoimmune diseases have been developed and validated by the University Hospital of Limoges, France, and have been made accessible via a website service since 2005 (https://pharmaco.chu-limoges.fr). Over the first 10 years, the service has handled approximately 55,000 requests from 121 different transplantation services worldwide (with a majority from France).

The impact of the service over the first 5 years was evaluated in a retrospective study of data obtained from 3311 adult kidney transplant recipients with at least two AUC requests, which looked at the efficacy of MMF dose adjustment based on MPA $AUC_{0-12 h}$ Bayesian estimation [61]. When the MMF dosage recommendations were actually carried out by the clinicians, $72-80\%$ of estimated MPA AUC values calculated on the occasion of the subsequent request were within the $30-60$ mg $\times$ h/L target range, as opposed to only $39-57\%$ within range when the dosage recommendations were not followed.

16.2.4.6 Clinical utility of mycophenolate mofetil TDM

A few prospective randomized trials evaluated the clinical utility of MMF TDM by comparing the outcome of renal transplant patients receiving, over the first year posttransplantation, either a fixed-dose (FD) regimen of MMF (1 g twice daily in adults) or a concentration-controlled (CC) regimen adjusted to achieve a target MPA $AUC_{0-12\ h}$. The fixed-dose concentration-controlled (FDCC) trial [168] enrolled adult and pediatric patients co-treated with CsA or Tac, allowed for different analytical methods for MPA measurement, employed MLR for AUC estimation, and let clinicians calculate the adjusted doses to reach a target of 45 mg $\times$ h/L. The trial did not show any difference between the two groups in terms of treatment failure (a composite of BPAR, graft loss, death, or MMF discontinuation) by 12 months posttransplantation. The authors attributed the lack of difference partly to the fact that physicians were reluctant to implement substantial dose changes. Indeed, retrospective analysis of the concentration-effect data showed a significant association between MPA AUC on Day Three and BPAR occurring in the first month, as well as in the first year posttransplantation. More specifically, later re-analysis showed that this statistical association was only true in patients with high risk of rejection (ie, patients with delayed graft function, second or third transplantation, panel reactive antibodies >15%, four or more human leukocyte antigen mismatches, or of black race) [169].

In the APOMYGRE study [142], only adult patients co-treated with CsA were enrolled. MPA measurements were performed by high-performance liquid chromatography, and a standalone computer program provided to each investigating center calculated the AUCs by Bayesian estimation [159], and provided the new dose (rounded up or down to feasible dosing) to be given to the patient based on the current dose and measured AUC. The median MPA AUCs were higher in the CC group at Day 14 (2698 $\pm$ 543 vs 2000 mg/d) and at Month One (2969 $\pm$ 780 vs 1960 $\pm$ 186 mg/d), and a significantly lower incidence of treatment failure (BPAR, graft loss, death, or MMF discontinuation) was found in this group compared to the FD group (29.2% vs 47.7%, $p = 0.03$), mainly due to a significantly lower incidence of BPAR (7.7% vs 24.6%, $p = 0.01$) and longer survival time without BPAR (Cox model, $p = 0.017$).

After a systematic literature search, Knight and Morris [170] concluded, "The current data regarding therapeutic monitoring of MMF is of limited quality. The most promising results to date come from LSS, with benefit seen in one prospective randomized trial. Further prospective trials and longer follow-up are required to investigate the optimum sampling strategy and subsets of patients who may benefit from monitoring, but the current evidence in favor of monitoring is weak." This seems a reasonable summary of current knowledge.

In summary, even if the routine use of MMF TDM has not been formally recommended based on the conflicting results of randomized studies, a recent retrospective analysis of a cohort of kidney transplant recipients showed that longitudinal exposure to MPA AUC is a better predictor of patient outcome than longitudinal CNI exposure in kidney transplant recipients receiving either CsA monitored on C_2 levels or Tac monitored on C_0 levels [146]. In addition, consensus conferences have recommended MPA monitoring based on the $AUC_{0-12\ h}$, with a target range of $30-60$ mg $\times$ h/L and adequate tools for AUC estimation using a limited sampling strategy, which are abundantly available in the literature and on the Internet.

16.3 OVERALL SUMMARY

Based on the literature so far, as described in the present chapter, individualizing immunosuppressive drug doses based on AUC targets may provide clinical benefits. Performing randomized clinical trials to support this statement is difficult and costly, but estimating individual AUCs can easily be achieved with the use of population models and computer tools. Still, the user interface needs to be adapted to the ordinary transplant physicians or clinical pharmacists for daily, and preferably bedside, use. In addition, experienced pharmacometricians are probably needed as well, to provide additional know-how for particularly difficult patients and also to continuously develop tools to satisfy future demands.

REFERENCES

[1] Mjörnstedt L, Sørensen SS, von Zur Muhlen B, Jespersen B, Hansen JM, Bistrup C, et al. Improved renal function after early conversion from a calcineurin inhibitor to everolimus: a randomized trial in kidney transplantation. Am J Transplant 2012;12(10):2744−53.

[2] Holdaas H, Midtvedt K, Asberg A. A drug safety evaluation of everolimus in kidney transplantation. Expert Opin Drug Saf 2012;11(6):1013−22.

[3] Lim WH, Eris J, Kanellis J, Pussell B, Wiid Z, Witcombe D, et al. A systematic review of conversion from calcineurin inhibitor to mammalian target of rapamycin inhibitors for maintenance immunosuppression in kidney transplant recipients. Am J Transplant 2014;14(9):2106−19.

[4] Bestard O, Crespo E, Stein M, Lucia M, Roelen DL, de Vaal YJ, et al. Cross-validation of IFN-gamma Elispot assay for measuring alloreactive memory/effector T cell responses in renal transplant recipients. Am J Transplant 2013;13(7):1880−90.

[5] van Besouw NM, Zuijderwijk JM, de Kuiper P, Ijzermans JN, Weimar W, van der Mast BJ. The granzyme B and interferon-gamma enzyme-linked immunospot assay as alternatives for cytotoxic T-lymphocyte precursor frequency after renal transplantation. Transplantation 2005;79(9):1062−6.

[6] Dinavahi R, Heeger PS. T-cell immune monitoring in organ transplantation. Curr Opin Organ Transplant 2008;13(4):419−24.

[7] Piccinini G, Gaspari F, Signorini O, Remuzzi G, Perico N. Recovery of blood mononuclear cell calcineurin activity segregates two populations of renal transplant patients with different sensitivities to cyclosporine inhibition. Transplantation 1996;61(10):1526−31.

[8] Yano I, Masuda S, Egawa H, Sugimoto M, Fukudo M, Yoshida Y, et al. Significance of trough monitoring for tacrolimus blood concentration and calcineurin activity in adult patients undergoing primary living-donor liver transplantation. Eur J Clin Pharmacol 2012;68(3):259−66.

[9] Yatscoff RW, Aspeslet LJ. The monitoring of immunosuppressive drugs: a pharmacodynamic approach. Ther Drug Monit 1998;20(5):459−63.

[10] Koefoed-Nielsen PB, Karamperis N, Jørgensen KA. Validation of the calcineurin phosphatase assay. Clin Chem 2004;50(12):2331−7.

[11] Hoerning A, Wilde B, Wang J, Tebbe B, Jing L, Wang X, et al. Pharmacodynamic monitoring of mammalian target of rapamycin inhibition by phosphoflow cytometric determination of p70S6 kinase activity. Transplantation 2015;99(1):210−19.

[12] Mahalati K, Belitsky P, Sketris I, West K, Panek R. Neoral monitoring by simplified sparse sampling area under the concentration-time curve: its relationship to acute rejection and cyclosporine nephrotoxicity early after kidney transplantation. Transplantation 1999;68(1):55−62.

[13]   Grant D, Kneteman N, Tchervenkov J, Roy A, Murphy G, Tan A, et al. Peak cyclosporine levels (C_{max}) correlate with freedom from liver graft rejection: results of a prospective, randomized comparison of neoral and sandimmune for liver transplantation (NOF-8). Transplantation 1999;67(8):1133−7.

[14]   Cantarovitch M, Elstein E, De Varennes B, et al. Clinical benefit of Neoral dose monitoring with cyclosporine 2-hr post-dose levels compared with trough levels in stable heart transplant patients. Transplantation 1999;68:1839−42.

[15]   Levy G, Thervet E, Lake J, Uchida K. Consensus on Neoral C(2): Expert Review in Transplantation (CONCERT) Group: Patient management by Neoral C(2) monitoring: an international consensus statement. Transplantation 2002;73(Suppl. 9):S12−18.

[16]   Bowles MJ, Waters JB, Lechler RI, et al. Do cyclosporine profiles provide useful information in the management of renal transplant recipients? Nephrol Dial Transplant 1996;11:1597−602.

[17]   Grevel J, Welsh MS, Kahan BD. Cyclosporine monitoring in renal transplantation: area under the curve monitoring is superior to trough-level monitoring. Ther Drug Monit 1989;11:246−8.

[18]   Kahan BD, Welsh M, Rutzky LP. Challenges in cyclosporine therapy: the role of therapeutic monitoring by area under the curve monitoring. Ther Drug Monit 1995;17:621−4.

[19]   Wada K, Takada M, Ueda T, Ochi H, Morishita H, Hanatani A, et al. Pharmacokinetic study and limited sampling strategy of cyclosporine in Japanese heart transplant recipients. Circ J 2006;70(10):1307−11.

[20]   Koristkova B, Grundmann M, Brozmanova H, Perinova I, Safarcik K. Validation of sparse sampling strategies to estimate cyclosporine A area under the concentration-time curve using either a specific radioimmunoassay or high-performance liquid chromatography method. Ther Drug Monit 2010;32(5):586−93.

[21]   Sarem S, Nekka F, Barrière O, Bittencourt H, Duval M, Teira P, et al. Limited sampling strategies for estimating intravenous and oral cyclosporine area under the curve in pediatric hematopoietic stem cell transplantation. Ther Drug Monit 2015;37(2):198−205.

[22]   Debord J, Risco E, Harel M, Le Meur Y, Büchler M, Lachâtre G, et al. Application of a gamma model of absorption to oral cyclosporin. Clin Pharmacokinet 2001;40(5):375−82.

[23]   Rousseau A, Léger F, Le Meur Y, Saint-Marcoux F, Paintaud G, Buchler M, et al. Population pharmacokinetic modeling of oral cyclosporin using NONMEM: comparison of absorption pharmacokinetic models and design of a Bayesian estimator. Ther Drug Monit 2004;26(1):23−30.

[24]   Saint-Marcoux F, Marquet P, Jacqz-Aigrain E, Bernard N, Thiry P, Le Meur Y, et al. Patient characteristics influencing ciclosporin pharmacokinetics and accurate Bayesian estimation of ciclosporin exposure in heart, lung and kidney transplant patients. Clin Pharmacokinet 2006;45(9):905−22.

[25]   Kim MG, Kim IW, Choi B, Han N, Yun HY, Park S, et al. Population pharmacokinetics of cyclosporine in hematopoietic stem cell transplant patients: consideration of genetic polymorphisms. Ann Pharmacother 2015;49(6):622−30.

[26]   Han K, Pillai VC, Venkataramanan R. Population pharmacokinetics of cyclosporine in transplant recipients. AAPS J 2013;15(4):901−12.

[27]   Monchaud C, Rousseau A, Leger F, David OJ, Debord J, Dantoine T, et al. Limited sampling strategies using Bayesian estimation or multilinear regression for cyclosporin AUC(0−12) monitoring in cardiac transplant recipients over the first year post-transplantation. Eur J Clin Pharmacol 2003;58(12):813−20.

[28]   Leger F, Debord J, Le Meur Y, Rousseau A, Büchler M, Lachâtre G, et al. Maximum a posteriori Bayesian estimation of oral cyclosporin pharmacokinetics in patients with stable renal transplants. Clin Pharmacokinet 2002;41(1):71−80.

[29]   Tokui K, Kimata T, Uchida K, Yuasa H, Hayashi Y, Itatsu T, et al. Dose adjustment strategy for oral microemulsion formulation of cyclosporine: population pharmacokinetics-based analysis in kidney transplant patients. Ther Drug Monit 2004;26(3):287−94.

[30]   Åsberg A, Falck P, Undset LH, Dørje C, Holdaas H, Hartmann A, et al. Computer-assisted cyclosporine dosing performs better than traditional dosing in renal transplant recipients: results of a pilot study. Ther Drug Monit 2010;32(2):152−8.

[31] Fruit D, Rousseau A, Amrein C, Rollé F, Kamar N, Sebbag L, et al. Ciclosporin population pharmacokinetics and Bayesian estimation in thoracic transplant recipients. Clin Pharmacokinet 2013;52(4):277−88.

[32] Wu G, Pea F, Cossettini P, Furlanut M. Effect of the number of samples on Bayesian and non-linear least-squares individualization: a study of cyclosporine treatment of haematological patients with multidrug resistance. J Pharm Pharmacol 1998;50(3):343−9.

[33] Charpiat B, Falconi I, Bréant V, Jelliffe RW, Sab JM, Ducerf C, et al. A population pharmacokinetic model of cyclosporine in the early postoperative phase in patients with liver transplants, and its predictive performance with Bayesian fitting. Ther Drug Monit 1998;20(2):158−64.

[34] Woillard JB, Lebreton V, Neely M, Turlure P, Girault S, Debord J, et al. Pharmacokinetic tools for the dose adjustment of ciclosporin in haematopoietic stem cell transplant patients. Br J Clin Pharmacol 2014;78(4):836−46.

[35] Marquet P. Clinical application of population pharmacokinetic methods developed for immunosuppressive drugs. Ther Drug Monit 2005;27(6):727−32.

[36] Internation Neoral Renal Transplantation Study Group. Randomized, international study of cyclosporine microemulsion absorption profiling in renal transplantation with basiliximab immunoprophylaxis. Am J Transplant 2002;2(2):157−66.

[37] Etienne I, Toupance O, Bénichou J, Thierry A, Al Najjar A, Hurault de Ligny B, et al. A 50% reduction in cyclosporine exposure in stable renal transplant recipients: renal function benefits. Nephrol Dial Transplant 2010;25(9):3096−106.

[38] Ekberg H, Bernasconi C, Noldeke J, Yussim A, Mjörnstedt L, Erken U, et al. Cyclosporine, tacrolimus and sirolimus retain their distinct toxicity profiles despite low doses in the Symphony study. Nephrol Dial Transplant 2010;25(6):2004−10.

[39] Nankivell BJ, Borrows RJ, Fung CL, O'Connell PJ, Allen RD, Chapman JR. The natural history of chronic allograft nephropathy. N Engl J Med 2003;349(24):2326−33.

[40] Schlickeiser S, Boes D, Streitz M, Sawitzki B. The use of novel diagnostics to individualize immunosuppression following transplantation. Transpl Int 2015;28(8):911−20.

[41] Saint-Marcoux F, Woillard JB, Jurado C, Marquet P. Lessons from routine dose adjustment of tacrolimus in renal transplant patients based on global exposure. Ther Drug Monit 2013;35(3):322−7.

[42] Staatz CE, Tett SE. Clinical pharmacokinetics and pharmacodynamics of tacrolimus in solid organ transplantation. Clin Pharmacokinet 2004;43(10):623−53.

[43] Størset E, Holford N, Hennig S, Bergmann TK, Bergan S, Bremer S, et al. Improved prediction of tacrolimus concentrations early after kidney transplantation using theory-based pharmacokinetic modelling. Br J Clin Pharmacol 2014;78(3):509−23.

[44] Størset E, Holford N, Midtvedt K, Bremer S, Bergan S, Åsberg A. Importance of hematocrit for a tacrolimus target concentration strategy. Eur J Clin Pharmacol 2014;70(1):65−77.

[45] Venkataramanan R, Swaminathan A, Prasad T, Jain A, Zuckerman S, Warty V, et al. Clinical pharmacokinetics of tacrolimus. Clin Pharmacokinet 1995;29(6):404−30.

[46] Nagase K, Iwasaki K, Nozaki K, Noda K. Distribution and protein binding of FK506, a potent immunosuppressive macrolide lactone, in human blood and its uptake by erythrocytes. J Pharm Pharmacol 1994;46(2):113−17.

[47] Chow FS, Piekoszewski W, Jusko WJ. Effect of hematocrit and albumin concentration on hepatic clearance of tacrolimus (FK506) during rabbit liver perfusion. Drug Metab Dispos 1997;25(5):610−16.

[48] Beysens AJ, Wijnen RM, Beuman GH, van der Heyden J, Kootstra G, van As H. FK 506: monitoring in plasma or in whole blood? Transplant Proc 1991;23(6):2745−7.

[49] Moller A, Iwasaki K, Kawamura A, Teramura Y, Shiraga T, Hata T, et al. The disposition of 14C-labeled tacrolimus after intravenous and oral administration in healthy human subjects. Drug Metab Dispos 1999;27(6):633−6.

[50] Li Y, Hu X, Cai B, Chen J, Bai Y, Tang J, et al. Meta-analysis of the effect of MDR1 C3435 polymorphism on tacrolimus pharmacokinetics in renal transplant recipients. Transpl Immunol 2012;27(1):12−18.

[51] Lunde I, Bremer S, Midtvedt K, Mohebi B, Dahl M, Bergan S, et al. The influence of CYP3A, PPARA, and POR genetic variants on the pharmacokinetics of tacrolimus and cyclosporine in renal transplant recipients. Eur J Clin Pharmacol 2014;70(6):685−93.

[52] Aouam K, Chadli Z, Hammouda M, Fredj NB, Aloui S, May ME, et al. Development of limited sampling strategies for the estimation of tacrolimus area under the curve in adult kidney transplant recipients according to the posttransplantation time. Ther Drug Monit 2015;37(4):524−30.

[53] Mardigyan V, Tchervenkov J, Metrakos P, Barkun J, Deschenes M, Cantarovich M. Best single time points as surrogates to the tacrolimus and mycophenolic acid area under the curve in adult liver transplant patients beyond 12 months of transplantation. Clin Ther 2005;27(4):463−9.

[54] Ekberg H, Tedesco-Silva H, Demirbas A, Vitko S, Nashan B, Gurkan A, et al. Reduced exposure to calcineurin inhibitors in renal transplantation. N Engl J Med 2007;357(25):2562−75.

[55] Ekberg H, Mamelok RD, Pearson TC, Vincenti F, Tedesco-Silva H, Daloze P. The challenge of achieving target drug concentrations in clinical trials: experience from the Symphony study. Transplantation 2009;87(9):1360−6.

[56] Benkali K, Rostaing L, Premaud A, Woillard JB, Saint-Marcoux F, Urien S, et al. Population pharmacokinetics and Bayesian estimation of tacrolimus exposure in renal transplant recipients on a new once-daily formulation. Clin Pharmacokinet 2010;49(10):683−92.

[57] Chen HY, Chen TC, Min DI, Fischer GW, Wu YM. Prediction of tacrolimus blood levels by using the neural network with genetic algorithm in liver transplantation patients. Ther Drug Monit 1999;21(1):50−6.

[58] Monchaud C, de Winter BC, Knoop C, Estenne M, Reynaud-Gaubert M, Pison C, et al. Population pharmacokinetic modelling and design of a Bayesian estimator for therapeutic drug monitoring of tacrolimus in lung transplantation. Clin Pharmacokinet 2012;51(3):175−86.

[59] Benkali K, Premaud A, Picard N, Rerolle JP, Toupance O, Hoizey G, et al. Tacrolimus population pharmacokinetic-pharmacogenetic analysis and Bayesian estimation in renal transplant recipients. Clin Pharmacokinet 2009;48(12):805−16.

[60] Saint-Marcoux F, Debord J, Parant F, Labalette M, Kamar N, Rostaing L, et al. Development and evaluation of a simulation procedure to take into account various assays for the Bayesian dose adjustment of tacrolimus. Ther Drug Monit 2011;33(2):171−7.

[61] Saint-Marcoux F, Vandierdonck S, Prémaud A, Debord J, Rousseau A, Marquet P. Large scale analysis of routine dose adjustments of mycophenolate mofetil based on global exposure in renal transplant patients. Ther Drug Monit 2011;33(3):285−94.

[62] Saint-Marcoux F, Guigonis V, Decramer S, Gandia P, Ranchin B, Parant F, et al. Development of a Bayesian estimator for the therapeutic drug monitoring of mycophenolate mofetil in children with idiopathic nephrotic syndrome. Pharmacol Res 2011;63(5):423−31.

[63] Woillard JB, de Winter BC, Kamar N, Marquet P, Rostaing L, Rousseau A. Population pharmacokinetic model and Bayesian estimator for two tacrolimus formulations—twice daily Prograf and once daily Advagraf. Br J Clin Pharmacol 2011;71(3):391−402.

[64] Åsberg A, Midtvedt K, van Guilder M, Størset E, Bremer S, Bergan S, et al. Inclusion of CYP3A5 genotyping in a nonparametric population model improves dosing of tacrolimus early after transplantation. Transpl Int 2013;26(12):1198−207.

[65] Undre NA, Stevenson P, Schafer A. Pharmacokinetics of tacrolimus: clinically relevant aspects. Transplant Proc 1999;31(7A):21S−24SS.

[66] Undre NA, van Hooff J, Christiaans M, Vanrenterghem Y, Donck J, Heeman U, et al. Low systemic exposure to tacrolimus correlates with acute rejection. Transplant Proc 1999;31(1−2):296−8.

[67] Laskow DA, Vincenti F, Neylan JF, Mendez R, Matas AJ. An open-label, concentration-ranging trial of FK506 in primary kidney transplantation: a report of the United States Multicenter FK506 Kidney Transplant Group. Transplantation 1996;62(7):900−5.

[68] Wallemacq P, Armstrong VW, Brunet M, Haufroid V, Holt DW, Johnston A, et al. Opportunities to optimize tacrolimus therapy in solid organ transplantation: report of the European consensus conference. Ther Drug Monit 2009;31(2):139−52.

[69] Robertsen I, Åsberg A, Ingerø AO, Vethe NT, Bremer S, Bergan S, et al. Use of generic tacrolimus in elderly renal transplant recipients: precaution is needed. Transplantation 2015;99(3):528−32.

[70] Størset E, Åsberg A, Skauby M, Neely M, Bergan S, Bremer S, et al. Improved tacrolimus target concentration achievement using computerized dosing in renal transplant recipients—a prospective, randomized study. Transplantation 2015;99(10):2158−66.

[71] Bergmann TK, Hennig S, Barraclough KA, Isbel NM, Staatz CE. Population pharmacokinetics of tacrolimus in adult kidney transplant patients: impact of CYP3A5 genotype on starting dose. Ther Drug Monit 2014;36(1):62−70.

[72] Hesselink DA, Bouamar R, Elens L, van Schaik RH, van Gelder T. The role of pharmacogenetics in the disposition of and response to tacrolimus in solid organ transplantation. Clin Pharmacokinet 2014;53(2):123−39.

[73] Andrews LM, Riva N, de Winter BC, Hesselink DA, de Wildt SN, Cransberg K, et al. Dosing algorithms for initiation of immunosuppressive drugs in solid organ transplant recipients. Expert Opin Drug Metab Toxicol 2015;11(6):921−36.

[74] Campbell S, Hawley C, Irish A, Hutchison B, Walker R, Butcher BE, et al. Pre-transplant pharmacokinetic profiling and tacrolimus requirements post-transplant. Nephrology 2010;15(7):714−19.

[75] Boughton O, Borgulya G, Cecconi M, Fredericks S, Moreton-Clack M, MacPhee IA. A published pharmacogenetic algorithm was poorly predictive of tacrolimus clearance in an independent cohort of renal transplant recipients. Br J Clin Pharmacol 2013;76(3):425−31.

[76] Musuamba FT, Mourad M, Haufroid V, Delattre IK, Verbeeck RK, Wallemacq P. Time of drug administration, CYP3A5 and ABCB1 genotypes, and analytical method influence tacrolimus pharmacokinetics: a population pharmacokinetic study. Ther Drug Monit 2009;31(6):734−42.

[77] Musuamba FT, Mourad M, Haufroid V, Demeyer M, Capron A, Delattre IK, et al. A simultaneous d-optimal designed study for population pharmacokinetic analyses of mycophenolic acid and tacrolimus early after renal transplantation. J Clin Pharmacol 2012;52(12):1833−43.

[78] Passey C, Birnbaum AK, Brundage RC, Oetting WS, Israni AK, Jacobson PA. Dosing equation for tacrolimus using genetic variants and clinical factors. Br J Clin Pharmacol 2011;72(6):948−57.

[79] Press RR, Ploeger BA, den Hartigh J, van der Straaten T, van Pelt J, Danhof M, et al. Explaining variability in tacrolimus pharmacokinetics to optimize early exposure in adult kidney transplant recipients. Ther Drug Monit 2009;31(2):187−97.

[80] Staatz CE, Willis C, Taylor PJ, Tett SE. Population pharmacokinetics of tacrolimus in adult kidney transplant recipients. Clin Pharmacol Ther 2002;72(6):660−9.

[81] Wang P, Mao Y, Razo J, Zhou X, Wong ST, Patel S, et al. Using genetic and clinical factors to predict tacrolimus dose in renal transplant recipients. Pharmacogenomics 2010;11(10):1389−402.

[82] Antignac M, Barrou B, Farinotti R, Lechat P, Urien S. Population pharmacokinetics and bioavailability of tacrolimus in kidney transplant patients. Br J Clin Pharmacol 2007;64(6):750−7.

[83] Hinchliffe E, Adaway J, Fildes J, Rowan A, Keevil BG. Therapeutic drug monitoring of ciclosporin A and tacrolimus in heart lung transplant patients using dried blood spots. Ann Clin Biochem 2014;51(Pt 1):106−9.

[84] Koster RA, Alffenaar JW, Greijdanus B, Uges DR. Fast LC-MS/MS analysis of tacrolimus, sirolimus, everolimus and cyclosporin A in dried blood spots and the influence of the hematocrit and immunosuppressant concentration on recovery. Talanta 2013;115:47−54.

[85] Capron A, Mourad M, De Meyer M, De Pauw L, Eddour DC, Latinne D, et al. CYP3A5 and ABCB1 polymorphisms influence tacrolimus concentrations in peripheral blood mononuclear cells after renal transplantation. Pharmacogenomics 2010;11(5):703−14.

[86] Lemaitre F, Antignac M, Fernandez C. Monitoring of tacrolimus concentrations in peripheral blood mononuclear cells: application to cardiac transplant recipients. Clin Biochem 2013;46(15):1538−41.

[87] Knops N, van den Heuvel LP, Masereeuw R, Bongaers I, de Loor H, Levtchenko E, et al. The functional implications of common genetic variation in CYP3A5 and ABCB1 in human proximal tubule cells. Mol Pharm 2015;12(3):758−68.

[88] Kirchner GI, Meier-Wiedenbach I, Manns MP. Clinical pharmacokinetics of everolimus. Clin Pharmacokinet 2004;43(2):83−95.

[89] Zaza G, Granata S, Tomei P, Masola V, Gambaro G, Lupo A. mTOR inhibitors and renal allograft: Yin and Yang. J Nephrol 2014;27(5):495−506.

[90] Lloberas N, Torras J, Alperovich G, Cruzado JM, Gimenez-Bonafe P, Herrero-Fresneda I, et al. Different renal toxicity profiles in the association of cyclosporine and tacrolimus with sirolimus in rats. Nephrol Dial Transplant 2008;23(10):3111−19.

[91] Shihab F, Christians U, Smith L, Wellen JR, Kaplan B. Focus on mTOR inhibitors and tacrolimus in renal transplantation: pharmacokinetics, exposure-response relationships, and clinical outcomes. Transpl Immunol 2014;31(1):22−32.

[92] Flechner SM, Gurkan A, Hartmann A, Legendre CM, Russ GR, Campistol JM, et al. A randomized, open-label study of sirolimus versus cyclosporine in primary de novo renal allograft recipients. Transplantation 2013;95(10):1233−41.

[93] Gude E, Gullestad L, Arora S, Simonsen S, Hoel I, Hartmann A, et al. Benefit of early conversion from CNI-based to everolimus-based immunosuppression in heart transplantation. J Heart Lung Transplant 2010;29(6):641−7.

[94] Muhlbacher F, Neumayer HH, del Castillo D, Stefoni S, Zygmunt AJ, Budde K, et al. The efficacy and safety of cyclosporine reduction in de novo renal allograft patients receiving sirolimus and corticosteroids: results from an open-label comparative study. Transpl Int 2014;27(2):176−86.

[95] Soliman K, Mogadam E, Laftavi M, Patel S, Feng L, Said M, et al. Long-term outcomes following sirolimus conversion after renal transplantation. Immunol Invest 2014;43(8):819−28.

[96] Budde K, Lehner F, Sommerer C, Reinke P, Arns W, Eisenberger U, et al. Five-year outcomes in kidney transplant patients converted from cyclosporine to everolimus: the randomized ZEUS study. Am J Transplant 2015;15(1):119−28.

[97] Chhabra D, Skaro AI, Leventhal JR, Dalal P, Shah G, Wang E, et al. Long-term kidney allograft function and survival in prednisone-free regimens: tacrolimus/mycophenolate mofetil versus tacrolimus/sirolimus. Clin J Am Soc Nephrol 2012;7(3):504−12.

[98] Klintmalm GB, Saab S, Hong JC, Nashan B. The role of mammalian target of rapamycin inhibitors in the management of post-transplant malignancy. Clin Transplant 2014;28(6):635−48.

[99] Kahan BD, Napoli KL, Kelly PA, Podbielski J, Hussein I, Urbauer DL, et al. Therapeutic drug monitoring of sirolimus: correlations with efficacy and toxicity. Clin Transplant 2000;14(2):97−109.

[100] Kahan BD, Stepkowski SM, Napoli KL, Katz SM, Knight RJ, Van Buren C. The development of sirolimus: the University of Texas-Houston experience. Clin Transpl 2000;145−58.

[101] Kovarik JM, Kahan BD, Kaplan B, Lorber M, Winkler M, Rouilly M, et al. Longitudinal assessment of everolimus in de novo renal transplant recipients over the first post-transplant year: pharmacokinetics, exposure-response relationships, and influence on cyclosporine. Clin Pharmacol Ther 2001;69(1):48−56.

[102] Kovarik JM, Sabia HD, Figueiredo J, Zimmermann H, Reynolds C, Dilzer SC, et al. Influence of hepatic impairment on everolimus pharmacokinetics: implications for dose adjustment. Clin Pharmacol Ther 2001;70(5):425−30.

[103] Budde K, Becker T, Arns W, Sommerer C, Reinke P, Eisenberger U, et al. Everolimus-based, calcineurin-inhibitor-free regimen in recipients of de-novo kidney transplants: an open-label, randomised, controlled trial. Lancet 2011;377(9768):837–47.

[104] Pham PT, Pham PC, Danovitch GM, Ross DJ, Gritsch HA, Kendrick EA, et al. Sirolimus-associated pulmonary toxicity. Transplantation 2004;77(8):1215–20.

[105] Moes DJ, Press RR, den Hartigh J, van der Straaten T, de Fijter JW, Guchelaar HJ. Population pharmacokinetics and pharmacogenetics of everolimus in renal transplant patients. Clin Pharmacokinet 2012;51(7):467–80.

[106] Emoto C, Fukuda T, Cox S, Christians U, Vinks AA. Development of a physiologically-based pharmacokinetic model for sirolimus: predicting bioavailability based on intestinal CYP3A content. CPT: Pharmacometrics Syst Pharmacol 2013;2:e59.

[107] Laplanche R, Meno-Tetang GM, Kawai R. Physiologically based pharmacokinetic (PBPK) modeling of everolimus (RAD001) in rats involving non-linear tissue uptake. J Pharmacokinet Pharmacodyn 2007;34(3):373–400.

[108] Zimmerman JJ, Ferron GM, Lim HK, Parker V. The effect of a high-fat meal on the oral bioavailability of the immunosuppressant sirolimus (rapamycin). J Clin Pharmacol 1999;39(11):1155–61.

[109] Kovarik JM, Hartmann S, Figueiredo J, Rordorf C, Golor G, Lison A, et al. Effect of food on everolimus absorption: quantification in healthy subjects and a confirmatory screening in patients with renal transplants. Pharmacotherapy 2002;22(2):154–9.

[110] Kovarik JM, Kalbag J, Figueiredo J, Rouilly M, Frazier OL, Rordorf C. Differential influence of two cyclosporine formulations on everolimus pharmacokinetics: a clinically relevant pharmacokinetic interaction. J Clin Pharmacol 2002;42(1):95–9.

[111] Kovarik JM, Noe A, Berthier S, McMahon L, Langholff WK, Marion AS, et al. Clinical development of an everolimus pediatric formulation: relative bioavailability, food effect, and steady-state pharmacokinetics. J Clin Pharmacol 2003;43(2):141–7.

[112] Amundsen R, Åsberg A, Ohm IK, Christensen H. Cyclosporine A- and tacrolimus-mediated inhibition of CYP3A4 and CYP3A5 in vitro. Drug Metab Dispos 2012;40(4):655–61.

[113] Brandhorst G, Tenderich G, Zittermann A, Oezpeker C, Koerfer R, Oellerich M, et al. Everolimus exposure in cardiac transplant recipients is influenced by concomitant calcineurin inhibitor. Ther Drug Monit 2008;30(1):113–16.

[114] Lamoureux F, Picard N, Boussera B, Sauvage FL, Marquet P. Sirolimus and everolimus intestinal absorption and interaction with calcineurin inhibitors: a differential effect between cyclosporine and tacrolimus. Fundam Clin Pharmacol 2012;26(4):463–72.

[115] Kirchner GI, Winkler M, Mueller L, Vidal C, Jacobsen W, Franzke A, et al. Pharmacokinetics of SDZ RAD and cyclosporin including their metabolites in seven kidney graft patients after the first dose of SDZ RAD. Br J Clin Pharmacol 2000;50(5):449–54.

[116] Lampen A, Zhang Y, Hackbarth I, Benet LZ, Sewing KF, Christians U. Metabolism and transport of the macrolide immunosuppressant sirolimus in the small intestine. J Pharmacol Exp Ther 1998;285 (3):1104–12.

[117] Neumayer HH, Paradis K, Korn A, Jean C, Fritsche L, Budde K, et al. Entry-into-human study with the novel immunosuppressant SDZ RAD in stable renal transplant recipients. Br J Clin Pharmacol 1999;48(5):694–703.

[118] Trepanier DJ, Gallant H, Legatt DF, Yatscoff RW. Rapamycin: distribution, pharmacokinetics and therapeutic range investigations: an update. Clin Biochem 1998;31(5):345–51.

[119] Yatscoff RW, Wang P, Chan K, Hicks D, Zimmerman J. Rapamycin: distribution, pharmacokinetics, and therapeutic range investigations. Ther Drug Monit 1995;17(6):666–71.

[120] Ferron GM, Mishina EV, Zimmerman JJ, Jusko WJ. Population pharmacokinetics of sirolimus in kidney transplant patients. Clin Pharmacol Ther 1997;61(4):416–28.

[121] MacDonald A, Scarola J, Burke JT, Zimmerman JJ. Clinical pharmacokinetics and therapeutic drug monitoring of sirolimus. Clin Ther 2000;22(Suppl. B):B101–21.

[122] Kahan BD. Sirolimus: a comprehensive review. Expert Opin Pharmacother 2001;2(11):1903–17.

[123] Cattaneo D, Cortinovis M, Baldelli S, Gotti E, Remuzzi G, Perico N. Limited sampling strategies for the estimation of sirolimus daily exposure in kidney transplant recipients on a calcineurin inhibitor-free regimen. J Clin Pharmacol 2009;49(7):773–81.

[124] Robertsen I, Åsberg A, Granseth T, Vethe NT, Akhlaghi F, Ghareeb M, et al. More potent lipid-lowering effect by rosuvastatin compared with fluvastatin in everolimus-treated renal transplant recipients. Transplantation 2014;97(12):1266–71.

[125] Robertsen I, Falck P, Andreassen AK, Næss NK, Lunder N, Christensen H, et al. Endomyocardial, intralymphocyte, and whole blood concentrations of ciclosporin A in heart transplant recipients. Transplant Res 2013;2(1):5.

[126] Bemelman FJ, de Maar EF, Press RR, van Kan HJ, ten Berge IJ, Homan van der Heide JJ, et al. Minimization of maintenance immunosuppression early after renal transplantation: an interim analysis. Transplantation 2009;88(3):421–8.

[127] Starling RC, Hare JM, Hauptman P, McCurry KR, Mayer HW, Kovarik JM, et al. Therapeutic drug monitoring for everolimus in heart transplant recipients based on exposure-effect modeling. Am J Transplant 2004;4(12):2126–31.

[128] Vitko S, Margreiter R, Weimar W, Dantal J, Viljoen HG, Li Y, et al. Everolimus (Certican) 12-month safety and efficacy versus mycophenolate mofetil in de novo renal transplant recipients. Transplantation 2004;78(10):1532–40.

[129] Vitko S, Tedesco H, Eris J, Pascual J, Whelchel J, Magee JC, et al. Everolimus with optimized cyclosporine dosing in renal transplant recipients: 6-month safety and efficacy results of two randomized studies. Am J Transplant 2004;4(4):626–35.

[130] Cattaneo D, Merlini S, Pellegrino M, Carrara F, Zenoni S, Murgia S, et al. Therapeutic drug monitoring of sirolimus: effect of concomitant immunosuppressive therapy and optimization of drug dosing. Am J Transplant 2004;4(8):1345–51.

[131] Kovarik JM, Tedesco H, Pascual J, Civati G, Bizot MN, Geissler J, et al. Everolimus therapeutic concentration range defined from a prospective trial with reduced-exposure cyclosporine in de novo kidney transplantation. Ther Drug Monit 2004;26(5):499–505.

[132] McAlister VC, Mahalati K, Peltekian KM, Fraser A, MacDonald AS. A clinical pharmacokinetic study of tacrolimus and sirolimus combination immunosuppression comparing simultaneous to separated administration. Ther Drug Monit 2002;24(3):346–50.

[133] Djebli N, Rousseau A, Hoizey G, Rerolle JP, Toupance O, Le Meur Y, et al. Sirolimus population pharmacokinetic/pharmacogenetic analysis and Bayesian modelling in kidney transplant recipients. Clin Pharmacokinet 2006;45(11):1135–48.

[134] Moes DJ, Swen JJ, den Hartigh J, van der Straaten T, van der Heide JJ, Sanders JS, et al. Effect of CYP3A4*22, CYP3A5*3, and CYP3A combined genotypes on cyclosporine, everolimus, and tacrolimus pharmacokinetics in renal transplantation. CPT: Pharmacometrics Syst Pharmacol 2014;3:e100.

[135] Picard N, Rouguieg-Malki K, Kamar N, Rostaing L, Marquet P. CYP3A5 genotype does not influence everolimus in vitro metabolism and clinical pharmacokinetics in renal transplant recipients. Transplantation 2011;91(6):652–6.

[136] Zochowska D, Wyzgal J, Paczek L. Impact of CYP3A4*1B and CYP3A5*3 polymorphisms on the pharmacokinetics of cyclosporine and sirolimus in renal transplant recipients. Ann Transplant 2012;17(3):36–44.

[137] Anglicheau D, Le Corre D, Lechaton S, Laurent-Puig P, Kreis H, Beaune P, et al. Consequences of genetic polymorphisms for sirolimus requirements after renal transplant in patients on primary sirolimus therapy. Am J Transplant 2005;5(3):595–603.

[138] Le Meur Y, Djebli N, Szelag JC, Hoizey G, Toupance O, Rerolle JP, et al. CYP3A5*3 influences sirolimus oral clearance in de novo and stable renal transplant recipients. Clin Pharmacol Ther 2006;80(1):51−60.

[139] Knight SR, Morris PJ. Does the evidence support the use of mycophenolate mofetil therapeutic drug monitoring in clinical practice? A systematic review 2008;85(11):1675−85.

[140] Kuypers DR, Le Meur Y, Cantarovich M, Tredger MJ, Tett SE, Cattaneo D, et al. Consensus report on therapeutic drug monitoring of mycophenolic acid in solid organ transplantation. Clin J Am Soc Nephrol 2010;5(2):341−58.

[141] Staatz CE, Tett SE. Clinical pharmacokinetics and pharmacodynamics of mycophenolate in solid organ transplant recipients. Clin Pharmacokinet 2007;46(1):13−58.

[142] Le Meur Y, Büchler M, Thierry A, Caillard S, Villemain F, Lavaud S, et al. Individualized mycophenolate mofetil dosing based on drug exposure significantly improves patient outcomes after renal transplantation. Am J Transplant 2007;7(11):2496−503.

[143] van Gelder T. Therapeutic drug monitoring for mycophenolic acid is value for (little) money. Clin Pharmacol Ther 2011;90(2):203−4.

[144] Daher Abdi Z, Essig M, Rizopoulos D, Le Meur Y, Prémaud A, Woillard JB, et al. Impact of longitudinal exposure to mycophenolic acid on acute rejection in renal transplant recipients using joint modeling approach. Pharmacol Res 2013;72:52−60.

[145] Byrne R, Yost SE, Kaplan B. Mycophenolate mofetil monitoring: is there evidence that it can improve outcomes? Clin Pharmacol Ther 2011;90(2):204−6. http://dx.doi.org/10.1038/clpt.2011.95. PMID:21772295.

[146] Daher Abdi Z, Prémaud A, Essig M, Alain S, Munteanu E, Garnier F, et al. Exposure to mycophenolic acid better predicts immunosuppressive efficacy than exposure to calcineurin inhibitors in renal transplant patients. Clin Pharmacol Ther 2014;96(4):508−15.

[147] van Gelder T, Hilbrands LB, Vanrenterghem Y, Weimar W, de Fijter JW, Squifflet JP, et al. A randomized double-blind, multicenter plasma concentration controlled study of the safety and efficacy of oral mycophenolate mofetil for the prevention of acute rejection after kidney transplantation. Transplantation 1999;68(2):261−6.

[148] Tett SE, Saint-Marcoux F, Staatz CE, Brunet M, Vinks AA, Miura M, et al. Mycophenolate, clinical pharmacokinetics, formulations, and methods for assessing drug exposure. Transplant Rev 2011;25 (2):47−57.

[149] Le Meur Y, Borrows R, Pescovitz MD, Budde K, Grinyo J, Bloom R, et al. Therapeutic drug monitoring of mycophenolates in kidney transplantation: report of the transplantation society consensus meeting. Transplant Rev 2011;25(2):58−64.

[150] Ting LS, Partovi N, Levy RD, Riggs KW, Ensom MH. Limited sampling strategy for predicting area under the concentration-time curve of mycophenolic acid in adult lung transplant recipients. Pharmacotherapy 2006;26(9):1232−40.

[151] Willis C, Taylor PJ, Salm P, Tett SE, Pillans PI. Evaluation of limited sampling strategies for estimation of 12-hour mycophenolic acid area under the plasma concentration-time curve in adult renal transplant patients. Ther Drug Monit 2000;22(5):549−54.

[152] Bruchet NK, Ensom MH. Limited sampling strategies for mycophenolic acid in solid organ transplantation: a systematic review. Expert Opin Drug Metab Toxicol 2009;5(9):1079−97.

[153] Abd Rahman AN, Tett SE, Staatz CE. How accurate and precise are limited sampling strategies in estimating exposure to mycophenolic acid in people with autoimmune disease? Clin Pharmacokinet 2014;53(3):227−45.

[154] Barraclough KA, Isbel NM, Franklin ME, Lee KJ, Taylor PJ, Campbell SB, et al. Evaluation of limited sampling strategies for mycophenolic acid after mycophenolate mofetil intake in adult kidney transplant recipients. Ther Drug Monit 2010;32(6):723−33.

[155] Le Guellec C, Bourgoin H, Büchler M, Le Meur Y, Lebranchu Y, Marquet P, et al. Population pharmacokinetics and Bayesian estimation of mycophenolic acid concentrations in stable renal transplant patients. Clin Pharmacokinet 2004;43(4):253−66.

[156] van Hest RM, van Gelder T, Vulto AG, Mathot RA. Population pharmacokinetics of mycophenolic acid in renal transplant recipients. Clin Pharmacokinet 2005;44(10):1083−96.

[157] Payen S, Zhang D, Maisin A, Popon M, Bensman A, Bouissou F, et al. Population pharmacokinetics of mycophenolic acid in kidney transplant pediatric and adolescent patients. Ther Drug Monit 2005;27(3):378−88.

[158] Prémaud A, Debord J, Rousseau A, Le Meur Y, Toupance O, Lebranchu Y, et al. A double absorption-phase model adequately describes mycophenolic acid plasma profiles in de novo renal transplant recipients given oral mycophenolate mofetil. Clin Pharmacokinet 2005;44(8):837−47.

[159] Prémaud A, Le Meur Y, Debord J, Szelag JC, Rousseau A, Hoizey G, et al. Maximum a posteriori Bayesian estimation of mycophenolic acid pharmacokinetics in renal transplant recipients at different postgrafting periods. Ther Drug Monit 2005;27(3):354−61.

[160] Musuamba FT, Rousseau A, Bosmans JL, Senessael JJ, Cumps J, Marquet P, et al. Limited sampling models and Bayesian estimation for mycophenolic acid area under the curve prediction in stable renal transplant patients co-medicated with ciclosporin or sirolimus. Clin Pharmacokinet 2009;48(11):745−58.

[161] Sherwin CM, Fukuda T, Brunner HI, Goebel J, Vinks AA. The evolution of population pharmacokinetic models to describe the enterohepatic recycling of mycophenolic acid in solid organ transplantation and autoimmune disease. Clin Pharmacokinet 2011;50(1):1−24.

[162] Colom H, Lloberas N, Andreu F, Caldés A, Torras J, Oppenheimer F, et al. Pharmacokinetic modeling of enterohepatic circulation of mycophenolic acid in renal transplant recipients. Kidney Int 2014;85(6):1434−43.

[163] Prémaud A, Weber LT, Tönshoff B, Armstrong VW, Oellerich M, Urien S, et al. Population pharmacokinetics of mycophenolic acid in pediatric renal transplant patients using parametric and nonparametric approaches. Pharmacol Res 2011;63(3):216−24.

[164] Dong M, Fukuda T, Vinks AA. Optimization of mycophenolic acid therapy using clinical pharmacometrics. Drug Metab Pharmacokinet 2014;29(1):4−11.

[165] de Winter BC, Mathot RA, Sombogaard F, Vulto AG, van Gelder T. Nonlinear relationship between mycophenolate mofetil dose and mycophenolic acid exposure: implications for therapeutic drug monitoring. Clin J Am Soc Nephrol 2011;6(3):656−63.

[166] Prémaud A, Rousseau A, Johnson G, Canivet C, Gandia P, Muscari F, et al. Inhibition of T-cell activation and proliferation by mycophenolic acid in patients awaiting liver transplantation: PK/PD relationships. Pharmacol Res 2011;63(5):432−8.

[167] Staatz CE, Tett SE. Maximum a posteriori Bayesian estimation of mycophenolic acid area under the concentration-time curve: is this clinically useful for dosage prediction yet?. Clin Pharmacokinet 2011;50(12):759−72.

[168] van Gelder T, Silva HT, de Fijter JW, Budde K, Kuypers D, Tyden G, et al. Comparing mycophenolate mofetil regimens for de novo renal transplant recipients: the fixed-dose concentration-controlled trial. Transplantation 2008;86(8):1043−51.

[169] van Gelder T, Tedesco Silva H, de Fijter JW, Budde K, Kuypers D, Arns W, et al. Renal transplant patients at high risk of acute rejection benefit from adequate exposure to mycophenolic acid. Transplantation 2010;89(5):595−9.

[170] Knight SR, Morris PJ. Does the evidence support the use of mycophenolate mofetil therapeutic drug monitoring in clinical practice? A systematic review. Transplantation 2008;85(12):1675−85.

INDIVIDUALIZING DOSAGE REGIMENS OF ANTINEOPLASTIC AGENTS

17

A. Aldaz and P. Schaiquevich

CHAPTER OUTLINE

17.1 HISTORY AND CURRENT STATUS

The clinical pharmacokinetics of anticancer drugs have been studied for over five decades, as reflected by many excellent scientific reports on different aspects in the field [1−31]. Older reports were based on the description of different methods to optimize the therapeutic scheme for translation into clinical practice. In addition, patients with different pathological conditions were identified to best adjust the dosage regimen of the anticancer treatment according to their physiological and pathological conditions [10,19]. Some of these populations include patients with renal or liver failure and obese patients [23−25,27,28,32−35]. Other reports have described the pharmacokinetic behavior of antineoplastic agents by grouping them based on data obtained from either clinical or research studies.

All these studies acknowledge the need for individualized dosage regimens using TDM in oncology, mainly based on the relationship between pharmacokinetic parameters of drug exposure (AUC or $C_{\max}$) and clinical endpoints, such as safety or efficacy (pharmacodynamics) [31,35−38]. Nonetheless, these reports also commented on the difficulties of performing TDM.

Among these limitations, the reports highlighted the issues in finding a therapeutic range especially for patients having solid tumors, and the lack of automated analytical methods that allow

Individualized Drug Therapy for Patients. DOI: http://dx.doi.org/10.1016/B978-0-12-803348-7.00017-4

for sample processing in a timely fashion. In addition, the difficulties are even more challenging with combination therapies and the sequence of administration of chemotherapies.

Current advances in analytical methodology—including the availability of commercial assay kits not only for methotrexate but also for 5-Fluorouracil (Saladax) or even for newer agents as in the case of paclitaxel, docetaxel, and monoclonal antibodies (bevacizumab, rituximab, or trastuzumab; eg, Theradiag)—will facilitate the implementation of routine TDM for these agents from the analytical perspective.

Still, most dose individualization in oncology is restricted to a small number of patients. A significant factor that has prevented progress is the absence of a correct definition of the therapeutic range due to a lack of short- and long-term results obtained in hospitals. Routine outpatient monitoring is performed on a daily or weekly basis, but the health professionals are usually overwhelmed by clinical demands. Many clinical, biochemical, and general observations are therefore not recorded, with loss of precious information for pharmacokinetic/pharmacodynamic (PK/PD) modeling.

Great efforts have been made in modeling hematological toxicities, including absolute neutrophil count related to the cytotoxic drug systemic exposure. However, these models became obsolete with the incorporation in the clinics of colony-stimulating growth factors. On the other hand, the limited available data on adverse events or efficacy has limited the development of PK/PD models to optimize the efficacy and safety of anticancer agents.

In oncology, it has been common to determine the clinical dose based on the maximum tolerable dose and the dose limiting toxicity that have been preestablished in clinical trials. However, based on the high interindividual variability in the pharmacokinetics of anticancer agents, the approximation of a fixed dose based on these two factors results in many patients being either underdosed, with subtherapeutic drug exposure, or overdosed, with toxicities. Dose adjustment performed in the framework of TDM has usually been intended to avoid severe toxicity during drug administration or in subsequent cycles of chemotherapy in patients with liver or renal failure or in obese patients. However, only in exceptional cases has an increase in the prescribed dose been suggested to patients.

The question is, why is dose reduction performed in cases of unacceptable toxicity, but conversely, why does a lack of toxicity generally not lead to an increase in the dose? Underdosed patients may well benefit from an increased dose, possibly improving their outcome and overall survival. Specifically, oncology patients greatly benefit from TDM for dose individualization as it provides a unique tool to guide the regimen and define the dose.

It is also important to emphasize the difference between clinical research and routine TDM. In the former, many—maybe hundreds—of preclinical and clinical PK/PD models have been published. Many of these population-based PK/PD reports on anticancer agents have involved complex models and over-parametrized systems that were never translated into the clinics, not even by the authors who published those reports. Additionally, some other models were made from studies funded by the pharmaceutical industry in Phase II/III clinical trials that also were not translated into the clinics. An important limitation of these models is that the validation techniques were constrained to simulations as there were no available data from other populations apart from those of the clinical trials. An interesting article that supports this concept is the one published by Brendel et al. [39]. They analyzed all PK and/or PD studies published between 2002 and 2004 and concluded that only around 30% of those models were adequately validated [39].

Oncology patients commonly receive a combination of multiple drugs, and the contribution of each single drug to the antitumor effect or toxicity is difficult to determine. In addition, the relationship between drug exposure and response may be modified by concomitant agents. Moreover, the incorporation of monoclonal antibodies in clinical protocols (FOLFOX, FOLFIRI) based on 5-FU treatment in colorectal cancer patients without performing a pharmacokinetic study for 5-FU made it more difficult to discern to which drug to attribute the clinical benefit or adverse events [40,41]. In this study [41], the authors could not draw any conclusions on the differences or similarities in 5-FU bioavailability in patients compared to those without concomitant medication as no pharmacokinetic studies were performed.

Despite all the limitations, TDM and individualized dosage of anticancer drugs are essential for clinical success. However, we are also facing a worldwide economic situation in the field of health care that warrants the measurement of the clinical results of drug treatments mainly in the area of high-cost agents such as the targeted anticancer drugs. This specific situation may encourage the search for new knowledge on the efficacy of therapeutic schemes in clinics, focusing on the pharmacokinetic parameters of drug exposure that best relate to the clinical outcome to provide new tools for routine TDM.

In addition to the functional status of cancer patients, genetic variability in enzymes or other molecular targets may explain some of the variability in response, safety pattern, and/or the disposition of the drug within a population. Pharmacogenetic testing of metabolic enzymes has proved its usefulness for 5-FU dose adjustment as explained later in this chapter. In addition, genetic changes in BCR-ABL and BRAF/MEK pathways are useful markers for dosing drug inhibitors for chronic myeloid leukemia (CML) and melanoma also detailed in following paragraphs. Despite great efforts and huge investments of money, very few biomarkers related to drug sensitivity have made their way to the clinics and their importance needs to be studied more to avoid under- or overdosing. This will be discussed later in the case of methotrexate in leukemia patients.

The pediatric population has special concerns that should be taken into account mainly based on the heterogeneity of the patients grouped as "pediatric." This group is subdivided into neonates, young infants, infants, toddlers, children, and adolescents as age determines the pharmacokinetics of anticancer agents. Children undergo developmental physiological changes throughout childhood, especially during the first week after birth, that affect the disposition, efficacy, and safety of chemotherapy. A detailed description of these changes has been published in a landmark report by Kearns et al. [42]. The large size differences among children are reflected in high interindividual variability in pharmacokinetic parameters that are a function of body size, such as clearance and volume of distribution. Weight and body surface area (BSA) are the most often accepted descriptors of morphology. Among other factors, the development of glomerular filtration and tubular secretion that affects renal drug elimination, qualitative and quantitative changes in plasma proteins with consequent changes in drug distribution mainly in newborns, and the reduced activity of enzymes of metabolism with marked differences in metabolic activity depending on age and compared to adults, all play significant roles. A clear example is the clinical experience with carboplatin dose adjustment based on renal function in newborns and infants as discussed in the following sections [43]. Nonetheless, there is a clear shortage of research and clinical progress in the treatment of pediatric cancer patients for several reasons. Clinical research in pediatrics requires a special design, mainly due to ethical and logistic reasons, including few and low-volume biological samples. Moreover, the availability of highly sensitive analytical methods is required for drug quantitation. Another reason is that the small number of enrolled pediatric patients weakens statistical power. Therefore, optimized limited-sampling strategies are central for any research in pediatric populations.

We wish to emphasize the significant need for development of a Unit of Pharmacokinetics, or of Individualized Drug Dosing, at the same clinical facility where the patients are hospitalized. The clinical center may define local priorities according to the characteristics of the patients, available facilities, and analytical methods. Thereby, the PK/PD behavior of the drugs used at the center can be modeled based on real and local data and thereafter validated using an external population. This type of model can easily be introduced into routine clinical practice.

Improved outcome of oncology patients subjected to TDM in comparative prospective studies has been well documented for carboplatin, methotrexate, taxanes, 5-fluorouracil, and some newer compounds including the tyrosine kinase inhibitors (TKI) as will be developed in the following sections of the present chapter. Therefore, the aim of the present chapter is to summarize the existing evidence from current TDM and clinical pharmacokinetic dosage adjustments of these antineoplastic agents. Other drugs including gemcitabine and capecitabine can occasionally be subjected to monitoring but are still mainly restricted to clinical research due to the requirements for the quantitation of intracellular active metabolites.

17.1.1 CARBOPLATIN

Carboplatin (1,1-cyclobutanedicarboxylate)platinum(II) is a second-generation platinum compound. Although it was first introduced in the 1980s and severe hematological toxicity has been a very frequent adverse event, it plays a key role in a broad spectrum of malignancies in adults and children including brain tumors, breast and ovarian cancer, lung, prostate, and head and neck cancer.

Carboplatin is a cell-cycle-phase nonspecific agent that causes intra- and inter-strand DNA and DNA-protein crosslinks, thus inhibiting cell replication. It forms strong platinum-nitrogen bonds mainly at position 7 of DNA guanine.

It is more stable and less reactive than other platinum derivatives such as cisplatin. It has a rate constant for aquation or interacting with water of 7.2×10^{-7} per s compared to 8×10^{-5} per s for cisplatin. In addition, the rates of binding to DNA are 81 and 6.3 mg Pt/g DNA/h for carboplatin and cisplatin, respectively [44]. Therefore, carboplatin shows less binding to DNA, resulting in a more favorable adverse-events profile, mainly devoid of nephro- and neurotoxicity. However, its use is still associated with significant myelosuppression (especially thrombocytopenia).

In plasma, free or unbound carboplatin can be found as two different entities, carboplatin itself and a decarboxylated product usually named ultrafiltrable platinum. *In vivo*, carboplatin is metabolized to diammino-platinum able to irreversibly interact with proteins and to nonplatinum carboxyl products.

The pharmacokinetics and pharmacodynamics of carboplatin have been extensively reviewed [45]. Free or nonprotein-bound platinum systemic exposure represented by the area under the concentration curve (AUC) is the main pharmacokinetic parameter that significantly correlates with hematological toxicity as well as antitumor activity in both children and adults. Conversely, dose estimation of carboplatin based on size covariates (weight or BSA) has been shown to be a poor descriptor of pharmacological response. Other authors proposed a threshold of 5 to 6 mg × min/mL for unbound platinum AUC as lower exposures correlate with higher probability of treatment failure in testicular cancer patients when combined with bleomycin and etoposide [46,47]. In addition, Jodrell et al. [48] supported the use of unbound platinum AUC as a biomarker of antitumor activity in patients with ovarian cancer showing a sigmoidal relationship between systemic exposure and response. They showed that AUC values higher than 5 mg × min/mL did not lead to significant changes in the response or in the percentage of complete response. On the other hand, other authors have suggested that the effective range can be higher than 5−7 mg × min/mL in ovarian cancer and could even reach 12 mg × min/mL [49]. However, AUC values higher than 8 mg × min/mL were associated with a 30% and 48% probability of grade III/IV leucopenia and thrombocytopenia, respectively, with a 100% risk at an AUC over 10 mg × min/mL. These observations agreed with those previously reported by others [50,51] who showed an increase in the risk of severe hematologic toxicity up to 33% and 62% at a plasma AUC of 7 and 8 mg × min/mL, respectively. Finally, there is much evidence that supports a nonlinear sigmoidal relationship between unbound carboplatin AUC and myelosuppression.

Carboplatin dose adjustment is therefore required to attain the target AUC and achieve efficacy while avoiding toxicity. TDM is of particular importance for patients in whom carboplatin exposure may be more difficult to predict and in whom pharmacokinetic variability may lead to life-threatening toxicity if the target AUC is exceeded. Among these special populations are pediatric cancer patients with renal failure receiving high-dose carboplatin regimens, and infants. The main route for carboplatin elimination is through renal filtration of unbound platinum. Interindividual variability is high. In this setting, dose adjustment is guided by following unbound carboplatin AUC and targeted to values between 5.2 and 7.8 mg × min/mL for each individual patient based on renal function. Moreover, based on the PK/PD data obtained on the first day of infusion, dosage adjustment can be then performed for subsequent infusions of the same cycle or remaining cycles of chemotherapy, a concept known as a *pharmacokinetically guided approach.*

Free or unbound platinum is usually measured using atomic absorption spectrophotometry. Although this is not a new technology, very few hospitals run routine assays using this instrument, which limits routine carboplatin monitoring. In addition, plasma samples have to be processed using special containers provided with a membrane, to separate the unbound fraction of the drug as the pharmacologically active specimen.

There are different strategies to guide carboplatin dose adjustment based on clinical and biochemical parameters [52−55] or using AUC estimation by means of *a priori* algorithms [56−60]. Among *a posteriori* methods for unbound carboplatin AUC estimation usually using limited-sampling strategies include multiple linear regression equations and Bayesian analysis [55,59,60].

The evaluation of renal function is based on the glomerular filtration rate (GFR), creatinine clearance, or anthropometric and biochemical parameters. In addition, GFR can be measured either as EDTA clearance, ^{99}Tc-DTPA (diethylentriaminepentaacetic acid) clearance, or as creatinine clearance (CCr). In the former cases, the prediction is based on radioisotopic determination of GFR. However, the use of radioisotopes to determine GFR and, thereafter, carboplatin clearance is controversial and not available in all countries and clinical facilities. For CCr, serum creatinine could be used, but it has been highly discouraged for GFR determination in patients with renal failure. Cystatin C has also been proposed as an alternative filtration marker for GFR estimation [33,61]. In cases in which creatinine clearance could be used, different indirect methods for the determination are available using the Cockcroft and Gault, Modification of Diet in Renal Disease (MDRD, [62]), and Jelliffe formulas [34]. Of note is the estimation of creatinine clearance in patients with unstable renal function based on age, gender, weight, and height as previously described by Jelliffe [34].

The most widely used model to estimate carboplatin exposure in adults is the algorithm published by Calvert et al. [32]:

$$Dose = Target\ AUC \times (GFR + 25)$$

Dose in mg, AUC in mg × min/mL, and GFR in mL/min.

The dose is estimated on a daily basis according to the protocol in which the target AUC is stated. In addition, in each protocol, the route of administration and the length of the infusion are usually described.

The widespread use of this formula is based on the ease of its calculation in the daily practice of adult cancer patients, giving an acceptable estimate of carboplatin exposure. Nevertheless, the main limitation of the Calvert formula concerns GFR estimation if calculated using CCr and the nonrenal factor of the equation (the number 25 in the given equation). If used for pediatrics, this estimation is neither accurate nor certain. The formula was developed based on the GFR determination using Cr-EDTA. As we previously discussed, isotopic determination of GFR is limited. Moreover, it has been reported that sub-therapeutic doses may be attained if using the Jelliffe GFR calculation for the Calvert formula [33].

Chatelut et al. [63] proposed an alternative equation that was derived from a population-based pharmacokinetic analysis of patient data considering biochemical and anthropometric covariates in the formula to calculate carboplatin clearance:

$$CL = 0.134 \times body\ weight + [218 \times body\ weight \times (1 - 0.314 \times gender) \times (1 - 0.00457 \times age)]/SCr$$

where CL is in mL/min, body weight in kg, SCr in μMol/L, and gender = 0 for male and 1 for female.

Then, the dose would be obtained by the following equation:

$$Dose\ (mg) = CL\ (mL/min) \times Target\ AUC\ (mg \times min/mL)$$

One of the limitations is related to the decision on what body weight descriptor to use in the formula for low-weight or obese patients. In the latter case, the use of this formula can lead to a significant increase in the incidence of toxicity [35,64,65]. Benezet, one of the researchers of the Group of Chatelut that developed this equation, proved that the formula overpredicts carboplatin clearance in obese patients.

Therefore, Benezet et al. [35] proposed a correction for body weight in obese patients suggesting the mean value between the actual and the ideal body weight, calculating the latter according to the Lorentz equation:

$$Ideal\ weight\ (kg)\ for\ males = Height\ (cm) - 100 - ((Height\ (cm) - 150)/4)$$

and for females it would be:

$$Ideal\ weight = Height\ (cm) - 100 - ((height(cm) - 150)/2)$$

The ASCO guidelines published in 2012 suggest that in obese patients the maximum creatinine clearance to be used is 125 mL/min without further assessment or corrections [24,25]. However, in obese patients with impaired renal function, a correction for body weight should also be applied. A common equation used in the clinical practice that calculates the adjusted body weight is (adjusted body weight − ideal body weight + 0.4 × [total body weight − ideal body weight]). Additionally, body weight has to be reconsidered in cachectic patients to avoid excessive toxicity [64]. The mean body weight between ideal and total weight should be used in these cases.

Despite numerous approximations, the discussion is centered on the predictive ability of the different methods for AUC estimation. Huitema et al. [59] used a Bayesian approximation based on a two-compartment model developed using the author's data. They compared the results with others previously published using a limited-sampling scheme and also, if calculated, using the Calvert and Chatelut algorithms. The main conclusion is that the most precise estimation of AUC is obtained by using Bayesian methods.

Finally, we would like to comment on a specific case in which carboplatin monitoring is recommended. The study reported by Picton et al. described carboplatin dose adjustment in a premature infant [66]. Renal function of newborns and infants changes continuously and significantly during the first week of life. The kidney of the newborn has a very low GFR, which doubles during the first 2 weeks of life in both term and preterm infants due to physiological development. Moreover, GFR in preterm infants is highly correlated with gestational age. Specifically, a pharmacokinetically guided dosing approach was reported to avoid excessive toxicity while attaining antitumor activity with carboplatin in a premature infant with a solid eye tumor using population estimates from children with solid tumors and an individualized Bayesian approach. Blood samples were obtained over the 3 days on which the target cumulative AUC was calculated. Each day the AUC and clearance was calculated to estimate the remaining exposure to be attained and the corresponding dose to achieve it for attaining the total accumulated AUC. Interestingly, the individual carboplatin clearance almost doubled over an interval of 7 weeks from the first to the third chemotherapy course, probably as GFR increased during this period while serum creatinine decreased 18% from the first to the second cycle and thereafter remained constant. Therefore, the implications of this approach for carboplatin dosing are clear and based on actual carboplatin clearance.

For all these reasons, carboplatin monitoring is not mandatory, and available equations may be used for routine dose adjustment. However, in specific populations including neonates, infants, obese, and cachectic patients as well as patients undergoing hemodialysis [56,67,68], carboplatin TDM and Bayesian individualization are the best tools for dose adjustment in order to maximize efficacy and avoid excessive toxicity.

17.1.2 METHOTREXATE

Methotrexate is a folate antagonist that exerts its antitumor effect through a potent and competitive inhibition of dihydrofolate reductase (DHFR), the enzyme responsible of intracellular conversion of dihydrofolic acid to the active form tetrahydrofolic acid. Tetrahydrofolic acid acts as a donor of a group with one carbon atom and is a coenzyme in *de novo* purine and phosphate thymidine synthesis and some protein synthesis. Therefore, methotrexate (MTX) interferes with purine and pyrimidine synthesis affecting cell development and division.

Some aspects of MTX pharmacokinetics that we would like to point out include that the drug enters the cell via the reduced folate carrier. Once in the cell, it undergoes accumulation as polyglutamates (MTX-PGs) that contribute to the intracellular permanence of MTX and therefore the enhanced pharmacological activity as inhibitors of DHFR. Glomerular filtration and active tubular secretion are the main renal elimination routes of MTX, with 70–90% of the dose renally excreted in the first 24 h after infusion. MTX can also be converted to 7-hydroxymethotrexate, and both compounds are poorly soluble at acidic pH and therefore can precipitate in the renal tubules, leading to renal toxicity [69].

In addition, MTX-PGs inhibit thymidylate synthase (TS) and can also interfere with the activity of methylenetetrahydrofolate reductase (MTHFR), contributing to the cytotoxic effects of MTX.

Treatment with MTX is complex due to several factors that affect the clinical outcome of the patient. Among those factors are type of tumor and stage; genetic polymorphisms of MTX target enzymes (MTHFR, DHFR, thymidylate synthase); polymorphisms of proteins involved in drug metabolism and transport, including the solute carrier organic anion transporter 1B1 or SLC01B1, the folate receptor, ABCB1, and ABCC2 [69,70]; the dose; the duration of MTX infusion; concomitant chemotherapeutics; and leucovorin rescue.

The current use of MTX in oncology is mainly centered on the treatment of acute lymphoblastic leukemia (ALL), non-Hodgkin lymphoma (NHL), and osteosarcoma. In these cases, MTX is used in high doses (HDMTX) or doses higher than 1 or 5 g/m^2 depending on the author with variations in the duration of the infusion.

Therefore, for ALL and NHL, the doses are usually between 1 and 5 g/m^2 infused over a 24 h-interval, delivering 10% of the total dose during the first 30 min of the infusion to achieve the goal steady state concentration more rapidly. Nonetheless, in osteosarcoma and Ewing sarcoma, the clinical dosages range from 8 to 12 g/m^2 and can be delivered during 4 or 6 h depending on the clinical protocol.

MTX treatment has substantially improved since the first introduction into the clinics in the 1970s. Research has been carried out by many groups around the world. However, the contribution made by St. Jude Children's Research Hospital (SJCRH) is noteworthy [71].

Previous reports have shown a relationship between plasma concentrations and systemic exposure with clinical response in ALL and in osteosarcoma. For HDMTX in ALL, we are in line with the SJCRH guideline of attaining a steady state plasma concentration (Cp^{ss}) of 33 μM (range, 23–43 μM) in low-risk B-lineage ALL and 65 μM (range, 55–75 μM) for high-risk T- or B-lineage ALL patients [72]. Of note, higher plasma MTX levels after HDMTX were associated with lower risk of relapse. However, higher than manageable exposures can also lead to increased probability of toxicity, dose adjustment to lower the dose, and delay in subsequent courses of chemotherapy. All these factors adversely affect the efficacy of the treatment.

For osteosarcoma, it was proposed that the pharmacokinetic parameter related to clinical outcome was the concentration at the end of the infusion (C_{peak}) with values of 1000 μM after the 4-h infusion and $C_{peak} = 700$ μM after the 6-h infusion [73–75]. Afterward, Aquerreta et al. showed that the AUC_{0-48} was the parameter of HDMTX exposure that best predicted the tumor response in terms of overall survival in a pediatric population after 12 years of follow-up [76]. The threshold for response was established at 4000 $\mu M \times h$, but patients who showed a better response attained a mean $AUC_{0-48} = 6253$ $\mu M \times h$ and $C_{peak} = 1000$ μM in agreement with previous findings by others [73]. Importantly, Aquerreta et al. not only confirmed the relationship between systemic exposure and disease-free survival but also emphasized the importance of avoiding delays between courses of therapy, and the determination of dose intensity defined as the weekly average dose of MTX. Dose intensity of MTX is a significant prognostic factor in osteosarcoma. A group of patients with a lower AUC_{0-48} (less than 4800 $\mu M*h$) showed better disease-free survival than those with higher exposures, probably due to the lack of delays in the chemotherapy scheme and the time interval between cycles that was 7 days less than for the rest of the patients. Other authors supported the importance of dose intensity for the clinical response in terms of disease-free survival in osteosarcoma [77]. Although routine monitoring of plasma MTX levels is currently performed as part of most osteosarcoma protocols, there are still controversies over which drug-exposure parameter should be followed and the target to be attained related to clinical outcome [78]. Another parameter to be considered is the percentage of tumor necrosis as surrogate of histological tumor response and well-documented prognostic factor of clinical outcome [74,76].

Although not well established yet, it was suggested that the target AUC for CNS lymphoma should be between 1000 to 1100 $\mu M \times h$ [79,80]. The authors also stressed the importance of the dose intensity during all four cycles of chemotherapy.

After discussing the relevant pharmacokinetic parameters and their values for improving clinical outcome in different tumors, the next aim is to control the severe toxicity derived from HDMTX administration. In this sense, the dose and the attained C_{peak} are related to toxicity. HDMTX toxicity includes nephrotoxicity, hepatotoxicity, mucositis, myelotoxicity, and neurotoxicity [81]. To prevent renal toxicity mainly from 7-OH-MTX precipitation in the renal tubules during HDMTX schemes, patients undergo urine alkalinization using $NaHCO_3$ combined with hyper-hydration. In addition, patients require monitoring of MTX plasma concentrations and a personalized rescue treatment with leucovorin, a reduced folic acid that counters MTX activity in the cell [82]. When excessive doses of leucovorin are administered, the efficacy of MTX may be diminished [78,83,84]. Although not all the results are clear yet, Cohen et al. concluded that there was not enough scientific evidence to limit leucovorin rescue as it would not jeopardize MTX efficacy based on available reports [85]. HDMTX-related neurotoxicity could be avoided by increasing leucovorin dosage from 150 to 180 mg/m^2. Leucovorin rescue usually starts 36−42 h after the start of the infusion for hematologic tumors, and at 24 h for osteosarcoma, respectively. However, a higher risk of MTX toxicity in ALL patients that receive MTX dosages of 5−6 g/m^2 could occur if leucovorin rescue starts after 36 h of the beginning of the infusion [86].

The first study that demonstrated the usefulness and superiority of individualized dosing for HDMTX treatment for preventing excessive toxicity was reported by Evans in 1998 [87]. HDMTX doses were adjusted during the 24-h infusion in a timely fashion so as to attain the targeted exposure [87]. However, this procedure cannot be performed in all clinical settings as it needs quite rapid feedback from the clinical laboratory. Thereafter, the doses should be adjusted according to the patient's requirements in terms of efficacy and safety. In addition, as we do not count on early clinical symptoms that can predict renal impairment, plasma MTX levels are an undisputed tool for preventing MTX toxicities. Therefore, patients that receive HDMTX undergo pharmacokinetically guided leucovorin rescue.

As mentioned previously, MTX is usually infused over 24 h for hematologic tumors. In these cases, it has been proposed that 42 h after the start of the infusion a MTX plasma concentration $>1 \mu M$ is associated with a higher risk of toxicity [88]. Nevertheless, in osteosarcoma patients, there is no consensus on the concentration associated with an increased incidence of toxicity, but it has been proposed to be >3.5 or $>5 \mu M$ 24 h after the end of the infusion (C_{24}) or $>10 \mu M$ from the beginning of the infusion depending on the report [89,90]. Interestingly, Aquerreta et al. [76] showed that in osteosarcoma, patients showing $C_{24} >3.5 \mu M$ had doubled the incidence of nephrotoxicity. In addition, for every $1\,\mu M$ increase in C_{24}, the risk of renal toxicity increased by 43%. They also observed differences in the incidence of hematologic toxicities according to a C_{24} more than or less than $3.5\,\mu M$. Although not explicitly mentioned but deduced from the reported graphs, Crews et al. [78] showed that nephrotoxicity developed in patients with a $C_{24} = 3.8\,\mu M$, in agreement with Aquerreta et al.'s report [76].

Clinical protocols for hematologic tumors generally agree to start leucovorin rescue between 36 and 42 h of the infusion start using $15\,mg/m^2$ every 6 h until MTX plasma concentration is $\leq 0.2\,\mu M$, while some authors propose to stop at a plasma concentration of $<0.1\,\mu M$ in situations of delayed excretion [91]. In this sense, Pauley et al. reported the use of five standard doses of leucovorin every 6 h beginning 42 h after the start of infusion (C_{42}) and doses (10 or $15\,mg/m^2$) were assigned according to the patient risk classification [72]. In addition, leucovorin doses were increased in patients with delayed excretion with MTX concentrations $>1\,\mu M$ at C_{42}, and antifolate administration was continued until the MTX concentration was <0.1 or $<0.03\,\mu M$ in patients who developed toxicity. Special care should be given to patients with a MTX concentration of $\geq 10\,\mu M$ at C_{42}, as these are patients at high risk of developing toxicities. The criterion of stopping leucovorin rescue at a fixed value of $0.2\,\mu M$ can be risky as MTX might have accumulated into a deeper or third compartment with extensive release, and thus prolonged TDM is advised [90,92]. There is no consensus on the strategy to stop leucovorin rescue in osteosarcoma patients. However, it is commonly performed as for hematologic tumors or until plasma MTX concentrations $<0.05\,\mu M$ are reached.

Altogether, the critical MTX concentration at which intensive leucovorin rescue needs to be started and the time to end antifolate rescue are still under debate.

More recently, carboxypeptidase-G2 or glucarpidase has become available for adult and pediatric patients with HDMTX-induced renal failure and delayed MTX elimination ($C_{42-48} > 10\,\mu M$). Glucarpidase is a recombinant form of a bacterial enzyme (carboxypeptidase-G2) that metabolizes circulating MTX to DAMPA (4-deoxy-4-amino-N(10)-methylpteroic acid), an inactive metabolite of MTX, providing an alternative nonrenal route for MTX elimination. Thus, it is highly effective for rapid reduction of MTX plasma concentrations, thereby limiting severe toxicity. Its main drawback of its use is its high cost, and thus, a careful selection of the patients that should receive the enzyme is performed before prescription. In these patients, however, good clinical results may also be achieved with high-dose leucovorin with hyper-hydration at a lower price [91,93−95].

The clinical importance of identifying the cycles at risk of delayed MTX elimination so as to individualize leucovorin rescue and minimize MTX toxicity has led to the development of population-based pharmacokinetic models using limited-sampling strategies and Bayesian approaches [72,89,96−99]. These approaches permit aggressive chemotherapy dosage schedules in solid tumors and hematological malignancies while controlling toxicity. However, high intra-patient variability of MTX pharmacokinetic parameters has been reported, and therefore, TDM would be of less help in dose adjustment of subsequent cycles based on previous knowledge. Nonetheless, TDM is mandatory to be able to manage the toxicity of MTX during the cycle of infusion, and if there are no significant variations in body composition or the patient homeostasis, TDM is still advisable for MTX from our perspective. The intelligent use of pharmacokinetic software BestDose [available at www.lapk.org] to analyze the data and develop maximally precise dosage regimens should also be a big help. Also, in situations where intrapatient variability is high, the use of the interacting multiple model (IMM) sequential Bayesian approach [100]— which permits the model parameters to change with each new dose or data point—in the

BestDose software, resulting in the most precise tracking of serum drug concentrations over time [101], should facilitate individualized drug dosing in highly unstable patients with high intrapatient variability.

Finally, we offer some comments on individualizing MTX treatment based on pharmacogenetic findings. Although MTX dosage assignment is performed in many centers around the world based on the polymorphisms of MTHFR, in our opinion, this decision has led to unexpected consequences for patients that should be taken into account when deciding the dose. Specifically, in the protocol of the Spanish Societies of Pediatric Hematology and Oncology (SEHOP, LAL/SEHOP-2005), it was decided to guide MTX dosage based on the pharmacogenetics of the drug and to disregard the pharmacokinetically guided approach. It was then stated that patients with Down syndrome and homozygous or double heterozygous for C77T and/or 1298C mutations were selected for a dose reduction of 3 g/m^2, while wild-type patients received the full dose of 5 g/m^2. The analysis of the results of that protocol showed a decrease in the survival rate of patients treated with 3 g/m^2 compared to those in the 5 g/m^2 dose group and, in particular, of intermediate-risk patients. Therefore, in the following protocol LAL/SEHOP- PETHEMA 2013, the proposed MTX dose was 5 g/m^2 for all patients without enrollment according to the MTHFR polymorphism. We believe these results indicate that the relationship between pharmacogenetics and pharmacokinetics should be further studied and validated before translation into clinical practice. Currently available clinical evidence indicates that the best results in terms of survival rate are attained using a pharmacokinetically guided approach for MTX dosing.

It should also be noted, as a general rule, that observing drug behavior directly, using TDM, takes into quantitative account all the known effects as well as all the as-yet-undiscovered effects of the genetic variations and the quantitative effects of all the known and as yet undiscovered drug interactions, to make a truly individualized model of drug behavior in each individual patient.

In conclusion, although controversy still exists on the efficacy of MTX exposure, TDM is mandatory with special emphasis on HDMTX infusions. The decrease in the mortality rate associated with HDMTX has been a consequence of TDM of MTX and supportive care including leucovorin rescue, hyper-hydration, and urine alkalinization until plasma MTX levels allow discontinuation of leucovorin.

17.1.3 TAXANES

Paclitaxel and docetaxel are chemotherapeutic agents that belong to the taxanes group and were incorporated into cancer therapeutics in the 1990s. Taxanes revolutionized breast cancer treatment, notably increasing patient survival. In addition, they are also active against ovarian, prostate, sarcoma, lung, and head and neck cancer among others. The mechanism of action involves a reversible union to the beta subunit of tubulin leading to stabilized and nonfunctional microtubules producing G_2-M cell cycle arrest [102].

The administration schedule is based on data obtained in Phase I, II, and III studies, although patients included in these studies do not reflect the general population that receives the drugs in routine clinical practice. Interestingly, the knowledge of docetaxel management has been gained from different studies of docetaxel pharmacokinetics in different groups of patients according to races and ages, among others [103–107].

Taxanes have poor solubility in water. Therefore, paclitaxel formulations include Cremophor EL, and docetaxel pharmaceutical forms include polysorbate 80 and ethanol 13% w/w. The presence of these solvents in the formulation influences the toxicity (eg, hypersensitivity) and efficacy. Specifically, Cremophor EL affects the concentration of free paclitaxel and determines the nonlinear pharmacokinetic behavior of the drug in this formulation [108].

Both docetaxel and paclitaxel belong to the taxanes family, but they are different cytostatic agents with respect to pharmacokinetics, toxicity, and activity [102,109−111]. In this sense, Sanli et al. showed different in vitro mechanisms of action and reported that the activity is concentration-dependent for docetaxel while it is time-dependent for paclitaxel [112]. In other words, docetaxel effect is related to the concentration of the drug at the site of action while the time interval that the concentration of the drug is above a certain threshold for producing the cytotoxic effect are time dependent effects related to paclitaxel activity.

Taxanes are good candidates for TDM due to their high interindividual but low intraindividual pharmacokinetic variability and the currently available analytical techniques. Sensitivity, specificity, and reproducibility are the basic analytical parameters used for a bioassay. A plus is the availability of commercial immunoassays for routine clinical practice [113−115]. Even though these methods are easy to use in the laboratory, generally the limit of quantitation is much higher than using HPLC or LC/MSMS, either of which is more sensitive. In all cases, adequate validation is required to perform the analytical technique on a daily basis.

The pharmacokinetics of both drugs have been extensively characterized, and population-based pharmacokinetic models are available [5,108,116]. Docetaxel pharmacokinetics can be described by a three-compartment linear model, while paclitaxel in Cremophor EL can be described also using three compartments but having a nonlinear distribution to the second compartment and nonlinear elimination from the central compartment. Moreover, after high dosages of docetaxel (300 mg/m^2), there is some evidence of nonlinearity in docetaxel distribution that should be taken into consideration when using these dosages [117,118]. Docetaxel distribution is highly influenced by plasma proteins, as it is extensively bound to beta-acid glycoprotein. It is well known that cancer patients have altered levels of beta-acid glycoprotein, and therefore, interindividual variation in plasma protein concentration may affect docetaxel distribution and systemic clearance.

Both docetaxel and paclitaxel are subject to extensive metabolic conversion in the liver mediated by cytochrome P4503A isoenzymes (CYP3A4 and CYP3A5) and CYP2C8 in the case of paclitaxel resulting in inactive metabolites. In addition, the efflux P-glycoprotein (encoded by the *ABCB1* gene) and the transporter encoded by the *MRP2* gene both mediate biliary excretion of taxanes and their metabolites. Therefore, fecal excretion is the main route of elimination of docetaxel and its metabolites [119−122].

Docetaxel dosage ranges from 60 to 100 mg/m^2 and is usually delivered as a 1-h intravenous infusion every 3 weeks. Paclitaxel is administered as an intravenous infusion over 1 or 3 h on a weekly basis depending on the protocol. Although taxane dosing is based on BSA in routine clinical practice, large interindividual variability in pharmacokinetics is observed, and patients may experience severe and life-threatening adverse events or lack of efficacy. Therefore, BSA normalization does not fully account for interindividual variability in docetaxel PK. Although in a study of a small sample, there was an advantage of docetaxel TDM using the systemic AUC compared to BSA-normalized dosing [121]. In this prospective study from Engels et al., patients were randomly allocated to receive either BSA-docetaxel individualized dosage or PK-guided dose based on the pharmacokinetic data obtained in the first cycle. All patients received a BSA-dosage for the first course of treatment. The authors showed that using a TDM approach, interindividual variability in docetaxel AUC was reduced by 35% albeit not attaining statistical significance when compared to the parameter calculated in the BSA-based dosing group. Therefore, while docetaxel guided dosage is feasible, the advantages over BSA-dosage treatment were not established, at least in this small sample size study. Interestingly, in both groups of patients the decrease in white blood cell count and absolute neutrophil count after the second course of docetaxel were similar. However, a possible explanation might be that the target AUC for the PK-guided arm was not adequate.

The pharmacokinetics of docetaxel are affected by several covariates including plasma albumin, alpha-acid glycoprotein, liver function, BSA, and concomitant administration of CYP3A4 inducers or inhibitors [118,123,124]. Interindividual variability in taxane pharmacokinetics may determine the variability observed in the occurrence of adverse events and efficacy. However, each patient's own sensitivity to the drugs (pharmacodynamics) also plays a role.

Strategies to individualize docetaxel administration schedules based on phenotypic or genotype-dependent differences in CYP3A expression are under way. Nonetheless, the impact of CYP3A isoform polymorphisms on docetaxel disposition and safety and efficacy in the clinical setting remain to be determined. An association of the ABCB1 C3435T polymorphism and docetaxel AUC has been reported to be of prognostic value in breast cancer [120,125]. The protein encoded by the *ABCB1* gene mediates the elimination of four inactive compounds resulting from CYP3A metabolism. Moreover, a higher risk of docetaxel-induced hematological toxicity has been reported in patients carrying an *ABCB1* variant allele [120].

The most notable adverse events of taxanes are severe hematologic (grade 3/4 neutropenia and febrile neutropenia) and neurologic toxicities. Several reports have shown a relationship between docetaxel plasma exposure and severe hematologic toxicity (neutropenia, febrile neutropenia), and efficacy [118,123,124,126,127]. In addition, Baker et al. described a relationship between the unbound docetaxel AUC and the grade of neutropenia and the development of neutropenic fever [128]. Nevertheless, the authors did not provide a therapeutic target of docetaxel exposure to avoid the severe myelotoxicity. In studies that focused on total AUC, the expected target to be avoided was not provided either, but one study reported a maximum AUC of 2.3 µg × h/mL to avoid hematological toxicity [103,126,129,130]. In a representative number of cancer patients receiving 75 to 100 mg/m^2, docetaxel clearance was inversely proportional to grade 4 neutropenia. Specifically, a 25% to 50% decrease in docetaxel clearance increased the odds of developing severe neutropenia and febrile neutropenia at least twofold [121]. Moreover, docetaxel plasma AUC has been documented to be related to severe adverse events in lung cancer patients treated with dosages of 100 mg/m^2. Two studies compared docetaxel safety in terms of incidence of neutropenia in patients randomized to receive docetaxel at a fixed dose or a dose normalized by BSA or based on CYP3A activity [121,131]. The BSA-normalized study considered a target exposure of 4.9 µg × h/mL at a dosage of 100 mg/m^2 and the one based on CYP3A enzyme activity, selected a dosage of 60 mg/m^2 that would result in an AUC of 2.7 µg × h/mL. Interestingly, both studies showed a comparable reduction in neutrophil count in both the BSA-normalized and the target-dosage group, probably due to lack of difference in mean AUC between groups. Moreover, they also showed that a significant reduction in the interindividual variability in docetaxel AUC could be attained using PK-guided dosing compared to BSA-normalized dosing.

Therefore, we stress the need for TDM considering the high interindividual variability of paclitaxel and docetaxel and thus the low probability of attaining an adequate pharmacological target based on a standard or BSA-normalized dosing.

Although data on the relationship between docetaxel systemic exposure and efficacy are inconclusive, there is some evidence of a trend toward higher survival rates when the AUC is increased. In addition, docetaxel AUC has been reported as a parameter related to efficacy expressed as time to progression and death in lung cancer patients.

In contrast to our previous observations, in 2010 the report of the French society of Pharmacology and Therapeutics concluded that there was not enough evidence to recommend docetaxel TDM in routine clinical practice [122]. Subsequently, Aramendia [132] proposed that in patients with breast cancer treated with four cycles of adriamycin plus cyclophosphamide followed by four cycles of docetaxel at 100 mg/m^2 every 3 weeks, the target exposure in each cycle is a maximum plasma concentration or C_{max} of 3.5 µg/mL and an AUC of 4.5 µg × h/mL per cycle of chemotherapy. Those targets are recommended as upper thresholds to avoid excessive toxicity that may lead to severe adverse effects and delay between cycles. We would also like to highlight that a 95.8% rate of overall survival was attained after 8.6 years using these C_{max} and AUC targets.

Most of the evidence published regarding paclitaxel is for the formulation that contains Cremophor EL. Therefore, the information provided here takes into account this commercial formulation. Nonetheless, we would like to comment on the existence of nanoparticles of albumin loaded with paclitaxel. Interestingly, nanoparticle albumin-bound paclitaxel has also shown a relation to paclitaxel pharmacokinetics and the incidence of neutropenia [133], specifically the time that paclitaxel plasma concentration is higher than 720 ng/mL. In this sense, a paclitaxel plasma concentration more than 720 ng/mL showed a significant correlation with the probability of developing a reduction in 50% of the absolute neutrophil count.

Previous reports showed an association between paclitaxel efficacy and hematologic toxicity (neutropenia) and the time that the plasma concentration remains above 0.05 µM (equivalent to 42.7 ng/mL), usually named $T_{>0.05}$ [108,116]. Years later, the authors proposed that targeting a $T_{>0.05}$ between 26 and 31 h allows a reduction of the incidence of severe neutropenia [134]. In addition, a recent report suggested that a single blood sample obtained between 18 and 30 h after the start of paclitaxel administration on a basis of weekly administration allowed one to predict $T_{>0.05}$. Moreover, the authors proposed an algorithm based on $T_{>0.05}$ obtained in the first cycle to correct the dose on the following cycles to control the incidence of peripheral neuropathy induced by chemotherapy [135]. Then, a dose reduction, increase, or no modification was suggested based on the time for $T_{>0.05}$ attained in the first cycle after paclitaxel infusion in a weekly fashion so as to reduce the incidence of neurotoxicity. Although $T_{>0.05}$ is commonly used, some authors suggested targeting a plasma concentration above 0.1 µM ($T_{>0.1}$) equivalent to 85.4 ng/mL [136]. Other proposals were published by Smorebong et al. showing that the systemic exposure of unbound paclitaxel was a valid pharmacokinetic parameter for guiding the dosage compared to the previously described threshold models based on a single target level [137]. Conversely, other authors refute the superiority of the models that take into account the exposure of unbound paclitaxel over the threshold models [138]. Finally, others reported the relationship between paclitaxel $T_{>0.05}$, paclitaxel unbound AUC, or total systemic exposure and peripheral neuropathy with only $T_{>0.05}$ remaining as a predictor variable of this adverse event in the final COX model [139].

In an interesting study, Kraff et al. developed a user-friendly tool for paclitaxel TDM with an Excel® program [140]. The aim was to develop a tool that is easy to use in clinical practice for targeting paclitaxel $T_{>0.05}$ with acceptable accuracy and precision.

Few studies have evaluated the relationship between paclitaxel pharmacokinetics and efficacy. However, de Jonge et al. [141] used a Bayesian algorithm for paclitaxel dose individualization to attain $T_{>0.1}$ for at least 15 h after starting the administration in nonsmall cell lung cancer (NSCLC) patients. In the first course of treatment, patients received a standard dose of 175 mg/m^2 over 3 h. Thereafter, dose increments were performed in 43% of the individualized cycles of chemotherapy infusion without increasing the incidence of hematological toxicity. Unfortunately, the authors did not analyze the relationship between paclitaxel exposure and the efficacy of the treatment.

Important data on paclitaxel dose adjustment based on TDM will become available soon for patients with NSCLC receiving concomitant carboplatin as the prospective CEPAC-TDM study has recently been finished.

17.1.4 5-FLUOROURACIL

Along with methotrexate, 5-fluorouracil (5-FU) is the most widely monitored chemotherapeutic agent in clinical practice. It belongs to the antimetabolite family and has several mechanisms of action. The metabolite 5-fluoro-2'-deoxyuridine-5'-monophosphate (FdUMP) mainly inhibits DNA synthesis by irreversible inhibition of thymidylate synthase. In addition, fluorodeoxyuridine triphosphate (FdUTP) and fluorouridine triphosphate (5-FUTP) interfere with DNA and RNA synthesis, respectively.

5-FU has a short elimination half-life highly dependent on the dose and infusion protocol. Because of this, it is usually given as a continuous intravenous infusion over several hours or even days according to various protocols. The predominant activity of 5-FU on DNA or RNA depends on how it is given (bolus vs continuous infusion).

Dihydropyrimidine dehydrogenase (DPD) is the rate-limiting enzyme in the metabolic pathway of 5-FU to 5-fluorodihydrouracil (5-FUH2). DPD is abundantly expressed in the liver, but it is also present in other tissues, including bone marrow, intestinal epithelium, and spleen. DPD enzyme activity is critical when evaluating severe toxicity to 5-FU as 60% to 90% of the administered 5-FU dose is metabolized by DPD in the liver. There is a well-known association between deficiency of DPD activity and reduced 5-FU metabolism with an increase in severe or even fatal toxicity following standard doses of 5-FU in such patients [142,143]. Molecular defects of the gene that encodes for DPD (DPYD) lead to decreased enzyme activity. A complete deficiency of DPD activity occurs in about 0.1% of patients. Knowledge of this deficiency may help prevent severe toxicity. The splice-site variant IVS12 + 1 G>A in DPYD results in a truncated DPD protein without a 5-FU binding site.

Another important point mutation is 2846 A>T, also associated with decreased DPD activity. Thus, DPYD genotyping is proposed as part of dosing guidelines for initializing 5-FU therapy and to recommend the avoidance of 5-FU treatment in homozygous patients having DYPD nonfunctional variants [144−146]. Nonetheless, there is not always a direct relationship between genotype and phenotype. Sometimes, decisions based only on genotyping may lead to avoidance of 5-FU treatment in patients who may have benefitted from this agent, specifically those with colorectal cancer. Because of this, it is necessary to determine not only DPD activity, but also the systemic exposure to 5-FU and the ratio of 5-FU to 5-FUH2 exposures. Although some patients do not present with decreased DPD activity, they may show a marked increase in the parent-to-metabolite concentration exposure ratio as a consequence of limited metabolic capacity [147]. Therefore phenotype, together with genotype—or phenotype as a sole tool—may be the best option for initial 5-FU dose adjustment according to the elimination capacity of the individual patient to optimize efficacy while preventing severe toxicity. An excellent position paper was published by Boisdrom et al., proposing an algorithm for 5-FU dose adjustment after the initial dose based on a combination of patient phenotype and DPD genotype to predict 5-FU catabolic deficiencies [148]. Direct estimation of the metabolism of 5-FU is currently possible through the determination of plasma uracil (U) and dihydrouracil (UH2) levels by HPLC. Therefore, the authors combined patient phenotype and DPD genotype in a dosing algorithm by measuring plasma uracil and dihydrouracil levels and UH2-to-U plasma level ratio along with the identification of DPYD mutations. This algorithm has been incorporated in clinical practice, together with the inverse ratio U-to-UH2 [149–151] or the ratio UH2-to-U, and 5-FU plasma levels for individualized dosing. Finally, the 5-FU dosing algorithm based on genotype, phenotype, and physiological and pathological parameters has become available in commercial software (ODPM Tox and ODPM Protocol, ODPM).

Polymorphisms in the genes that code for other enzymes that participate in 5-FU metabolism, including MTHFR and TS have also been proposed, but so far with inconsistent results and lack of translation to clinical practice.

In oncology, there are few examples of TDM being prospectively evaluated using pharmacokinetically guided dosage compared to BSA-normalized dosage documented as for 5-FU [152,153]. However, two randomized trials compared the performance of pharmacokinetically guided 5-FU dosage adjustment versus BSA-dosing. A significant reduction in the incidence of severe hematological toxicity and improvement in the objective response rate were observed in the PK-guided groups compared to standard BSA-adjusted dosing. Moreover, years ago, it was reported that almost 50% of the patients would be outside the target range if dosed according to BSA. 5-FU has been subjected to TDM due to its nonlinear pharmacokinetics, wide interindividual variability pharmacokinetics, and numerous studies that have shown a relationship between 5-FU disposition and clinical efficacy and safety [154,155]. There is a clear relationship between 5-FU systemic exposure and efficacy measured as overall survival and progression-free survival, and the clinical benefits in terms of efficacy and safety of 5-FU pharmacokinetically guided dosing have been well established in cancer patients [156–159].

Recently, Yang et al. published a metaanalysis designed to compare the efficacy and toxicity observed with dosing by use of pharmacokinetic parameters versus BSA-based dose adjustment. The PK-based 5-FU dosage confirmed a superior overall response rate and improved toxicities [160].

The studies by Milano and Gamelin [153,158,161] set the basis for defining the therapeutic range of 5-FU in head and neck and colorectal cancer patients, respectively. In each cycle independently of the infusion length, a therapeutic range for 5-FU systemic exposure of 20 to 30 µg × h/mL has been proposed. We would like to emphasize that 5-FU dose adjustment is performed based on the pharmacokinetic parameters obtained in the first cycle to achieve the target systemic exposure in the following cycles of chemotherapy. Additionally, at Clínica Universidad de Navarra we previously observed that up to 24% of the patients who received 5-FU in the first cycle of its treatment were under the lower target range of 20 µg × h/mL, supporting the concept of routine TDM [162]. Rapid analytical turnaround in the measurement of 5-FU and the UH2-to-U concentration ratio contribute to the ease of performing TDM for 5-FU.

At Clínica Universidad de Navarra, in patients with a UH2-to-U ratio between 4 and 6 and a plasma concentration of uracil higher than 13.9 ng/mL (considered as potential risk patients), a plasma sample is obtained during the infusion in order to quantitate 5-FU. If patients are treated under FOLFIRI, FOLFOX-6, and FOLFIRINOX (regimens consisting of the combination of 5-FU and irinotecan/leucovorin, oxaliplatin/leucovorin, and irinotecan/leucovorin and oxaliplatin, respectively) the sample for 5-FU quantitation is obtained after 20 to 24 h of the start of the infusion. Otherwise, a sample is obtained between 9 to 11 h of starting 5-FU treatment under a FLOT regimen (5-FU concomitant to leucovorin, oxaliplatin, and docetaxel). Thereafter, we perform a Bayesian estimation of systemic 5-FU using the USC-*PACK software that allows attaining a systemic exposure of 30 µg × h/mL [163−165]. Individualized Bayesian estimations are performed after the first blood samples and depending on the estimated AUC, different strategies are followed according to each patient's pathological situation and the desired target systemic exposure. Thus, 5-FU infusion can be stopped sooner than originally planned, but after reaching the target AUC calculated by Bayesian estimation the infusion rate can be reduced and thereafter, the end of the infusion based on individualized requirements. Therefore, patients showing high uracil concentrations and low UH2-to-U ratio are followed closely using earlier and serial concentration assessments of 5-FU to prevent severe adverse events. Although the recommended therapeutic range is 20 to 30 µg × h/mL, the systemic exposure has to be individualized for each patient as some will be able to tolerate even higher exposures than previously mentioned.

We would also like to emphasize the time for blood sampling for TDM analysis. If the collection time is close to the initiation of the infusion (2 h after start), a significantly lower estimation of the AUC would be obtained as previously described by Kaldate et al. [166].

Lastly, we would like to highlight potential drug interactions, specifically with alternative medicines stressing the importance of 5-FU TDM [167,168]. One case report we observed at Clínica Universidad de Navarra was a pharmacokinetic interaction between 5-FU and garlic tablets. In this case, the patient showed an increase in his clearance that could lead to underexposure. Thus, it was recommended to stop the alternative medicine. Following this, the clearance was normalized in the following cycle.

In situations of toxicity, uridine triacetate can be administered, although its availability in routine clinical settings is currently a complex process since it is only an investigational drug at present [169].

17.1.5 TARGETED THERAPIES

Irinotecan (CPT-11), a potent topoisomerase-I inhibitor, is a prodrug that is converted to the active metabolite SN-38 (7-ethyl-10-hydroxycamptothecin) by carboxylesterases. Glucuronidation is the main metabolic pathway of SN-38, mediated by the uridine diphosphate glucuronosyltransferase (UGT) family of enzymes. SN-38 then undergoes biliary excretion as the inactive glucuronide SN-38-G [170]. Polymorphic variants of UGT impair SN-38 excretion. Since the systemic exposure of SN-38 has been associated with the efficacy and severity of irinotecan toxicity (severe neutropenia and diarrhea), it is highly recommended to test for the most common UGT variants (UGT1A1*28) to identify those patients with decreased glucuronidation of SN-38 who are therefore at risk for severe neutropenia and Gilbert syndrome among others.

Also, pharmacogenetic testing is a useful tool to identify patients with normal function of metabolizing enzymes, who therefore, can benefit from increasing irinotecan dose. Patients homozygous for UGT1A1*28 should receive a reduced dose when starting treatment. This is a clear and routinely performed pharmacogenetic testing in the clinical routine treatment of cancer patients. In children with solid tumors, irinotecan is used in a protracted schedule of 5 daily doses for 2 consecutive weeks [171].

Despite a trend toward higher SN-38 systemic exposure in patients homozygous to UGT1A1*28 genotyping, TDM and the clinical status of each individual patient are necessary to identify patients at increased risk of severe toxicity. Thus, for special populations, irinotecan TDM should always be performed along with genotyping.

We would also like to comment about the importance of CYP3A4 mediated metabolism of irinotecan to APC (7-ethyl-10-[4-N-(5-aminopentanoic acid)-1-piperidino]carbonyloxy camptothecin) and NPC (7-ethyl-10-(4-amino-1-piperidino)carbonyloxy camptothecin) [172]. Despite the production of inactive metabolites, this route of metabolism is important if irinotecan is concomitantly administered with CYP3A4 inhibitors such as ketoconazole, fluconazole, or voriconazole. In this case, the formation of APC and NPC is impaired, and thus, there is an increased metabolism from irinotecan to SN-38 potentially causing severe toxicity. Therefore, irinotecan is at risk of drug-drug interactions when concomitantly administered with CYP3A4 inhibitors.

Previous reports have shown the relationship between diarrhea and the product of plasma CPT-11 AUC and the plasma AUC ratio of SN-38 to the SN-38 glucuronide known as biliary index AUCCPT-11 × (AUC SN-38/AUCSN-38G) [173]. The biliary index has been correlated with SN-38 biliary concentrations, and in those cases of high indices, patients developed severe diarrhea. We have identified a threshold of 3.48 μg × h/mL for developing grade III/IV diarrhea [174]. Interestingly, in that study, the mean (SD) biliary index for patients that developed grade III and IV diarrhea was 5.3 ± 3.4 and 2.4 ± 1.3 μg × h/mL, respectively, close to those values previously reported by Gupta et al. [173].

TKI have become first-line treatments for Philadelphia- positive CML. They also play an important role in NSCLC and breast cancer. Specifically, the BCR-ABL1 gene encodes a tyrosine kinase enzyme that is central to the pathogenesis of CML.

Adverse events to imatinib include edema, skin rash, and neutropenia that may lead to poor compliance and thus, decrease efficacy. TDM is a useful tool to assess compliance related to suboptimal response, and also to monitor for toxicities that may lead to clinical decisions about reducing the dose or even switching to other TKIs. In addition, TKI are subjected to drug-drug, food-drug and herbal-drug interactions, making TDM mandatory for this class of agents [175]. Imatinib trough concentrations (C_0) are monitored every week during the first month of treatment to target levels higher than 1000 ng/mL. Thereafter, C_0 are obtained once or every three months after three months of treatment, along with assessment of the clinical response based on the levels.

TDM of another potent inhibitor of BCR-ABL1, dasatinib, is recommended to avoid pleural effusions but also, there is a risk of developing BCR-ABL mutations at lower systemic exposures. Usually, dasatinib maximum concentration is monitored. Finally, in the clinical routine of nilotinib, dose-adjustments are also based on C_0 levels, but in maintenance patients, it is also recommended to adjust according to UGT1A1 polymorphisms to maintain the exposure in the desired values.

17.2 CONCLUSIONS

While the present chapter was not intended to cover all available chemotherapy agents, we believe we have shown that TDM is a mandatory tool for optimizing treatment with anticancer agents.

REFERENCES

[1] Alnaim L. Therapeutic drug monitoring of cancer chemotherapy. J Oncol Pharm Pract 2007;13:207−21.
[2] Bardin C, et al. Therapeutic drug monitoring in cancer − are we missing a trick? Eur J Cancer 2014;50:2005−9.
[3] Canal P, Chatelut E. Dose optimization in clinical oncology: pharmacokinetic-pharmacodynamic relationship. Bull Cancer 1996;83:256−65.
[4] De Jonge ME, et al. Individualised cancer chemotherapy: strategies and performance of prospective studies on therapeutic drug monitoring with dose adaptation: a review. Clin Pharmacokinet 2005;44:147−73.
[5] Van den Bongard HJ, et al. Pharmacokinetically guided administration of chemotherapeutic agents. Clin Pharmacokinet 2000;39:345−67.
[6] Gao B, et al. Evidence for therapeutic drug monitoring of targeted anticancer therapies. J Clin Oncol 2012;30:4017−25.
[7] Gotta V, et al. Therapeutic drug monitoring of imatinib: Bayesian and alternative methods to predict trough levels. Clin Pharmacokinet 2012;51:187−201.
[8] Robert S, Mancini PB. Chemotherapy administration sequence: a review of the literature and creation of a sequencing chart. J Hematol Oncol Pharm 2011;1.
[9] Judson IR. Pharmacokinetic modelling−a prelude to therapeutic drug monitoring for all cancer patients? Eur J Cancer 1995;31A:1733−5.
[10] Kobayashi K, Ratain MJ. Individualizing dosing of cancer chemotherapy. Semin Oncol 1993;20:30−42.
[11] Lennard L. Therapeutic drug monitoring of antimetabolic cytotoxic drugs. Br J Clin Pharmacol 1999;47:131−43.
[12] Lennard L. Therapeutic drug monitoring of cytotoxic drugs. Br J Clin Pharmacol 2001;52(Suppl. 1):75S−87S.
[13] McDonald GB, Frieze D. A problem-oriented approach to liver disease in oncology patients. Gut 2008;57:987−1003.
[14] Nieto Y, Vaughan WP. Pharmacokinetics of high-dose chemotherapy. Bone Marrow Transplant 2004;33:259−69.
[15] Paci A, et al. Review of therapeutic drug monitoring of anticancer drugs part 1 − cytotoxics. Eur J Cancer 2014;50:2010 −19.
[16] Ranson MR, Scarffe JH. Population and Bayesian pharmacokinetics in oncology. Clin Oncol (R Coll Radiol) 1994;6:254−60.
[17] Ribba B, Holford N, Mentré F. The use of model-based tumor-size metrics to predict survival. Clin Pharmacol Ther 2014;96:133−5.
[18] Rousseau A, Marquet P. Application of pharmacokinetic modelling to the routine therapeutic drug monitoring of anticancer drugs. Fundam Clin Pharmacol 2002;16:253−62.
[19] Saleem M, et al. Target concentration intervention in oncology: where are we at? Ther Drug Monit 2012;34:257−65.
[20] Tranchand B, et al. Pharmacology of anticancer drugs in the elderly: tools for dose-adjustment. Bull Cancer 2008;95 FMC Onc:F21−7.

[21] Widmer N, et al. Review of therapeutic drug monitoring of anticancer drugs part two − targeted therapies. Eur J Cancer 2014;50:2020−36.

[22] Brenner DE, Wiernik PH, Wesley M, Bachur NR. Acute doxorubicin toxicity. Relationship to pretreatment liver function, response, and pharmacokinetics in patients with acute nonlymphocytic leukemia. Cancer 1984;53:1042−8.

[23] Donelli MG, Zucchetti M, Munzone E, D'Incalci M, Crosignani A. Pharmacokinetics of anticancer agents in patients with impaired liver function. Eur J Cancer 1998;34:33−46.

[24] Griggs JJ, et al. Appropriate chemotherapy dosing for obese adult patients with cancer: American Society of Clinical Oncology clinical practice guideline. J Clin Oncol 2012;30:1553−61.

[25] Hall RG, Jean GW, Sigler M, Shah S. Dosing considerations for obese patients receiving cancer chemotherapeutic agents. Ann Pharmacother 2013;47:1666−74.

[26] Hon YY, Evans WE. Making TDM work to optimize cancer chemotherapy: a multidisciplinary team approach. Clin Chem 1998;44:388−400.

[27] Janus N, Thariat J, Boulanger H, Deray G, Launay-Vacher V. Proposal for dosage adjustment and timing of chemotherapy in hemodialyzed patients. Ann Oncol 2010;21:1395−403.

[28] Kintzel PE, Dorr RT. Anticancer drug renal toxicity and elimination: dosing guidelines for altered renal function. Cancer Treat Rev 1995;21:33−64.

[29] Superfin D, Iannucci AA, Davies AM. Commentary: oncologic drugs in patients with organ dysfunction: a summary. Oncologist 2007;12:1070−83.

[30] Zandvliet AS, Schellens JHM, Beijnen JH, Huitema ADR. Population pharmacokinetics and pharmacodynamics for treatment optimization in clinical oncology. Clin Pharmacokinet 2008;47:487−513.

[31] Kloft C, Wallin J, Henningsson A, Chatelut E, Karlsson MO. Population pharmacokinetic-pharmacodynamic model for neutropenia with patient subgroup identification: comparison across anticancer drugs. Clin Cancer Res 2006;12:5481−90.

[32] Calvert AH, et al. Carboplatin dosage: prospective evaluation of a simple formula based on renal function. J Clin Oncol 1989;7:1748−56.

[33] Schmitt A, et al. A universal formula based on cystatin C to perform individual dosing of carboplatin in normal weight, underweight, and obese patients. Clin Cancer Res 2009;15:3633−9.

[34] Jelliffe R. Estimation of creatinine clearance in patients with unstable renal function, without a urine specimen. Am J Nephrol 2002;22:320−4.

[35] Bénézet S, et al. How to predict carboplatin clearance from standard morphological and biological characteristics in obese patients. Ann Oncol 1997;8:607−9.

[36] Friberg LE, Henningsson A, Maas H, Nguyen L, Karlsson MO. Model of chemotherapy-induced myelosuppression with parameter consistency across drugs. J Clin Oncol 2002;20:4713−21.

[37] Testart-Paillet D, et al. Contribution of modelling chemotherapy-induced hematological toxicity for clinical practice. Crit Rev Oncol Hematol 2007;63:1−11.

[38] Wallin JE, Friberg LE, Karlsson MO. A tool for neutrophil guided dose adaptation in chemotherapy. Comput Methods Programs Biomed 2009;93:283−91.

[39] Brendel K, et al. Are population pharmacokinetic and/or pharmacodynamic models adequately evaluated? A survey of the literature from 2002 to 2004. Clin Pharmacokinet 2007;46:221−34.

[40] Rinaldi F, George E, Adler AI. NICE guidance on cetuximab, bevacizumab, and panitumumab for treatment of metastatic colorectal cancer after first-line chemotherapy. Lancet Oncol 2012;13:233−4.

[41] Douillard J-Y, et al. Panitumumab-FOLFOX4 treatment and RAS mutations in colorectal cancer. N Engl J Med 2013;369:1023−34.

[42] Kearns GL, et al. Developmental pharmacology − drug disposition, action, and therapy in infants and children. N Engl J Med 2003;349:1157−67.

[43] Picton SV, et al. Therapeutic monitoring of carboplatin dosing in a premature infant with retinoblastoma. Cancer Chemother Pharmacol 2009;63:749−52.

[44] Knox RJ, Friedlos F, Lydall DA, Roberts JJ. Mechanism of cytotoxicity of anticancer platinum drugs: evidence that cis-diamminedichloroplatinum(II) and cis-diammine-(1,1-cyclobutanedicarboxylato)-platinum(II) differ only in the kinetics of their interaction with DNA. Cancer Res 1986;46:1972−9.

[45] Van der Vijgh WJ. Clinical pharmacokinetics of carboplatin. Clin Pharmacokinet 1991;21:242−61.

[46] Horwich A, et al. Effectiveness of carboplatin, etoposide, and bleomycin combination chemotherapy in good-prognosis metastatic testicular nonseminomatous germ cell tumors. J Clin Oncol 1991;9:62−9.

[47] Childs WJ, Nicholls EJ, Horwich A. The optimisation of carboplatin dose in carboplatin, etoposide and bleomycin combination chemotherapy for good prognosis metastatic nonseminomatous germ cell tumours of the testis. Ann Oncol 1992;3:291−6.

[48] Jodrell DI, et al. Relationships between carboplatin exposure and tumor response and toxicity in patients with ovarian cancer. J Clin Oncol 1992;10:520−8.

[49] Calvert AH, et al. Carboplatin and granulocyte colony-stimulating factor as first-line treatment for epithelial ovarian cancer: a phase I dose-intensity escalation study. Semin Oncol 1994;21:1−6

[50] Reyno LM, et al. Impact of cyclophosphamide on relationships between carboplatin exposure and response or toxicity when used in the treatment of advanced ovarian cancer. J Clin Oncol 1993;11:1156−64.

[51] Lind MJ, et al. Phase I study of pharmacologically based dosing of carboplatin with filgrastim support in women with epithelial ovarian cancer. J Clin Oncol 1996;14:800−5.

[52] Taguchi J, et al. Prediction of hematologic toxicity of carboplatin by creatinine clearance rate. Jpn J Cancer Res 1987;78:977−82.

[53] Fish RG, et al. A dosing scheme for carboplatin in adult cancer patients based upon pre-infusion renal function and platelet count. Anticancer Drugs 1994;5:527−32.

[54] Egorin MJ, et al. Modeling toxicity and response in carboplatin-based combination chemotherapy. Semin Oncol 1994;21:7−19.

[55] Egorin MJ, et al. Prospective validation of a pharmacologically based dosing scheme for the cis-diammine-dichloroplatinum(II) analogue diamminecyclobutanedicarboxylatoplatinum. Cancer Res 1985;45:6502−6.

[56] Hulin A, Chatelut E, Royer B, Le Guellec C. Level of evidence for therapeutic drug monitoring of carboplatin. Therapie 2010;65:157−62.

[57] Ghazal-Aswad S, Calvert AH, Newell DR. A single-sample assay for the estimation of the area under the free carboplatin plasma concentration versus time curve. Cancer Chemother Pharmacol 1996;37:429−34.

[58] Sørensen BT, Strömgren A, Jakobsen P, Jakobsen A. A limited sampling method for estimation of the carboplatin area under the curve. Cancer Chemother Pharmacol 1993;31:324−7.

[59] Huitema AD, et al. Validation of techniques for the prediction of carboplatin exposure: application of Bayesian methods. Clin Pharmacol Ther 2000;67:621−30.

[60] De Jonge ME, et al. Accuracy, feasibility, and clinical impact of prospective Bayesian pharmacokinetically guided dosing of cyclophosphamide, thiotepa, and carboplatin in high-dose chemotherapy. Clin Cancer Res 2005;11:273−83.

[61] Inker LA, et al. Estimating glomerular filtration rate from serum creatinine and cystatin C. N Engl J Med 2012;367:20−9.

[62] Botev R, et al. Estimating glomerular filtration rate: Cockcroft -Gault and Modification of Diet in Renal Disease formulas compared to renal inulin clearance. Clin J Am Soc Nephrol 2009;4(5):899−906.

[63] Chatelut E, et al. Prediction of carboplatin clearance from standard morphological and biological patient characteristics. J Natl Cancer Inst 1995;87:573−80.

[64] Herrington JD, Tran HT, Riggs MW. Prospective evaluation of carboplatin AUC dosing in patients with a BMI > or = 27 or cachexia. Cancer Chemother Pharmacol 2006;57:241−7.

[65] Loh GW, Ting LSL, Ensom MHH. A systematic review of limited sampling strategies for platinum agents used in cancer chemotherapy. Clin Pharmacokinet 2007;46:471−94.

[66] Picton SV, et al. Therapeutic monitoring of carboplatin dosing in a premature infant with retinoblastoma. Cancer Chemother Pharmacol 2009 Mar;63(4):749−52.

[67] Kamei K, et al. Pharmacokinetics of carboplatin in a one-year-old anuric boy undergoing hemodialysis and a review of the literature. Ther Apher Dial 2015;19(5):491–6.

[68] Van Gorp F, et al. Dosing of carboplatin in a patient with amputated legs: a case report. J Oncol Pharm Pract 2014;20:473–5.

[69] Rau T, et al. High-dose methotrexate in pediatric acute lymphoblastic leukemia: impact of ABCC2 polymorphisms on plasma concentrations. Clin Pharmacol Ther 2006;80:468–76.

[70] Treviño LR, et al. Germline genetic variation in an organic anion transporter polypeptide associated with methotrexate pharmacokinetics and clinical effects. J Clin Oncol 2009;27:5972–8.

[71] Evans WE, et al. Clinical pharmacodynamics of high-dose methotrexate in acute lymphocytic leukemia. Identification of a relation between concentration and effect. N Engl J Med 1986;314:471–7.

[72] Pauley JL, et al. Between-course targeting of methotrexate exposure using pharmacokinetically guided dosage adjustments. Cancer Chemother Pharmacol 2013;72:369–78.

[73] Graf N, Winkler K, Betlemovic M, Fuchs N, Bode U. Methotrexate pharmacokinetics and prognosis in osteosarcoma. J Clin Oncol 1994;12:1443–51.

[74] Bacci G, et al. Predictive factors of histologic response to primary chemotherapy in osteosarcoma of the extremity: study of 272 patients preoperatively treated with high-dose methotrexate, doxorubicin, and cisplatin. J Clin Oncol 1998;16:658–63.

[75] Kwong DL, et al. Multidisciplinary management of osteosarcoma: experience in Hong Kong. Pediatr Hematol Oncol 1998;15:229–36.

[76] Aquerreta I, Aldaz A, Giráldez J, Sierrasesúmaga L. Methotrexate pharmacokinetics and survival in osteosarcoma. Pediatr Blood Cancer 2004;42:52–8.

[77] Hegyi M, et al. Clinical relations of methotrexate pharmacokinetics in the treatment for pediatric osteosarcoma. J Cancer Res Clin Oncol 2012;138:1697–702.

[78] Crews KR, et al. High-dose methotrexate pharmacokinetics and outcome of children and young adults with osteosarcoma. Cancer 2004;100:1724–33.

[79] Ferreri AJM, et al. Area under the curve of methotrexate and creatinine clearance are outcome-determining factors in primary CNS lymphomas. Br J Cancer 2004;90:353–8.

[80] Joerger M, Huitema ADR, Illerhaus G, Ferreri AJM. Rational administration schedule for high-dose methotrexate in patients with primary central nervous system lymphoma. Leuk Lymphoma 2012;53:1867–75.

[81] Zelcer S, Kellick M, Wexler LH, Gorlick R, Meyers PA. The memorial sloan kettering cancer center experience with outpatient administration of high dose methotrexate with leucovorin rescue. Pediatr Blood Cancer 2008;50:1176–80.

[82] Zelcer S, et al. Methotrexate levels and outcome in osteosarcoma. Pediatr Blood Cancer 2005;44:638–42.

[83] Borsi JD, Wesenberg F, Stokland T, Moe PJ. How much is too much? Folinic acid rescue dose in children with acute lymphoblastic leukaemia. Eur J Cancer 1991;27:1006–9.

[84] Skärby TVC, et al. High leucovorin doses during high-dose methotrexate treatment may reduce the cure rate in childhood acute lymphoblastic leukemia. Leukemia 2006;20:1955–62.

[85] Cohen IJ. Challenging the clinical relevance of folinic acid over rescue after high dose methotrexate (HDMTX). Med Hypotheses 2013;81:942–7.

[86] Cohen IJ, Wolff JE. How long can folinic acid rescue be delayed after high-dose methotrexate without toxicity? Pediatr Blood Cancer 2014;61:7–10.

[87] Evans WE, et al. Conventional compared with individualized chemotherapy for childhood acute lymphoblastic leukemia. N Engl J Med 1998;338:499–505.

[88] Relling MV, et al. Patient characteristics associated with high-risk methotrexate concentrations and toxicity. J Clin Oncol 1994;12:1667–72.

[89] Aquerreta I, Aldaz A, Giráldez J, Sierrasesúmaga L. Pharmacodynamics of high-dose methotrexate in pediatric patients. Ann Pharmacother 2002;36:1344–50.

[90] Sims PJ. Applied pharmacokinetics and pharmacodynamics. Principles of therapeutic drug monitoring. Am J Pharm Educ 2006;70(6):148.

[91] Cavone JL, Yang D, Wang A. Glucarpidase intervention for delayed methotrexate clearance. Ann Pharmacother 2014;48:897−907.

[92] Wright KD, et al. Delayed methotrexate excretion in infants and young children with primary central nervous system tumors and postoperative fluid collections. Cancer Chemother Pharmacol 2015;75:27−35.

[93] Widemann BC, et al. Efficacy of glucarpidase (carboxypeptidase g2) in patients with acute kidney injury after high-dose methotrexate therapy. Pharmacotherapy 2014;34:427−39.

[94] Scott JR, et al. Comparable efficacy with varying dosages of glucarpidase in pediatric oncology patients. Pediatr Blood Cancer 2015;62:1518−22.

[95] Flombaum CD, Meyers PA. High dose leucovorin as sole therapy for methotrexate toxicity. J Clin Oncol 1999;17:1589−94.

[96] Dombrowsky E, Jayaraman B, Narayan M, Barrett JS. Evaluating performance of a decision support system to improve methotrexate pharmacotherapy in children and young adults with cancer. Ther Drug Monit 2011;33:99−107.

[97] Pignon T, et al. Dosage adjustment of high-dose methotrexate using Bayesian estimation: a comparative study of two different concentrations at the end of 8-h infusions. Ther Drug Monit 1995;17:471−8.

[98] Johansson ÅM, et al. A population pharmacokinetic/pharmacodynamic model of methotrexate and mucositis scores in osteosarcoma. Ther Drug Monit 2011;33:711−18.

[99] Aumente D, et al. Population pharmacokinetics of high-dose methotrexate in children with acute lymphoblastic leukaemia. Clin Pharmacokinet 2006;45:1227−38.

[100] Bayard D, Jelliffe R. A Bayesian approach to tracking patients having changing pharmacokinetic parameters. J Pharmacokin Pharmacodyn 2004;31(1):75−107.

[101] Macdonald I, Staatz C, Jelliffe R, Thomson A. Evaluation and comparison of simple multiple model, richer data multiple model, and sequential interacting multiple model (IMM) Bayesian analyses of gentamicin and vancomycin data collected from patients undergoing cardiothoracic surgery. Ther Drug Monit 2008;30:67−74.

[102] Gligorov J, Lotz JP. Preclinical pharmacology of the taxanes: implications of the differences. Oncologist 2004;9(Suppl. 2):3−8.

[103] Ozawa K, Minami H, Sato H. Population pharmacokinetic and pharmacodynamic analysis for time courses of docetaxel-induced neutropenia in Japanese cancer patients. Cancer Sci 2007;98:1985−92.

[104] Kenmotsu H, Tanigawara Y. Pharmacokinetics, dynamics and toxicity of docetaxel: why the Japanese dose differs from the Western dose. Cancer Sci 2015;106:497−504.

[105] Ten Tije AJ, et al. Prospective evaluation of the pharmacokinetics and toxicity profile of docetaxel in the elderly. J Clin Oncol 2005;23:1070−7.

[106] Minami H, et al. Comparison of pharmacokinetics and pharmacodynamics of docetaxel and cisplatin in elderly and non-elderly patients: why is toxicity increased in elderly patients? J Clin Oncol 2004;22:2901−8.

[107] Minami H, et al. Population pharmacokinetics of docetaxel in patients with hepatic dysfunction treated in an oncology practice. Cancer Sci 2009;100:144−9.

[108] Gianni L, et al. Nonlinear pharmacokinetics and metabolism of paclitaxel and its pharmacokinetic/pharmacodynamic relationships in humans. J Clin Oncol 1995;13:180−90.

[109] Eisenhauer EA, Vermorken JB. The taxoids. Comparative clinical pharmacology and therapeutic potential. Drugs 1998;55:5−30.

[110] Rivera E, et al. Phase 3 study comparing the use of docetaxel on an every-3-week versus weekly schedule in the treatment of metastatic breast cancer. Cancer 2008;112:1455−61.

[111] Yonemori K, et al. Efficacy of weekly paclitaxel in patients with docetaxel-resistant metastatic breast cancer. Breast Cancer Res Treat 2005;89:237—41.

[112] Sanli UA, et al. Which dosing scheme is suitable for the taxanes? An in vitro model. Arch Pharm Res 2002;25:550—5.

[113] López LZ, Pastor AA, Beitia JMA, Velilla JA, Deiró JG. Determination of docetaxel and paclitaxel in human plasma by high-performance liquid chromatography: validation and application to clinical pharmacokinetics. Ther Drug Monit 2006;199—205.

[114] Vergniol JC, Bruno R, Montay G, Frydman A. Determination of Taxotere in human plasma by a semi--automated high-performance liquid chromatographic method. J Chromatogr 1992;582:273—8.

[115] Huizing MT, et al. Quantification of paclitaxel metabolites in human plasma by high-performance liquid chromatography. J Chromatogr B Biomed Appl 1995;674:261—8.

[116] Joerger M, et al. Population pharmacokinetics and pharmacodynamics of paclitaxel and carboplatin in ovarian cancer patients: a study by the European organization for research and treatment of cancer-pharmacology and molecular mechanisms group and new drug development group. Clin Cancer Res 2007;13:6410—18.

[117] Mc Leod HL, Kearns CM, Kuhn JG, Bruno R. Evaluation of the linearity of docetaxel pharmacokinetics. Cancer Chemother Pharmacol 1998;42(2):155—9.

[118] Bruno R, et al. Population pharmacokinetics/pharmacodynamics of docetaxel in phase II studies in patients with cancer. J Clin Oncol 1998;16:187—96.

[119] Baker SD, Sparreboom A, Verweij J. Clinical pharmacokinetics of docetaxel: recent developments. Clin Pharmacokinet 2006;45:235—52.

[120] Kim H-J, et al. ABCB1 polymorphism as prognostic factor in breast cancer patients treated with docetaxel and doxorubicin neoadjuvant chemotherapy. Cancer Sci 2015;106:86—93.

[121] Engels FK, et al. Therapeutic drug monitoring for the individualization of docetaxel dosing: a randomized pharmacokinetic study. Clin Cancer Res 2011;17:353—62.

[122] Gerritsen-van Schieveen P, Royer B. Level of evidence for therapeutic drug monitoring of taxanes. Fundam Clin Pharmacol 2011;25:414—24.

[123] Nieto Y, et al. Phase I and pharmacokinetic study of gemcitabine administered at fixed-dose rate, combined with docetaxel/melphalan/carboplatin, with autologous hematopoietic progenitor-cell support, in patients with advanced refractory tumors. Biol Blood Marrow Transplant 2007;13:1324—37.

[124] Slaviero KA, Clarke SJ, McLachlan AJ, Blair EYL, Rivory LP. Population pharmacokinetics of weekly docetaxel in patients with advanced cancer. Br J Clin Pharmacol 2004;57:44—53.

[125] Bosch TM, et al. Pharmacogenetic screening of CYP3A and ABCB1 in relation to population pharmacokinetics of docetaxel. Clin Cancer Res 2006;12:5786—93.

[126] Charles KA, et al. Predicting the toxicity of weekly docetaxel in advanced cancer. Clin Pharmacokinet 2006;45:611—22.

[127] Veyrat-Follet C, Bruno R, Olivares R, Rhodes GR, Chaikin P. Clinical trial simulation of docetaxel in patients with cancer as a tool for dosage optimization. Clin Pharmacol Ther 2000;68:677—87.

[128] Baker SD, et al. Relationship of systemic exposure to unbound docetaxel and neutropenia. Clin Pharmacol Ther 2005;77:43—53.

[129] Bruno R, Vivier N, Veyrat-Follet C, Montay G, Rhodes GR. Population pharmacokinetics and pharmacokinetic-pharmacodynamic relationships for docetaxel. Invest New Drugs 2001;19:163—9.

[130] Puisset F, et al. Clinical pharmacodynamic factors in docetaxel toxicity. Br J Cancer 2007;97:290—6.

[131] Yamamoto N, et al. Randomized pharmacokinetic and pharmacodynamic study of docetaxel: dosing based on body-surface area compared with individualized dosing based on cytochrome P450 activity estimated using a urinary metabolite of exogenous cortisol. J Clin Oncol 2005;23:1061—9.

[132] Aramendia B.J.M. Pharmacokinetic-pharmacodynamic relationships of docetaxel in breast cancer. Doctoral Thesis, University of Navarra, 2011.

[133] Chen N, et al. Pharmacokinetics and pharmacodynamics of nab-paclitaxel in patients with solid tumors: disposition kinetics and pharmacology distinct from solvent-based paclitaxel. J Clin Pharmacol 2014;54:1097—107.

[134] Joerger M, et al. Evaluation of a pharmacology-driven dosing algorithm of 3-weekly paclitaxel using therapeutic drug monitoring: a pharmacokinetic-pharmacodynamic simulation study. Clin Pharmacokinet 2012;51:607−17.

[135] Kraff S, et al. Pharmacokinetically based dosing of weekly paclitaxel to reduce drug-related neurotoxicity based on a single sample strategy. Cancer Chemother Pharmacol 2015;75:975−83.

[136] Danesi R, et al. Pharmacokinetics and pharmacodynamics of combination chemotherapy with paclitaxel and epirubicin in breast cancer patients. Br J Clin Pharmacol 2002;53:508−18.

[137] Smorenburg CH, et al. Randomized cross-over evaluation of body-surface area-based dosing versus flat-fixed dosing of paclitaxel. J Clin Oncol 2003;21:197−202.

[138] Egorin MJ. Horseshoes, hand grenades, and body-surface area-based dosing: aiming for a target. J Clin Oncol 2003;21:182−3.

[139] Mielke S, et al. Association of paclitaxel pharmacokinetics with the development of peripheral neuropathy in patients with advanced cancer. Clin Cancer Res 2005;11.4043 50.

[140] Kraff S, Lindauer A, Joerger M, Salamone SJ, Jaehde U. Excel-based tool for pharmacokinetically-guided dose adjustment of paclitaxel. Ther Drug Monit 2015;37(6):725−32.

[141] De Jonge ME, et al. Bayesian pharmacokinetically guided dosing of paclitaxel in patients with non--small cell lung cancer. Clin Cancer Res 2004;10:2237−44.

[142] Ploylearmsaeng S, Fuhr U, Jetter A. How may anticancer chemotherapy with fluorouracil be individualised? Clin Pharmacokinet 2006;45:567−92.

[143] Van Kuilenburg ABP, et al. Evaluation of 5-fluorouracil pharmacokinetics in cancer patients with a c.1905 + 1G > A mutation in DPYD by means of a Bayesian limited sampling strategy. Clin Pharmacokinet 2012;51:163−74.

[144] Morel A, et al. Clinical relevance of different dihydropyrimidine dehydrogenase gene single nucleotide polymorphisms on 5-fluorouracil tolerance. Mol Cancer Ther 2006;5:2895−904.

[145] Swen JJ, et al. Pharmacogenetics: from bench to byte−an update of guidelines. Clin Pharmacol Ther 2011;89:662−73.

[146] Caudle KE, et al. Clinical pharmacogenetics implementation consortium guidelines for dihydropyrimidine dehydrogenase genotype and fluoropyrimidine dosing. Clin Pharmacol Ther 2013;94:640−5.

[147] Di Paolo A, et al. Relationship between plasma concentrations of 5-fluorouracil and 5-fluoro-5,6-dihydrouracil and toxicity of 5-fluorouracil infusions in cancer patients. Ther Drug Monit 2002;24:588−93.

[148] Boisdron-Celle M, et al. 5-Fluorouracil-related severe toxicity: a comparison of different methods for the pretherapeutic detection of dihydropyrimidine dehydrogenase deficiency. Cancer Lett 2007;249:271−82.

[149] Jiang H, Lu J, Ji J. Circadian rhythm of dihydrouracil/uracil ratios in biological fluids: a potential biomarker for dihydropyrimidine dehydrogenase levels. Br J Pharmacol 2004;141:616−23.

[150] Ciccolini J, et al. A rapid and inexpensive method for anticipating severe toxicity to fluorouracil and fluorouracil-based chemotherapy. Ther Drug Monit 2006;28:678−85.

[151] Yang CG, et al. DPD-based adaptive dosing of 5-FU in patients with head and neck cancer: impact on treatment efficacy and toxicity. Cancer Chemother Pharmacol 2011;67:49−56.

[152] Fety R, et al. Clinical impact of pharmacokinetically-guided dose adaptation of 5-fluorouracil: results from a multicentric randomized trial in patients with locally advanced head and neck carcinomas. Clin Cancer Res 1998;4:2039−45.

[153] Gamelin E, et al. Individual fluorouracil dose adjustment based on pharmacokinetic follow-up compared with conventional dosage: results of a multicenter randomized trial of patients with metastatic colorectal cancer. J Clin Oncol 2008;26:2099−105.

[154] Terret C, et al. Dose and time dependencies of 5-fluorouracil pharmacokinetics. Clin Pharmacol Ther 2000;68:270−9.

[155] De Bruijn EA, et al. Non-linear pharmacokinetics of 5-fluorouracil as described by in vivo behaviour of 5,6 dihydro-5-fluorouracil. Biochem Pharmacol 1986;35:2461−5.

[156] Gamelin E, Boisdron-Celle M. Dose monitoring of 5-fluorouracil in patients with colorectal or head and neck cancer—status of the art. Crit Rev Oncol Hematol 1999;30:71−9.

[157] Gusella M, et al. Predictors of survival and toxicity in patients on adjuvant therapy with 5-fluorouracil for colorectal cancer. Br J Cancer 2009;100:1549−57.

[158] Santini J, et al. 5-FU therapeutic monitoring with dose adjustment leads to an improved therapeutic index in head and neck cancer. Br J Cancer 1989;59:287−90.

[159] Milano G, et al. Relationship between fluorouracil systemic exposure and tumor response and patient survival. J Clin Oncol 1994;12:1291−5.

[160] Yang R, Zhang Y, Zhou H, et al. Individual 5-fluororacil dose adjustment via pharmacokinetic monitoring versus conventional body-area surface method: a meta-analysis. Ther Drug Monit 2016;38(1):79−86.

[161] Milano G, Etienne MC. Potential importance of dihydropyrimidine dehydrogenase (DPD) in cancer chemotherapy. Pharmacogenetics 1994;4:301−6.

[162] Egüés A, et al. Pharmacokinetically Guided Dose Adjustment of 5-Fluorouracil (5-FU) in Gastrointestinal Cancer Patients. Eur J Hosp Pharm 2013;20:A132.

[163] Roman O, et al. A pilot study of oxaliplatin, irinotecan and PK-adjusted 5-fluorouracil within a multidisciplinary approach in locally advanced pancreatic cancer patients. J Clin Oncol 33 2015 (suppl; abstr e15220)

[164] Fusco JP, et al. A retrospective analysis of preoperative FOLFOX chemotherapy for locally advanced colon cancer patients with pharmacokinetic-guided dose adjustments of 5-FU. Ann Oncol 2014;25 (suppl 2):ii83−4.

[165] Determinación de pirimidinas endógenas y monitorización de 5-fluorouracilo. Claves para la eficacia y seguridad. II congreso de Oncología médica y Farmacia Oncológica. in Tendiendo puentes (2014).

[166] Kaldate RR, Haregewoin A, Grier CE, Hamilton SA, McLeod HL. Modeling the 5-fluorouracil area under the curve versus dose relationship to develop a pharmacokinetic dosing algorithm for colorectal cancer patients receiving FOLFOX6. Oncologist 2012;17:296−302.

[167] Helsby NA, Lo WY, Thompson P, Laking GR. Do 5-fluorouracil therapies alter CYP2C19 metaboliser status?. Cancer Chemother Pharmacol 2010;66:405−7.

[168] Aldaz A, et al. Utilidad de la monitorizacion farmacocinética de 5-FU para detectar interacciones farmacológicas: a propósito de un caso. In: Tendiendo Puentes; 2014.

[169] Andreica IW, Pfeifer E, Rozov M, et al. Fluorouracil overdose: clinical manifestations and comprehensive management during and after hospitalization. J Hematol Oncol Pharm 2015;5(2):43−7.

[170] Mathijssen RH, et al. Clinical pharmacokinetics and metabolism of irinotecan (CPT-11). Clin Cancer Res 2001;7:2182−94.

[171] Stewart CF, et al. UGT1A1 promoter genotype correlates with SN-38 pharmacokinetics, but not severe toxicity in patients receiving low-dose irinotecan. J Clin Oncol 2007;25(18):2594−600.

[172] Santos A, et al. Metabolism of irinotecan (CPT-11) by CYP3A4 and CYP3A5 in humans. Clin Cancer Res 2000;6:2012−20.

[173] Gupta E, et al. Metabolic fate of irinotecan in humans: correlation of glucuronidation with diarrhea. Cancer Res 1994;54:3723−5.

[174] Castellanos C, Aldaz A, Zufia L, et al. Biliary index accurately predicts the severity of the topoisomerase inhibitor irinotecan (CPT-11) induced diarrhea in colorectal cancer patients. Proc Am Soc Clin Oncol 2003;22:162.

[175] Haouala A, et al. Drug interactions with the tyrosine kinase inhibitors imatinib, dasatinib, and nilotinib. Blood 2011;117(8):e75−87.

[176] Cox LA. A biomathematical model of hematotoxicity. Environ Int 1999;25:805−17.

CONTROLLING BUSULFAN THERAPY IN CHILDREN

18

M. Neely, M. Philippe, N. Bleyzac and S. Goutelle

CHAPTER OUTLINE

18.1 INTRODUCTION

Allogeneic hematopoietic stem cell transplantation (HSCT) remains the major treatment for numerous pediatric disorders including leukemia, severe hemoglobinopathies, and immune deficiencies. However the overall survival of these patients is affected by a high rate of transplantation-related mortality (TRM).

Apart from infections due to immunosuppression, one of the most frequent complications that accounts for TRM is venoocclusive disease (VOD) of the liver due to myeloablative treatment before transplantation [1]. The incidence of VOD varies between 20% and 50% depending on the types of pathologies requiring HSCT [1]. The introduction of intravenous busulfan has helped to decrease this incidence, although it remains around 10−20%. Once VOD develops, the mortality rate is high due to associated multiorgan failure.

Among the cytotoxic agents used in the pretransplant conditioning regimen, busulfan is well known to be associated with liver toxicity and VOD. Busulfan is an alkylating agent mostly used in combination with cyclophosphamide before transplantation in myeloablative conditioning regimens. Dosing by intravenous administration is now the preferred route in many centers. Despite intravenous dosing, numerous studies have documented highly variable pharmacokinetics (PK) and plasma exposures between patients [2−5]. Moreover, there is a considerable body of evidence that the target exposure for busulfan is quite narrow, such that there is a small difference between higher plasma concentrations associated with increased risk of toxicity [6,7] and lower concentrations associated with increased risk of graft failure due to residual host immune cells [8−10].

The administration of standard dose regimens leads to quite variable responses, from inefficacy to toxicity. Controlling this variability with individualized dosing can be helpful to reduce a part of

Individualized Drug Therapy for Patients. DOI: http://dx.doi.org/10.1016/B978-0-12-803348-7.00018-6

TRM and improve clinical outcome of the transplanted patients. Nguyen et al. reported that in children, IV busulfan clearance correlates with body weight [4]. This finding led to the development of a weight-based dosing nomogram in children that was then approved for inclusion in the package leaflet in Europe. Simulations based on the nonlinear weight-based dosing strategy from Nguyen and colleagues predicted a 75% probability of achieving the target AUC range of $900-1500 \, \mu mol \cdot min/L/dose$, which was significantly better than various other dosing methods, but still leaves room for improvement [11]. In the United States, initial busulfan dosing, according to the FDA-approved package insert, is 0.8 mg/kg IV every 6 h for patients >12 kg, and 1.1 mg/kg for those ≤12 kg. However, as reported in the insert, based on population modeling and simulated probability of target attainment (PTA, described later in this chapter), this dosing is expected to achieve the proper exposure in only 60% of patients. Therefore, whatever initial dosing is used, a nonnegligible proportion of patients remains under- or overdosed. Busulfan therapeutic drug monitoring and management (TDM) is therefore routinely recommended and practiced at pediatric transplantation centers to maximize chances of successful therapy within the narrow exposure range for all the patients.

To adjust dosing, most centers appear to use several measured busulfan concentrations obtained after the first dose, anywhere between four and nine samples [12]. From these, a common approach is to estimate the $AUC_{0-\infty}$ or steady-state AUC_{0-t}, where t is the dosing interval, by noncompartmental methods, including trapezoidal approximation. From this estimate, dosing is adjusted by simple proportionality according to the equation $Dose_{new} = Dose_{given} \times AUC_{desired}/AUC_{measured}$ [13].

A major problem with calculation of AUC from the first dose will arise if accumulation of drug until steady state is neglected, which underestimates the total AUC and therefore overestimates required dosages [14]. Another problem with this approach is the large number of blood samples that must be obtained during a single dosing interval to estimate AUC. The package insert recommends a minimum of three, and preferably four (or more). Some centers, including the Children's Hospital Los Angeles (CHLA, where MN works) have used nine samples to precisely calculate AUC within a 6-h window. This is very burdensome to nurses, phlebotomists, laboratory personnel, and the patients, who must be dedicated to obtaining the required results in a timely enough fashion to permit any necessary dose adjustments. For this reason, centers are beginning to turn toward population modeling (a.k.a. pharmacometrics) and the techniques discussed in this book as a means to tailor initial dosing more finely than available in the US and European package inserts and to adjust subsequent dosing to achieve the target exposure with fewer blood samples.

To apply pharmacometrics to calculate doses for any drug, including busulfan, one must have a population model. Several population models of busulfan PK have been published in the last 3 years [15−21], and alternative methods for calculating the initial dose of busulfan have been proposed, based on these models [11,22]. Recently the group from the University of San Francisco has begun to develop a tool to use a model for dose optimization [15]. The lack of good software tools is a barrier to the application of pharmacometrics to the bedside, as we have discussed previously [23,24]. However, this group's tool is an Excel spreadsheet that currently is only designed to choose the initial dose based on the mean population parameter values and the patient's age and weight. We feel that while this is better than noncompartmental methods, to truly optimize therapy, we must use an approach and a tool that can tailor the dose to an individual based on measured responses, updating estimates of the ideal dose as knowledge of the patient is gained.

In the past, we have used maximum a posteriori (MAP) Bayesian techniques as implemented in our older USC*PACK software [25] to successfully manage busulfan therapy. With such dose optimization, we have been able to increase the number of patients within the therapeutic AUC range and improve outcome of patients [14]. We based our estimates of Bayesian posterior (individual) parameter estimates on only 2 (IV busulfan) or 3 (oral busulfan) plasma concentration measurements. Our first report included 29 children who received an oral busulfan-based conditioning regimen, with doses given every 6 h [26]. We adjusted the doses to reach a target mean 6-hourly AUC between 4 and 6 $\mu g \cdot h/mL$. We evaluated the performance of the Bayesian adaptive individualized regimens by comparing the incidence of toxicity, chimerism (incomplete engraftment), and VOD-free survival with historically matched patients conditioned with standard doses of busulfan. The incidence of VOD was 3.4% versus 24.1% ($p = .022$) in the control group, while the incidence of stomatitis was not significantly different, despite a trend to be less severe. Engraftment was successful in all patients with individualized busulfan dose regimens, while 12% graft failure was observed in others ($p = .010$). The 90-day VOD-free survival was significantly higher in patients with individualized busulfan doses: 97% versus 76% ($p = .026$). Overall survival was 83% in patients with individualized busulfan doses versus 65% in others ($p = .031$).

Our second report focused on IV busulfan [14]. This study included 138 children receiving busulfan in 16 doses with the first dose assigned based on weight and subsequent doses adjusted to a local AUC target range of 980−1250 $\mu mol \cdot min/L$. Busulfan TDM combined with model-based dose adjustment was associated with an increased probability of AUC target attainment, for both target range: 90.8% versus 74.8% for the conventional target range, 66.2% versus 43.9% for the local target range ($p < .001$). Event-free survival was 88.5%, overall survival was 91.5%, with a median follow-up of 54 months, and VOD occurred in 18.3% of patients.

More recently, we have used nonparametric population modeling and multiple model (MM), Bayesian adaptive control, as discussed extensively in this book, to develop and validate a model for intravenous busulfan that can be used to optimize individual therapy with two samples after any dose change to confirm predicted plasma drug exposure. In the remainder of this chapter, we describe this process in detail.

Populations for model building and validation. To build a population model, it is ideal to have some subjects who can be included in the model-building population, and another group or groups who can be used to check the generalizability of the model. In other words, can the model predict concentrations in more than one group of patients?

For our model-building population, since patients at CHLA have such intensive sampling, we had a lot of data available to us to build a robust, rich population model. We included the records of 53 children for whom we happened to have assembled complete data over a period from 2011 to 2013. After developing the model, we used an additional 11 patients admitted in the latter part of 2013, who were not included in the model-building cohort, to form an external validation group. This means that we used them to test how well the model could predict their concentrations even though they had not been included when the model was built.

As another validation cohort, we also used the busulfan dosing history and measured concentrations from 105 pediatric patients who had been cared for at the University Hospitals of Lyon (Hospices Civils de Lyon), France, from 2006 to 2012.

Finally, to validate the application of the model in our BestDose software for MM Bayesian adaptive control of therapeutic drug dosing [23,27–29], we used an additional 20 patients admitted to CHLA from the end of 2013 through 2014, who were not part of any other cohort.

The characteristics of the various populations used in this project are shown in Table 18.2. The model-building and validation populations were similar in age and weight, but the French cohort had far fewer busulfan blood samples per patient, since they were managed with USC*PACK, as we described earlier. The BestDose cohort was heavier than the others, because the pharmacy and laboratory deliberately selected patients with a wide range of weights for the validation.

We will describe shortly exactly how we used these varied populations.

Data needed to make a population model. Of course, when one builds a population model, all relevant information must be captured in the data file so that the algorithm can fit the data to the model equations to estimate the distributions of the model parameters for all subjects in the population. These relevant data include dose amounts, times of doses, routes of doses, infusion times of intravenous doses, times and measured concentrations (or other outputs such as effects), and subject covariate values, such as weight. Recall that a covariate is a subject factor that may be associated with some model parameter, such as weight with volume of distribution. Again, we have summarized some of this information in Tables 18.1 and 18.2.

As far as the samples per patient available to us, the standard protocol at CHLA is to collect nine blood samples for measurement of plasma busulfan with the first dose and every dose that is different from the previous dose. The samples are collected just prior to, and 0, 0.25, 0.5, 1, 1.5, 2.5, 3.5, and 4 h after the end of a 2-h infusion. In the Lyon cohort, two blood samples were drawn 0.5 and 2 h after the end of the first busulfan infusion in each patient.

Sample analysis and assay error. As you have read in other chapters (especially see Chapter 4, Optimizing Laboratory Assay Methods for Individualized Therapy), knowing the characteristics of the assays used to measure your samples is a crucial part of a population modeling project. The certainty (or uncertainty) of each measurement, captured by the error or estimated standard deviation (SD) of any value, is used to appropriately weight data in the model-fitting process. Values that come from a range where the assay is less precise (higher SD) will carry

Table 18.1 Different PK Targets Used in the Clinical TDM of Busulfan in Children

Target Type (Units)	Time Span (h)	Target Range
AUC ($\mu M \times$ min)		
AUC_{0-6}	0–6	877–1315
AUC_{24}	0–24	3508–5260
AUC_{96}	0–96	14,032–21,048
AUC (mg $\times$ h/L)		
AUC_{0-6}	0–6	3.6–5.4
AUC_{24}	0–24	14.4–21.6
AUC_{96}	0–96	57.6–86.1
C_{ave} (ng/mL)	0–96	600–900

AUC, area under the time-concentration curve; C_{ave}, average concentration.

Table 18.2 Characteristics of the Patient Cohorts Described in This Chapter

Cohort	Model-Building	Validation 1	Validation 2	BestDose
Source	CHLA	Lyon	CHLA	CHLA
Number	53	105	11	20
Age (years)	7.8 (0.2−19.0)	5.6 (0.1−21)	5.8 (0.5−14.2)	10.2 (0.25−18)
Weight (kg)	26.5 (5.6−78.0)	20.3 (3.4−59.6)	22.7 (5.2−53.4)	46.4 (5.2−110.9)
All doses (mg/kg)	1.1 (0.7−1.8)	1.2 (0.6−5.2)	1.2 (0.9−1.5)	0.83 (0.5−1.3)
Samples/patient	16.7 (6−26)	3.3 (1−13)	15.9 (8−26)	25.2 (17−26)
C_{ave}(ng/mL)	750 (390−1190)	750 (390−1860)	780 (550−950)	714 (564−914)

Data are presented as mean (range).
CHLA, Children's Hospital Los Angeles; C_{ave}, average concentration over 96 h.

less weight than more precise measurements. Therefore, here we describe the assays for our busulfan project.

All samples from CHLA are assayed for busulfan in the Special Chemistry Laboratory using a validated HPLC assay [30]. In this sense, validated usually means that the assay is able to report values for a range of known concentrations within a certain percent coefficient of variation (CV%) for replicate samples on different days (interday) or on the same day (intraday). Usually a CV% ≤15% is considered acceptable, but of course, this is arbitrary, as we have discussed in Chapter 4, Optimizing Laboratory Assay Methods for Individualized Therapy. Busulfan plasma concentrations from Lyon were measured by HPLC with UV detection for data before 2010 [31], and by an updated, cross-validated liquid chromatography−tandem mass spectrometry method after 2010 [32]. All the assays used were linear from 20 to 2000 ng/mL with a reported interday imprecision of <10%.

During the fitting procedure, we weight the concentrations with their Fisher information of $1/$Var, where Var is the variance. Var is, of course, the SD squared. To estimate the SD of any measured concentration, we used an error polynomial of the form $SD = \sqrt{Var} = 0.0019 + 0.021 \times$ [conc] $+ 0.017 \times$ [conc]^2, where conc is the busulfan concentration. So, in this case $C_0 = 0.0019$, $C_1 = 0.021$, $C_2 = 0.017$, and $C_3 = 0$. Again, see Chapter 4 for details and to review assay error polynomial equations in more detail. We estimated the coefficient values from the reported intraassay standard concentrations and SDs of six replicates of the assay used at CHLA [30], fitted to zero- to third-degree polynomials with the *makeErrorPoly* function in Pmetrics. For the Lyon cohort, the polynomial was $SD = \sqrt{Var} = 0.0007 + 0.056 \times$ [conc] $- 0.019 \times$ [conc]^2, based on their assays [32]. Both second-degree polynomials fitted their respective assay validation data with an R^2 of >.99.

You can see what the output of the *makeErrorPoly* function looks like in Fig. 18.1. There are three curves in the plot, corresponding to the first-, second-, and third-degree polynomial equations. We selected the curve that was the best combination of R^2 and parsimony. In other words, the second-degree polynomial had an almost perfect R^2, had one fewer term than the third degree, and did not rapidly increase beyond a concentration of 2 mg/L (2000 ng/mL).

Additionally, during the modeling process, we allowed Pmetrics to fit a fixed but unknown additive lambda term, such that concentrations were weighted by $\left((SD+\lambda)^2\right)^{-1}$, where lambda is

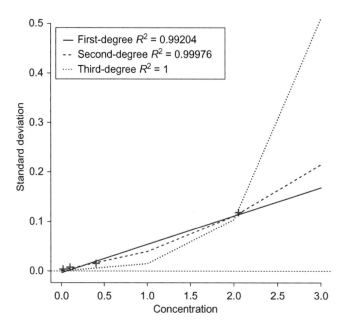

FIGURE 18.1

Relationship between (top) K_eS (elimination adjusted allometrically for body size) and (bottom) VS (volume adjusted allometrically for body size) and age. Equations for the polynomials are shown in the legend for Table 18.4.

representative of additional noise such as errors in sample timing or model misspecification. The final cycle value of lambda was 0.058, about half of the lowest measured concentration (0.11 mg/L), indicating very low error beyond measurement noise and very low model misspecification.

Population modeling. Because we ultimately wanted to use the model for MM Bayesian adaptive control in BestDose, we constructed a nonparametric population model using the nonparametric adaptive grid [33,34] algorithm in Pmetrics [35] and the individual patient busulfan dosing history, concentrations, and covariates, as we have just described.

As is typical, we started with the simplest model and gradually added complexity as suggested by the data. First, we tested one-compartment models consisting of an infusion into a central compartment with volume V and elimination K_e, with differing initial ranges for both parameters. A good starting range for rate transfer constants such as K_e is 0−5, which corresponds to a half-life of $\ln(2)/K_e$, which is infinity to 8.3 min, a very broad range. For volume terms, we typically research what is known about the drug and choose a suitable range, such as 0−100 L. Of course, a drug cannot have a 0 volume, just as it cannot have an infinite half-life. These are simply boundaries beyond which NPAG will not estimate. We also tested models with an additional peripheral compartment and transfer of drug to the peripheral compartment from the central (KCP) and the reverse (KPC).

For each compartmental model, we explored the effect of including covariates. As we mentioned earlier, covariates are subject-specific factors that might be associated with model parameter values. For models that include children, we have found that allometric scaling is usually the best way to relate weight to model parameters [36]. In allometry, one scales V and K_e for body size by using fixed exponents on body weight of -0.25 for K_e and of 1 for V. For example, $K_e = K_e0*$ $\text{wt}^{-0.25}$ and $V = V0*\text{wt}$. Allometry is similar, but slightly superior to body surface area scaling, and more consistent with observed drug behavior than parameters scaled by body weight. There are many ways to use allometric scaling when adjusting for size, whether from animals to humans or within mixed adult-pediatric populations. Some argue that it is best to fix the exponents (-0.25 for rate constants, 1 for volumes, and 0.75 for clearances) [37], while others equally strongly argue that the exponents should be fitted terms [38]. We have usually fixed the terms and allowed variability to be present in other model parameters. For busulfan, we used the lesser of actual body weight (ABW) or ideal bodyweight (IBW) calculated using the Traub and Johnson formula [39] in our allometric sizing.

Once we accounted for body size with allometric scaling, we then tested for the effect of other covariates, particularly age for pediatric datasets, on model parameters by comparing likelihood and predictions with and without age included in the model. Busulfan is not eliminated in the urine, so we did not include a renal function descriptor. Although some data have suggested that genetic polymorphisms of busulfan metabolizing enzyme may influence the drug PK, this was not investigated, as we did not have any pharmacogenomic patient data available to us [40].

In Fig. 18.2 you can see how age relates to both busulfan elimination and volume of distribution, once both parameters were adjusted for size by allometry. It is important to adjust for size before age, because the two are obviously highly correlated. Based on the shape of trend curve, we used Pmetrics to fit zero- to third-order polynomials to the median posterior values of elimination and volume, adjusted for size, for each patient and their age. We did this in exactly the same way as we described for the previous assay error, using *makeErrorPoly* in Pmetrics. The plots of these polynomials are included in Fig. 18.2. This is one approach to age inclusion in a population model. Long-Boyle exemplified another approach to include age in their population model of busulfan [15]. They estimated a breakpoint age, below which the slope of the age−clearance relationship was one value and above which the slope was a different value. Finally, yet another approach is to model the age relationship as a nonlinear sigmoidal function, such that maturation $= 1/[1 + (\text{age}/\text{age50})^{-\text{Hill}}]$, where age50 is the age at which maturation is 50% complete and $-$Hill controls the steepness of the relationship [11]. All of these approaches are empirical, in that they are not trying to recapitulate true underlying mechanisms of maturation in drug disposition, but simply to reproduce the behavior in a mathematical and predicable manner. We chose our approach to minimize the number of additional parameters that needed to be fitted. If the model had not predicted well, particularly in the context of BcstDose, we would have revised our inclusion of age to one of the other models.

Choosing the final model is as much art and opinion as it is science and statistics. The choice of the "final" model always should be influenced by the purpose of the modeling project. For example, if the goal is to be as accurate and precise as possible with the very first dose, a larger range of included covariates may be helpful. Remember, that before the first concentration is measured, all patients who have the same set of covariate values will have the same optimal dose amount calculated for a particular target. That is because the same set of model parameter values is used when there is no information (ie, measured concentrations) available to calculate the Bayesian posterior parameter values for the patient. The only way, then, to individualize the first dose is to

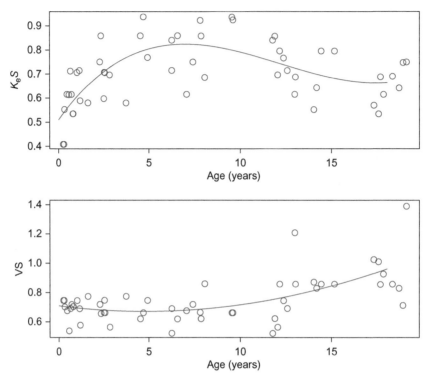

FIGURE 18.2

Output from the makeErrorPoly function in Pmetrics to estimate assay error coefficients from busulfan assay validation data. Each curve is a polynomial fit to standard concentrations and the SD of the found concentrations obtained during routine assay validation. The equation for the first-order polynomial is $SD = -0.0029 + 0.057 \times$ [drug], where SD is the standard deviation and [drug] is the measured concentration. For the second-order polynomial, the equation is $SD = 0.0019 + 0.021 \times$ [drug] $+ 0.017 \times$ [drug]^2. As described in the text, this was the equation we settled upon for our busulfan model. Finally, the third-order polynomial equation is $SD = 0.00033 + 0.059 \times$ [drug] $- 0.085 \times$ [drug]$^2 + 0.041 \times$ [drug]^3. Note that for both the first- and third-order, there are concentrations that could cause SD to be estimated as a negative number, which will cause a problem during fitting in Pmetrics or use of BestDose, and must be avoided.

use individual covariates (eg, weight, age, sex, genotype) to modify the values of the model parameters.

On the other hand, if the goal is simply to control therapy as accurately and precisely as possible, and there is time to obtain measured concentrations to generate Bayesian posterior parameter value distributions for our patient, we have often found that too many covariates in a model can actually hamper performance, as the model is too constrained by overly burdensome covariate equations. In reality, we are probably fitting noise, even if statistically this is not apparent during the model-building process. This can become a problem when we try to use such a complex model in new patients.

Table 18.3 Comparison of Candidate Models, All After 100 Cycles

Model #	Comp	Parameters	−2*LL	AIC	Bias	Imprecision
1	1	K_e, V	−1944	−1938	0.003	0.076
2	2	K_e, V, KCP, KPC	−2172	−2162	0.000	0.072
3	1	#1 + allometric	−1982	−1976	−0.001	0.069
4	2	#2 + allometric	−2370	−2360	−0.012	0.058
5	**1**	**#3 + age**	**−2012**	**−2006**	**−0.003**	**0.070**
6	2	#4 + age	−2436	−2426	−0.008	0.056

Bold indicates the model that was selected.
Comp, number of compartments; K_m, elimination from central compartment; V, volume of central compartment; KCP, transfer rate from central to peripheral compartment; KPC, transfer rate from peripheral to central compartment; LL, log likelihood; AIC, Akaike Information Criterion.
Bias and Imprecision are calculated as reported in the text, based on the median population parameter values for each model.
Models are reported in order of complexity, with allometric indicating allometric scaling of model parameter values for body size, and age indicating the addition of an age polynomial to allometrically scaled models, as described in the text. Based on the discussion in the text, we chose model #5, in bold, to develop further.

Since we were most interested in being able to control overall busulfan exposure, with time to obtain samples from our individual patients who would be managed with BestDose, we chose the final model primarily to minimize the bias and imprecision of the predictions versus observations. Bias was the mean error of the difference between predictions (pred$_i$) and observations (obs$_i$), ie, Bias $= \frac{1}{N}\sum_{i=1}^{N}\left(\text{pred}_i - \text{obs}_i\right)$, where N is the total number of observations. Imprecision was the square root of variance of prediction error, ie, bias-adjusted root mean squared error calculated by

$$\sqrt{\left[\frac{1}{N}\sum_{i=1}^{N}\left(\text{pred}_i - \text{obs}_i\right)^2\right] - \text{Bias}^2}.$$

Model comparisons are shown in Table 18.3. Considering all six candidate models divided into three pairs of one- and two-compartment models without covariates, with size scaling, and with size plus age scaling, respectively, within each model pair, the two-compartment model had the best (lowest) likelihood and AIC. Overall, the pair of one- or two-compartment allometric + age models were the most likely. Within this pair, the two-compartment model was more likely. However, as we said, we were primarily concerned with minimal prediction bias and imprecision, so we chose the one-compartment, allometrically and age-scaled model (#5 in Table 18.3) as the final structural model, with equations and population parameter values shown in Table 18.4.

Indeed, predicted busulfan concentrations, based either on population or on Bayesian posterior medians, were well matched to their corresponding measured concentrations, as shown in Fig. 18.3. The Bayesian posterior bias (mean prediction error) was −3.2 ng/mL with an imprecision (root mean bias-adjusted squared error) of 70 ng/mL. To put these in context, the mean observed concentration was 758 ng/mL; therefore the mean bias is only 0.42% of this, with an imprecision of 9.2%.

As we did for voriconazole [27], we summarized parameter values in the final model as weighted medians for central tendencies of a nonparametric distribution with a 95% confidence interval (95% CI) around the median, and the median absolute weighted deviation (MAWD) from

Table 18.4 Population Parameter Value Summaries in the Final Model

Parameter	Median (95% CI)	MAWD (95% CI)	Range
K_eS	1.01 (0.93–1.07)	0.084 (0.050–0.13)	0.76–1.16
VS	1.01 (0.98–1.04)	0.052 (0.021–0.11)	0.74–1.55

MAWD is the median absolute weighted deviation, analogous to variance for a normal distribution (see text). In the model, $K_e = KeS * \text{ibw}^{-0.25} * (C_0 + C_1 * [\text{age}] + C_2 * [\text{age}]^2 + C_3 * [\text{age}]^3)$ and $V = VS * \text{ibw} * (C_0 + C_1 * [\text{age}] + C_2 * [\text{age}]^2)$, where K_e is the elimination rate constant from the central compartment in per h; K_eS is the scaled K_e; ibw is ideal bodyweight in kg, calculated using the Traub and Johnson formula [39]; V is the volume of the central compartment in L; and VS is the scaled volume. $C_0, \ldots, C_3$ are the coefficients describing the age dependence of K_e and V, which were fixed in the final model. For K_e, $C_0 = 0.51$, $C_1 = 0.10$, $C_2 = -0.010$, $C_3 = 0.00029$. For V, $C_0 = 0.71$, $C_1 = -0.016$, $C_2 = 0.0017$.

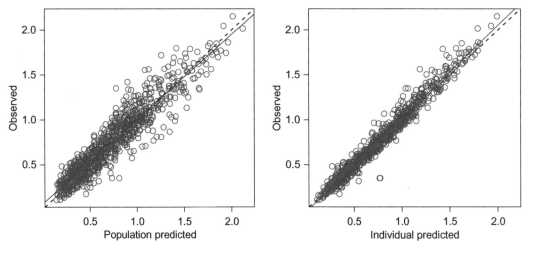

FIGURE 18.3

Observed versus predicted plots for busulfan. Predictions were based on the median population parameter values (left) or the medians of the individual Bayesian posterior parameter values (right).

the median as a measure of the variance of a nonparametric distribution, with its 95% CI. These estimates correspond to weighted mean, 95% CI of the mean, variance, and 95% CI of the variance, respectively, for a sample from a normal distribution.

Validation against external cohorts. As we described earlier in the chapter, we used separate groups of subjects to test how well the model could also predict their busulfan concentrations. This is a common method of "validating" a model. Of course, one way to look at this is that if indeed we are able to predict measured concentrations with minimal bias, in fact we are validating that the second population is similar to the first. Nevertheless, there is value in this exercise, as it gives us some confidence that our model represents the population of interest. If the second population is not well served by the model, one approach is to combine the two populations if possible to make a

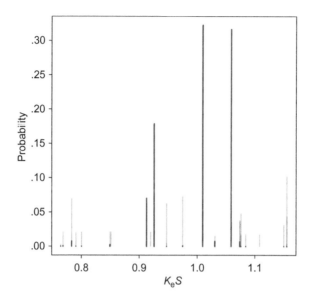

FIGURE 18.4

Probability distribution for the model parameter K_eS (also known as a marginal plot) for a single subject, where K_eS is the size- and age-adjusted elimination rate constant of busulfan. The light gray spikes represent values for K_eS and their probabilities in the population model, ie, the Bayesian prior distribution. The red (dark gray in print versions) spikes are the probabilities of each point in the Bayesian posterior distribution for subject 105. You can see that the values of the points have not changed, only the probabilities, as described in the text. Some points in the Bayesian prior have become so improbable in the Bayesian posterior that they do not have any red (dark gray in print versions) value at all.

more diverse model, and use a third population to test the generalizability. Unfortunately this may not always be possible to do, eg, when the second population is very sparsely sampled and unlikely to contribute much to estimates of the parameter value distributions in the population of interest.

In our case, using what we hoped would be the final model, we calculated the nonparametric Bayesian posterior parameter value distributions for each of the 105 French patients and the 11 additional CHLA patients using their own busulfan dosing, concentrations, and weights. This is known as a zero-cycle run in Pmetrics, because we are not using NPAG to estimate new points for the validation populations. For each subject in the validation population, Pmetrics simply recalculates the probability of each support point in the population model based on how well it predicts the measured concentrations for the patient's administered doses, times of doses and samples, and covariate values. Support points whose model parameter values result in concentrations that closely match the patient's become more likely, and those with poor predictions become less likely. The parameter values for each support point don't change—only the probability of the support point. In this way, we have a new probability distribution of the support points, individualized to our single patient for whom we are trying to predict or control. You can see an example of this in Fig. 18.4. This again is the Bayesian posterior parameter value distribution that is the foundation of individual therapy.

We calculated bias, imprecision, and linear regression descriptors for the observations versus predictions, with predictions for each subject based on the median of his Bayesian posterior parameter value distribution. For the French cohort ($n = 105$), the bias was -4.6 ng/mL, and imprecision was 124 ng/mL. The intercept of the regression line for observations versus predictions was 21.4 (95% CI $-9.3-52.1$), and the slope was 0.98 (95% CI $0.94-1.01$), indicating that neither were significantly different from their ideal values of 0 and 1, respectively. The regression coefficient of determination (R^2) was .89. For the CHLA validation cohort ($n = 11$), prediction bias was 16.4 ng/mL, and imprecision was 119 ng/mL. The intercept of the regression line for observations versus predictions was -6.9 (95% CI $-46.0-32.2$) and the slope was 1.03 (95% CI $0.99-1.08$). R^2 was .92.

These statistics are very good. The ideal intercept of the regression line is 0, and the ideal slope is 1, as is the R^2, known as the coefficient of determination. Of course, in reality, one never achieves those ideals, but we can look at the statistical tests to determine whether our predictions significantly depart from the ideal. For these intercepts and slopes, the 95% confidence intervals all span the ideal, and thus none are significantly different from the ideal. There is no test for the coefficient of determination, but one generally hopes to see $R^2 > 90\%$ for the Bayesian posterior predictions in the model-building population and $>80\%$ for a validation population.

Using the model to calculate general starting doses and optimal, limited sampling times. First, we describe the application of a powerful simulation technique, called PTA, to use the model for the purpose of estimating a general starting dose. Second, we describe how we can use the model to calculate a small set of optimally timed samples that are designed to provide the most amount of information about our patients with the fewest blood draws.

For the initial dose PTA, from the final model, we used Pmetrics to simulate 1000 time−concentration profiles for several dosage amounts of busulfan, all administered every 6 h for 96 h, that is, 16 total doses, which matches the clinically used regimen. By simulation, we mean that we can randomly draw one set of values for each parameter in the model from the probability distribution of those parameter values in the population. To that set of parameter values, we can calculate what the busulfan concentration is at frequent intervals (eg, every 15 min) for any dosage regimen. We can do this repeatedly—10, 100, 1000, or any other number of times—to generate a set of time−concentration profiles.

For each set of profiles, corresponding to one dosage regimen, we determined the proportion of the 1000 simulated 96-h average concentrations (C_{ave}) that were between 600 and 900 ng/mL. This proportion is the PTA, where the target is a C_{ave} of 600−900 ng/mL. For other drugs, different targets might be appropriate, such as the ratio of peak to threshold, or percent of dosing interval above a threshold. In this way, we select the dosage with the highest success proportion as a reasonable initial dose. Simulations of doses of 4, 4.5, 5, 5.5, and 6 mg per age-adjusted, allometrically scaled kg resulted in target attainment rates of 68%, 77%, 64%, 46%, and 27%, respectively. This is shown in Fig. 18.5. Since 4.5 had the highest PTA, we calculated the dose in mg/kg for all combinations of weights from 0 to 100 kg in 2.5 kg increments, and ages from 0 to 18 years in 1-year increments. We used CDC growth tables (http://www.cdc.gov/growthcharts/1977charts.htm) to ensure that our weights and ages were properly correlated. We excluded weight-for-age combinations $<$5th percentile and $>$95th percentile by CDC criteria. The range of doses was 0.88−1.24 mg/kg, with the highest doses in the lightest 5−6 year olds and the lowest doses in the heaviest teenagers. The mean dose in those $\leq$12 kg was 1.1 mg/kg and in those $>$12 kg was 1.0 mg/kg, with 67% and 76% predicted to achieve a 96-h C_{ave} of 600−900 ng/mL, respectively. These doses can be considered as reasonable starting doses in the absence of a tool like BestDose, which we describe later.

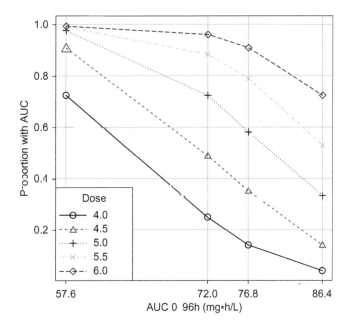

FIGURE 18.5

Probability of target attainment for various size- and age-adjusted doses of busulfan given as sixteen 2-h infusions every 6 h over a total of 96 h. The range of the targets for area under the time-concentration curve (AUC) over the entire 96 h is 57.6 mg*h/L, which represents the lower threshold for efficacy, to 86.4 mg*h/L, which represents an upper threshold for safety. Two intermediate targets are shown as well. Each point represents the proportion of 1000 possible time−concentration profiles for a given dose, generated by simulation as described in the text. The dose of 4.5 has the largest difference between upper and lower AUC thresholds, and it was the dose we chose to set as the best initial dose when a tool like BestDose is not used, as it will maximize the chances of any given patient to be within a therapeutic AUC range, recognizing that the probabilities of efficacy and safety are not constant throughout the whole range.

With pharmacometrics, it is possible to not only use the model to calculate the dose that achieves our target concentration with maximum accuracy and precision, but we can also calculate the times to most informatively sample a new patient. Our multiple model optimal (MMopt) sampling algorithm chooses the sample times that minimize the risk of choosing the wrong Bayesian posterior for the patient, ie, choosing the wrong probabilities for the support points in the Bayesian posterior, thereby estimating the wrong set of PK parameters for the patient [41]. For example, if we were to only sample at the pre-dose trough, we could very easily choose the wrong volume of distribution because we have no information about the peak concentration, which is most closely related to volume of distribution. Conversely, if we were to only sample at the time of a peak concentration, we would have almost no information about the elimination of the drug. The solution is to find the sample times that provide the most information about the patient. For this analysis, we used the latest version of our algorithm, which is a weighted MMopt (wMMopt), tuned in this case to specifically ensure that we could estimate a patient's busulfan AUC most reliably.

For a one-sample strategy, the wMMopt time was 2.25 h after starting a 2-h infusion, or 15 min after the end of the infusion. For the two-sample strategy, the wMMopt times were 2.25 and 6 h after the start of the infusion, or 15 min and 4 h after the end of the infusion, ie, a peak and trough.

Busulfan software dosing controller construction and validation. To truly validate the model for clinical use, we used it in our MM Bayesian adaptive dosing controller [23,28,42], which we call a software "cartridge" in our BestDose computer program for individual patient therapeutic drug dose optimization. The busulfan cartridge included the structural model equations relating input (busulfan dosing and patient's covariates) to output (busulfan plasma concentrations), and the discrete joint probability distribution of the values of the equation pharmacokinetic parameters in the population, consisting of support points in the final model. BestDose uses the cartridge and each patient's covariates (eg, weight and age) and busulfan dosing and concentration data to find the least biased and most precise dosage regimen relative to a target patient drug exposure (ie, busulfan AUC) as we have described in Chapter 14: Controlling Antiretroviral Therapy in Children and Adolescents With HIV infection.

To validate the busulfan dosing strategy (BestDose cartridge), for the 20 patients who were not part of any other cohort, the CHLA laboratory provided all busulfan concentrations and the patients' ideal/actual body weights. All 20 patients had a prespecified C_{ave} target, either 700 ($N = 4$) or 800 ($N = 16$) ng/mL. We were also provided the doses each patient had actually received. All patients except for two had three sets of nine samples; the remaining two patients had only two such sets. Our task was to use BestDose to make three dose recommendations to achieve the overall target C_{ave}: (1) for Doses 3−16 based on sampling after Dose 1 and the first 2 doses given; (2) for Doses 7−16 based on sampling after Doses 1 and 5 and the first 6 doses given; and (3) for Doses 11−16 based on sampling after Doses 1, 5, and 9 and the first 10 doses given. We first used all available concentrations for a given patient to generate the Bayesian posterior from which we used BestDose to calculate the doses that achieved the target C_{ave}. In BestDose, it is possible to directly target an AUC, so in each case we used AUC_{0-96} as the target and divided it by 96 to get C_{ave}. We then repeated this process using only the samples at the one or two wMMopt times in each sampling period to generate the Bayesian posteriors for dose calculations.

The exact same data and targets were sent to a reference center in the United States for busulfan dose calculation based on noncompartmental analysis of busulfan AUC using WinNonLin and proportional dosing [13]. We were blinded to their dose recommendations when generating BestDose recommendations from either the full set of measured concentrations for each patient (18−27 samples) or the reduced MMopt set (4−6 samples). After generating all the BestDose recommendations, we computed percentage bias (%bias) and imprecision, analogous to those used in the modeling process previously described, compared to the reference (REF) dose recommendations. We defined %bias as (BestDose − REF)/REF, and mean percent bias as $MPB = \frac{1}{D} \sum_{i=1}^{D} \%bias_i$, where D is the total number of dose recommendations. This means that a positive %bias indicates BestDose recommendations were higher than REF recommendations. Imprecision was the square root of variance in %bias (root mean bias-adjusted percent squared error),

ie, $\sqrt{\left(\frac{1}{D} \sum_{i=1}^{D} \%bias_i^2\right) - MPB^2}$.

Table 18.5 shows the summaries of dose recommendations from the reference center compared to the BestDose recommendations using the full set of concentrations or the wMMopt subsets to

Table 18.5 Bias and Imprecision of Dose Calculations Made With BestDose, Multiple-Model Adaptive Control, and the Final Population Model, Compared to Recommendations Made by the Seattle Cancer Care Alliance Pharmacokinetics Laboratory (SCCAPL) Using Noncompartmental Estimation of Busulfan Area Under the Time-Concentration Curve (AUC)

	SSCAPL	Full	MMopt1	MMopt2
Dose 3				
Mean (range) dose (mg)	35.7 (6.0–60.0)	35.7 (6.1 to 63.0)	32.3 (6.1 to 58.0)	36.5 (6.1 to 68)
Mean (95% CI) bias	–	0.2% (−2.4 to 2.9, p = .85)	−9.2% (−16.7 to −1.5, **p = .02**)	1.9% (−0.3 to 4.2, p = .08)
Imprecision	–	5.5%	15.7%	4.6%
Dose 7				
Mean (range) dose (mg)	32.1 (4.8–57.0)	31.9 (4.5 to 61.0)	29.1 (3.9 to 57.5)	32.1 (4.6 to 61.5)
Mean (95% CI) bias	–	−1.3% (−6.1 to 3.5, p = .57)	−10.8% (−18.6 to −3.0, **p = .01**)	−0.7% (−5.5 to 4.0, p = .75)
Imprecision	–	9.9%	16.4%	9.9%
Dose 11				
Mean (range) dose (mg)	31.3 (4.8–66.0)	32.4 (4.6 to 82.0)	28.7 (3.6 to 73.6)	32.7 (4.8 to 81.6)
Mean (95% CI) bias	–	1.6% (−4.0 to 7.3, p = .55)	−11.1% (−21.8 to −0.6, **p = .04**)	4.0% (−1.8 to 9.9, p = .16)
Imprecision	–	11.6%	22.1%	12.1%

A negative bias indicates that the BestDose calculation was less than the SCCAPL dose. Full, all data points were used to generate the individual patient's Bayesian posterior parameter value distribution from the population model; MMopt1, only the concentrations 15 min after the end of the infusion were used to generate the Bayesian posterior; MMopt2, only concentrations 15 min and 4 h after the end of the infusion (ie, a peak and trough) were used to generate the Bayesian posterior.

generate the Bayesian posteriors, as well as the bias and imprecision. Using all available data to generate the Bayesian posterior resulted in dose calculations by BestDose that had negligible overall bias across all dose recommendations of 0.1%, relative to the REF dose calculations and a very low imprecision of 9.0%. The one-sample wMMopt schedule tended toward low dose recommendations, with an average bias of −10.3% and with greater imprecision of 18.1%. The two-sample wMMopt dose recommendations also had very low bias of only 1.7% and an imprecision of 8.8%.

18.2 DISCUSSION

Controlling busulfan therapy with Bayesian techniques can achieve target concentrations with the fewest number of samples. Furthermore, based on our earlier work with MAP-Bayesian control, we know that we can also improve outcomes of busulfan therapy, with reduced incidence of VOD and better engraftment.

In this chapter we have provided a detailed description of our latest project to develop a nonparametric population pharmacokinetic model of intravenous busulfan in children of diverse ages and weights, and use of that model in the MM Bayesian control algorithm in BestDose. As for our MAP-Bayesian model, a one-compartment model with age and weight dependence adequately described the data in the model-building population. For the average age in the current population of 8 years and an ideal body weight of 26.7 kg, K_e was 0.36 per h, V was 0.69 L/kg, and clearance was 4.14 mL/min/kg, which agree well with clearance and volume in the US package insert of 0.64 L/kg and 3.37 mL/min/kg, respectively as well as in other reports [18,43,44].

Our nonparametric model includes weight and age as significant covariates that are independently associated with busulfan PK across the entire pediatric age range. Other models have included an age function only in the youngest children [11,17], while the model of Long-Boyle et al. also included age effects across the entire pediatric age range, defined by an increasing rate of allometrically scaled clearance up to a fixed age of 12 years, after which clearance declined [15]. We did not fix our age function in any way, preferring to simply fit a continuous age-related polynomial to avoid a uniform maturation breakpoint applied to all patients. Investigating age-related changes resulting from maturation of physiological processes is one of the biggest challenges in pediatric PK modeling, and weight and maturation are of course highly correlated [45]. By first scaling weight allometrically, we were able to discern the additional age relationship to busulfan elimination and volume of distribution, but despite the quality of the model fit, it is an empiric fit, and mechanistic interpretation of the polynomial relationship between age and PK parameters is limited. Without further data in adults, this model should only be used for the pediatric population up to age 18 years.

We have verified the ability of the model to closely predict busulfan concentrations in nearly 120 additional children who were not included in the model-building dataset. Most importantly, we then incorporated that model as a software cartridge in the BestDose computer program for optimizing target-oriented doses of busulfan using our MM Bayesian adaptive control algorithm. In a blinded comparison, we have shown that with only two optimally timed samples using our MMopt algorithm, this model can very closely match busulfan dose recommendations based on noncompartmental analysis that requires 6—9 concentrations. We are the only group to propose a two-sample strategy for IV busulfan in pediatrics. Dupuis et al. recommended a three-sample strategy to calculate AUC with an acceptable level of precision and a lack of bias [46]. However, their strategy was based on multiple linear regression after the first dose only, and its applicability after that is unknown. Our wMMopt times (15 min and 4 h after the end of any infusion, ie, a peak and trough) are easy to remember, fit well into common drug monitoring paradigms, and could reduce problems related to the timing of the blood samples. Even one sample, should the other be lost or contaminated, is sufficient to make a reasonable estimate of AUC. Furthermore, Bayesian approaches are generally more accurate than nomograms [47,48], and they are robust enough to provide interpretable results when sample times deviate from a schedule, which is not true for nomograms. The implementation of the tools and limited sampling strategies presented in this work in clinical practice can greatly reduce the burden and cost of the traditional approach of busulfan monitoring in many centers treating stem-cell transplant children, while preserving accurate estimation of drug exposure and dose requirements.

We have also provided initial busulfan dose recommendations based on weight $\leq$12 kg or >12 kg. With 1.1 mg/kg IV every 6 h for 16 doses, 67% of the lighter patients are expected to be within a C_{ave} of 600−900 ng/mL. For the heavier patients, 76% will be in this range with 1.0 mg/kg IV every 6 h for 16 doses. Our dose recommendations are very similar but somewhat simpler than those of Long-Boyle et al. [15], and we also found that older, heavier individuals need a slightly higher dose on average than in the package insert. Zao et al. found that of 111 pediatric patients, 66% of the patients achieved a C_{ave} within the prespecified target range after the first dose [49]. They also noted that existing algorithms may be less applicable in very overweight or very young populations, both of which were represented in our cohorts (Table 18.2).

However, we must emphasize that targeted exposures may need to be more tailored than this broad range, and it is impossible to know beforehand whether a patient lies within the 24−33% who will be outside the therapeutic range. For this drug, TDM clearly remains mandatory.

We must also emphasize that it is better to use a tool like BestDose than a fixed dose regimen, even to plan the initial regimen before any concentrations are measured. Under these circumstances, even though the dose for everyone is based on the same weighted mean model parameter values, stratification by patient covariates is still possible. For example, if the weighted mean volume of distribution is 1.0 L/kg, each patient will still have their own volume of distribution based on their weight, before any measured concentrations are available to calculate the Bayesian posterior (ie, update the model for the individual patient) and truly personalize the predictions and dose calculations.

18.3 CONCLUSION

TRM in children can be significantly decreased by using population pharmacokinetic models and Bayesian individualization of dose regimens for drugs such as busulfan. It may well be the same for any other drug that has a narrow therapeutic range, where toxicity or inefficacy are responsible for potentially lethal events.

REFERENCES

[1] Frisk P, Lönnerholm G. Disease of the liver following bone marrow transplantation in children: incidence, clinical course and outcome in a long-term perspective. Acta Paediatr 1998;87(5):579−83.

[2] Vassal G, Michel G, Espérou H, Gentet JC, Valteau-Couanet D, Doz F, et al. Prospective validation of a novel IV busulfan fixed dosing for paediatric patients to improve therapeutic AUC targeting without drug monitoring. Cancer Chemother Pharmacol 2008;61(1):113−23.

[3] Schechter T, Finkelstein Y, Doyle J, Verjee Z, Moretti M, Koren G, et al. Pharmacokinetic disposition and clinical outcomes in infants and children receiving intravenous busulfan for allogeneic hematopoietic stem cell transplantation. Biol Blood Marrow Transplant 2007;13(3):307−14.

[4] Nguyen L, Fuller D, Lennon S, Leger F. IV busulfan in pediatrics: a novel dosing to improve safety/efficacy for hematopoietic progenitor cell transplantation recipients. Bone Marrow Transplant 2004;33(10):979−87.

[5] Cremers S, Schoemaker R, Bredius R, den HJ, Ball L, Twiss I, et al. Pharmacokinetics of intravenous busulfan in children prior to stem cell transplantation. Br J Clin Pharmacol 2002;53(4):386−9 PMCID: PMC1874261.

[6] Dix SP, Wingard JR, Mullins RE, Jerkunica I, Davidson TG, Gilmore CE, et al. Association of busulfan area under the curve with veno-occlusive disease following BMT. Bone Marrow Transplant 1996;17 (2):225−30.

[7] Grochow LB, Jones RJ, Brundrett RB, Braine HG, Chen TL, Saral R, et al. Pharmacokinetics of busulfan: correlation with veno-occlusive disease in patients undergoing bone marrow transplantation. Cancer Chemother Pharmacol 1989;25(1):55−61.

[8] McCune JS, Gooley T, Gibbs JP, Sanders JE, Petersdorf EW, Appelbaum FR, et al. Busulfan concentration and graft rejection in pediatric patients undergoing hematopoietic stem cell transplantation. Bone Marrow Transplant 2002;30(3):167−73.

[9] Bolinger AM, Zangwill AB, Slattery JT, Risler LJ, Sultan DH, Glidden DV, et al. Target dose adjustment of busulfan in pediatric patients undergoing bone marrow transplantation. Bone Marrow Transplant 2001;28(11):1013−18.

[10] Slattery JT, Sanders JE, Buckner CD, Schaffer RL, Lambert KW, Langer FP, et al. Graft-rejection and toxicity following bone marrow transplantation in relation to busulfan pharmacokinetics. Bone Marrow Transplant 1995;16(1):31−42.

[11] McCune JS, Bemer MJ, Barrett JS, Scott Baker K, Gamis AS, Holford NHG. Busulfan in infant to adult hematopoietic cell transplant recipients: a population pharmacokinetic model for initial and Bayesian dose personalization. Clin Cancer Res 2014;20(3):754−63 PMCID: PMC3946385.

[12] McCune JS, Baker KS, Blough DK, Gamis A, Bemer MJ, Kelton-Rehkopf MC, et al. Variation in prescribing patterns and therapeutic drug monitoring of intravenous busulfan in pediatric hematopoietic cell transplant recipients. J Clin Pharmacol 2013;53(3):264−75.

[13] Maheshwari S, Kassim A, Yeh RF, Domm J, Calder C, Evans M, et al. Targeted busulfan therapy with a steady-state concentration of 600−700 ng/mL in patients with sickle cell disease receiving HLA-identical sibling bone marrow transplant. Bone Marrow Transplant 2013;49(3):366−9.

[14] Phillipe M, Bleyzac N, Goutelle S. Pharmacokinetic and analytical issues in busulfan area under the curve estimation and simulation. Biol Blood Marrow Transplant 2016;22(1):185.

[15] Long-Boyle JR, Savic R, Yan S, Bartelink I, Musick L, French D, et al. Population pharmacokinetics of busulfan in pediatric and young adult patients undergoing hematopoietic cell transplant: a model-based dosing algorithm for personalized therapy and implementation into routine clinical use. Ther Drug Monit 2015;37(2):236−45 PMCID: PMC4342323.

[16] Diestelhorst C, Boos J, McCune JS, Hempel G. Population pharmacokinetics of intravenous busulfan in children: revised body weight-dependent NONMEM® model to optimize dosing. Eur J Clin Pharmacol 2014;70(7):839−47.

[17] Savic RM, Cowan MJ, Dvorak CC, Pai S-Y, Pereira L, Bartelink IH, et al. Effect of weight and maturation on busulfan clearance in infants and small children undergoing hematopoietic cell transplantation. Biol Blood Marrow Transplant 2013;19(11):1608−14 PMCID: PMC3848313.

[18] Veal GJ, Nguyen L, Paci A, Riggi M, Amiel M, Valteau-Couanet D, et al. Busulfan pharmacokinetics following intravenous and oral dosing regimens in children receiving high-dose myeloablative chemotherapy for high-risk neuroblastoma as part of the HR-NBL-1/SIOPEN trial. Eur J Cancer 2012;48(16):3063−72.

[19] Bartelink IH, van Kesteren C, Boelens JJ, Egberts TCG, Bierings MB, Cuvelier GDE, et al. Predictive performance of a busulfan pharmacokinetic model in children and young adults. Ther Drug Monit 2012;34(5):574−83.

[20] Bartelink IH, Boelens JJ, Bredius RGM, Egberts ACG, Wang C, Bierings MB, et al. Body weight-dependent pharmacokinetics of busulfan in paediatric haematopoietic stem cell transplantation patients. Clin Pharmacokinet 2012;51(5):331−45.

[21] Paci A, Vassal G, Moshous D, Dalle J-H, Bleyzac N, Neven B, et al. Pharmacokinetic behavior and appraisal of intravenous busulfan dosing in infants and older children: the results of a population pharmacokinetic study from a large pediatric cohort undergoing hematopoietic stem-cell transplantation. Ther Drug Monit 2012;34(2):198−208.

[22] Bleyzac N. The use of pharmacokinetic models in paediatric onco-haematology: effects on clinical outcome through the examples of busulfan and cyclosporine. Fundam Clin Pharmacol 2008;22(6):605−8.

[23] Neely M, Jelliffe R. Practical therapeutic drug management in HIV-infected patients: use of population pharmacokinetic models supplemented by individualized Bayesian dose optimization. J Clin Pharmacol 2008;48(9):1081−91 PMCID: PMC2724306.

[24] Neely M, Jelliffe R. Practical, individualized dosing: 21st century therapeutics and the clinical pharmacometrician. J Clin Pharmacol 2010;50(7):842−7.

[25] Jelliffe R, Schumitzky A, Bayard D, Van Guilder M, Leary RH. The USC*PACK programs for parametric and nonparametric population PK/PD modeling, for multiple model adaptive control of drug dosage regimens, and for IMM Bayesian posterior individual models with changing parameter distributions during the period of data. Paris, France: Population Analysis Group in Europe; 2002.

[26] Bleyzac N, Souillet G, Magron P, Janoly A, Martin P, Bertrand Y, et al. Improved clinical outcome of paediatric bone marrow recipients using a test dose and Bayesian pharmacokinetic individualization of busulfan dosage regimens. Bone Marrow Transplant 2001;28(8):743−51.

[27] Neely M, Margol A, Fu X, Van Guilder M, Bayard D, Schumitzky A, et al. Achieving target voriconazole concentrations more accurately in children and adolescents. Antimicrob Agents Chemother 2015;59(6):3090−7 PMCID: PMC4432122.

[28] Jelliffe R, Bayard D, Milman M, Van Guilder M, Schumitzky A. Achieving target goals most precisely using nonparametric compartmental models and "multiple model" design of dosage regimens. Ther Drug Monit 2000;22(3):346−53.

[29] Jelliffe RW, Schumitzky A, Bayard D, Milman M, Van Guilder M, Wang X, et al. Model-based, goal-oriented, individualised drug therapy. Linkage of population modelling, new "multiple model" dosage design, Bayesian feedback and individualised target goals. Clin Pharmacokinet 1998;34(1):57−77.

[30] Peris JE, Latorre JA, Castel V, Verdeguer A, Esteve S, Torres-Molina F. Determination of busulfan in human plasma using high-performance liquid chromatography with pre-column derivatization and fluorescence detection. J Chromatogr B Biomed Sci Appl 1999;730(1):33−40.

[31] Bleyzac N, Barou P, Aulagner G. Rapid and sensitive high-performance liquid chromatographic method for busulfan assay in plasma. J Chromatogr B Biomed Sci Appl 2000;742(2):427−32.

[32] Reis dos EO, Vianna-Jorge R, Suarez-Kurtz G, Lima ELDS, Azevedo D de A. Development of a rapid and specific assay for detection of busulfan in human plasma by high-performance liquid chromatography/electrospray ionization tandem mass spectrometry. Rapid Commun Mass Spectrom 2005;19(12):1666−74.

[33] Yamada WM, Bartroff J, Bayard DS, Burke J, Van Guilder M, Jelliffe RW, et al. The nonparametric adaptive grid algorithm for population pharmacokinetic modeling [internet]. Report No.: TR-2014-1. Retrieved from: <http://www.lapk.org/techReports.php>; 2014.

[34] Tatarinova T, Neely M, Bartroff J, Van Guilder M, Yamada W, Bayard D, et al. Two general methods for population pharmacokinetic modeling: non-parametric adaptive grid and non-parametric Bayesian. J Pharmacokinet Pharmacodynam 2013;40(2):189−99 PMCID: PMC3630269.

[35] Neely MN, van Guilder MG, Yamada WM, Schumitzky A, Jelliffe RW. Accurate detection of outliers and subpopulations with Pmetrics, a nonparametric and parametric pharmacometric modeling and simulation package for R. Ther Drug Monit 2012;34(4):467—76 PMCID: PMC3394880.

[36] Anderson BJ, Holford NHG. Mechanistic basis of using body size and maturation to predict clearance in humans. Drug Metab Pharmacokinet 2009;24(1):25—36.

[37] Anderson BJ, Holford NHG. Mechanism-based concepts of size and maturity in pharmacokinetics. Annu Rev Pharmacol Toxicol 2008;48(1):303—32.

[38] Mahmood I. Dosing in children: a critical review of the pharmacokinetic allometric scaling and modelling approaches in paediatric drug development and clinical settings. Clin Pharmacokinet 2014;53 (4):327—46.

[39] Traub SL, Johnson CE. Comparison of methods of estimating creatinine clearance in children. Am J Hosp Pharm 1980;37(2):195—201.

[40] Brink ten MH, Zwaveling J, Swen JJ, Bredius RGM, Lankester AC, Guchelaar HJ. Personalized busulfan and treosulfan conditioning for pediatric stem cell transplantation: the role of pharmacogenetics and pharmacokinetics. Drug Discov Today 2014;19(10):1572—86.

[41] Bayard DS, Jelliffe RW, Neely MN. Bayes risk as an alternative to Fisher Information in determining experimental designs for nonparametric models. In: PODE 2012. Windlesham, Surrey, UK; 2013.

[42] Bayard DS, Milman MH, Schumitzky A. Design of dosage regimens: a multiple model stochastic control approach. Int J Bio-Med Comput 1994;36(1—2):103—15.

[43] Wall DA, Chan KW, Nieder ML, Hayashi RJ, Yeager AM, Kadota R, et al. Safety, efficacy, and pharmacokinetics of intravenous busulfan in children undergoing allogeneic hematopoietic stem cell transplantation. Pediatr Blood Cancer 2010;54(2):291—8.

[44] Gaziev J, Nguyen L, Puozzo C, Mozzi AF, Casella M, Perrone Donnorso M, et al. Novel pharmacokinetic behavior of intravenous busulfan in children with thalassemia undergoing hematopoietic stem cell transplantation: a prospective evaluation of pharmacokinetic and pharmacodynamic profile with therapeutic drug monitoring. Blood 2010;115(22):4597—604.

[45] Meibohm B, Laer S, Panetta JC, Barrett JS. Population pharmacokinetic studies in pediatrics: issues in design and analysis. AAPS J 2005;7(2):E475—87 PMCID: PMC2750985.

[46] Dupuis LL, Sibbald C, Schechter T, Ansari M, Gassas A, Théorêt Y, et al. IV busulfan dose individualization in children undergoing hematopoietic stem cell transplant: limited sampling strategies. Biol Blood Marrow Transplant 2008;14(5):576—82.

[47] Sime FB, Roberts MS, Roberts JA. Optimization of dosing regimens and dosing in special populations. Clin Microbiol Infect 2015;21(10):886—93.

[48] Hennig S, Holthouse F, Staatz CE. Comparing dosage adjustment methods for once-daily tobramycin in paediatric and adolescent patients with cystic fibrosis. Clin Pharmacokinet 2015;54(4):409—21.

[49] Zao JH, Schechter T, Liu WJ, Gerges S, Gassas A, Egeler RM, et al. Performance of busulfan dosing guidelines for pediatric hematopoietic stem cell transplant conditioning. Biol Blood Marrow Transplant 2015;21(8):1471—8.

INDIVIDUALIZING ANTIEPILEPTIC THERAPY FOR PATIENTS

19

I. Bondareva

CHAPTER OUTLINE

19.1 INTRODUCTION

The goal of antiepileptic drug (AED) therapy is seizure freedom without side effects. There are a number of reasons why this goal still is not achieved for all epileptic patients: incorrect AED selection as a result of incorrect diagnosis of seizure type, wide interindividual variability in dose response, AED tolerability, compliance with prescribed regimens, and others. The treatment of epilepsy should be individualized for each patient with respect to correct drug choice and appropriate drug dosage (adequate dose and frequency of AED dosing) [1]. Many of these problems can be solved with the help of therapeutic drug monitoring (TDM) and dosage individualization to achieve desired target serum concentrations [2−8].

Individualized Drug Therapy for Patients. DOI: http://dx.doi.org/10.1016/B978-0-12-803348-7.00019-8

Much is now known about the efficacy, safety, pharmacokinetics, adverse reactions, and drug—drug interactions of different AEDs. Several investigators report different peak times and corresponding peak concentrations and different values of pharmacokinetic (PK) parameters. Many authors have demonstrated wide variability in patient response and great differences in serum concentrations observed in patients receiving the same dosage, especially with polytherapy [9—14]. Although the therapeutic ranges of serum concentrations of the main anticonvulsants are well known, the dosages required to achieve a target therapeutic goal have been quite variable. Side effects also have been associated with a wide range of serum levels. Because of considerable inter-individual variation in the relationship between control of seizures and the serum concentration, *therapeutic ranges of serum drug concentrations should be used only as an initial guide* to further individualize the dose in order to further improve its effect or reduce toxicity for each individual patient. Therapeutic ranges cannot guarantee freedom of seizures to all patients. Seizures may be controlled at relatively lower levels for some patients, while toxic effects may appear at concentrations within the proposed therapeutic ranges for adults and children. Many investigators support the conclusion that for better seizure control individualizing of anticonvulsant dosage regimens is necessary. There is a general movement away from rigid therapeutic ranges to so-called individual therapeutic concentration among physicians concerned with epilepsy management [7].

Clinical experience has shown that careful and individualized dose adjustments aided by TDM can improve the treatment of epilepsy and help most patients to be controlled satisfactorily with monotherapy [9,10,12,14]. This is very important for long-term anticonvulsant therapy, which usually continues for years, and often for a lifetime. With modern analytical procedures such as gas chromatography and high-performance liquid chromatography, it is possible to measure drugs with high sensitivity and specificity. These techniques enable practitioners to monitor drug levels in body fluids routinely. TDM is especially useful for drugs for which a relationship between plasma level and clinical therapeutic effect has been established, as for AEDs [7,9,10]. The lack of direct measured markers for clinical efficacy or for the most common manifestations of AED toxicity, such as adverse central nervous system effects can also be an argument for TDM of AEDs [5,7].

While there is a consensus that TDM is an aid to individualize AED dosage, there are only two published randomized studies to date comparing treatment outcome with or without the use of TDM [15,16]. They have not provided evidence that TDM improves the outcome of drug treatment for epilepsy in terms of improved seizure control and reduced adverse drug effects in patients with newly diagnosed epilepsy [17]. The possible reason for this is the study design. For example, in the more recent Jannuzzi et al. (2000) study, 180 patients with partial or idiopathic generalized nonabsence epilepsy (a history of at least two seizures in the previous month), aged 6 to 65 years, requiring initiation of treatment with carbamazepine (CBZ), valproate (VPA), phenytoin (PHN), phenobarbital (PHB), or primidone (PRM) were randomly allocated to two groups according to an open, prospective, unblinded parallel-group design. All participants were prescribed the AED selected as the most appropriate by their physician. In one group, dosage was adjusted to achieve serum AED concentrations within a target range (10—20 µg/mL for PHN, 15—40 µg/mL for PHB, 4—11 µg/mL for CBZ, and 40—100 µg/mL for VPA) during a period of 3 months or less, whereas in the other group, dosage was adjusted on clinical grounds to achieve optimal seizure control over the shortest reasonable period. Blood samples for determination of AED levels were collected in both groups, but the TDM data were available for clinical decision making only in one of the groups. Patients were followed up for 24 months or until a change in therapeutic strategy was clinically indicated. The study failed to demonstrate a difference between the groups with and without TDM in the primary efficacy endpoint (the proportion of patients achieving complete seizure remission during the previous 12 months of follow-up) and in the secondary efficacy endpoints. However, in this study, the average therapeutic ranges and not the individual patient's optimal drug concentrations were used as a common target goal for all patients in the TDM group.

AEDs have widely varying pharmacokinetic and pharmacodynamic patient responses and so need careful management. TDM based only on measurement of serum drug concentrations without software for adaptive control of dosage has often been ineffective, even for drugs with well-known therapeutic ranges. Therapeutic ranges cannot guarantee freedom from seizures in all patients. It is only a statistical concept that is not rigidly applicable to all patients. However, selection of a specific therapeutic goal based on each individual patient's clinical need for the drug, the acceptable risk of toxicity to achieve it, and the possibility now of being able to calculate optimal dosage regimens to achieve this individualized goal are very important for effective therapy.

This problem can be addressed, first, using *population pharmacokinetic modeling* [18−21]. This is useful to develop the initial dosage regimen. Following this, TDM is used, and the regimen is appropriately adjusted to best achieve the desired target goal for that particular patient.

Many investigators agree that appropriate rational utilization of TDM with Bayesian feedback dosage adjustment facilitates epilepsy treatment with AEDs by increasing the seizure control and safety, as well as by reducing treatment costs.

Even though TDM data reflect the great variety in individual patient responses in clinically realistic conditions, such data are seldom used for processing because of their poor quality. Usually their quality is poor because each patient has only one or very few measured trough serum levels, usually at steady state. There has been an opinion that at steady state sampling prior to the next dose provides trough levels that are easily comparable [5].

Several *methods and programs* based on population modeling, which can handle sparse data, have been proposed in recent years. They permit use of TDM data for evaluation of drug pharmacokinetic parameters, drug interactions, kinetic linearity, and other pharmacokinetic aspects [22]. However, population modeling based mostly on data of steady-state trough samples can result only in estimation of clearance (CL) and its variability. In the steady state, the rate of drug administration equals the rate of drug elimination. Such models are based on the well-known relationships between dose (D), average concentration at steady state (Css), and apparent clearance (CL/F, where F equals bioavailability). If drug PK behavior can be described by linear kinetics, the ratio between maintenance dose and the Css is equal to the apparent clearance.

Without TDM (no feedback), the dose (D) to reach the target steady-state concentration (Css) can be calculated on the basis of the mean population CL/F value. If for an individual patient Css is measured at a given dose, his individual clearance value can be calculated from this relationship. Then this relationship with the estimated CL/F value might be used to calculate the maintenance dose needed to achieve a new desired Css. Using trough levels as average Css means that an individual target goal should be expressed in terms of trough levels at steady state without taking into consideration possible fluctuations of AED serum levels within the dosing interval.

This approach is widely used to determine population values of AED clearance and factors that contribute to its variability in different population of epileptic patients, as well to optimize AED dosage regimens based on trough TDM data. Even for the traditional linear one-compartment model, the use of mostly steady-state trough levels precludes identification of the individual volume of distribution and the elimination rate constant values separately. Such a sampling strategy does not allow estimation of the absorption rate constant (K_{abs}). Using a fixed population (K_{abs}) value from the literature instead of the identified individual parameter values makes simulation of the individual PK profile and visualization of the individual fluctuations of AED concentrations during dosing interval impossible. This information can help to prevent concentration-dependent adverse events or seizures known to appear at regular time intervals within a dosing interval.

In numerous earlier published studies, the nonlinear mixed effects population modeling program (NONMEM) has been used to evaluate covariates that influence clearance of AEDs [23−31]. Usually patients' age, body weight, and co-administration of enzyme inducers were considered as important factors of interindividual PK variability. Among other factors, patients' race, gender, smoking status, and drug formulation have been found to affect clearance of some AEDs. The majority of these multiple regression models for AED clearance estimated from sparse TDM data (trough steady-state sampling strategy mostly only on one occasion) reported linear or nonlinear clearance/AED dosage relationships. Different explanations for such a relationship were discussed, such as changes in bioavailability or changes in clearance and volume of distribution related to changes in protein binding. It is interesting that in some studies, for example in two studies of Blanco-Serrano et al. [23,24], both K_a and VS1 were held fixed so that all variation had to be attributed to variation in clearance. Because of this, their conclusions may not have been realistic.

Taking into consideration the wide interindividual variability in the pharmacokinetic behavior of drugs in the population, this possible clearance/dose relationship can be assessed in a PK study where at least a majority of patients had several serum concentration measurements made during periods of changing dosage on different occasions. Often in population studies, patients who receive higher doses are those who have been insensitive to lower doses. One reason for the observed linear or nonlinear clearance to dose relationship in population studies with sparse TDM data might be that in clinical practice the higher doses are often prescribed to individuals with higher drug clearance [24]. Typical population studies based on sparse TDM data have no information for estimation of intraindividual changes in CL values due to changes in dosage.

Identification of the factors that contribute to CL variability of AEDs and use of regression models can help in individualization of the therapy and in choosing the initial dosing regimen of a drug or modifying dosing regimens without the patient's TDM data. However, the magnitude of the residual and interindividual variability usually remaining in these final regression models for drug clearance shows the need for and justifies TDM and Bayesian adaptive control for optimization and adjustment of individualized dosage regimens for the patients. Bayesian approaches for concentration prediction based on optimal sampling strategies to get TDM measurements are also preferable.

The long-established so-called older AEDs (carbamazepine, valproate, phenytoin, and phenobarbital), still quite frequently used in epilepsy, will continue to be a factor in epilepsy treatment for the foreseeable future and will continue to demand the attention of clinicians. These AEDs have PK characteristics that increase the risk of toxicity: a relatively narrow therapeutic index, wide interindividual PK variability, frequent clinically significant drug−drug interactions, nonlinear metabolism of phenytoin, nonlinear concentration-dependent protein binding of valproate, and auto-induction of carbamazepine, for example. For these drugs, clinical effect correlates better with serum levels than with administered doses [5]. The intensity of pharmacodynamic effect of AEDs is linearly related to the serum levels at lower concentrations.

The aim of this chapter is to present the main results of our laboratory (see below) in population modeling of the older AEDs based on TDM data and to demonstrate methods of interpretation and usefulness of TDM of AEDs with Bayesian feedback dosage adjustment in real clinical settings.

19.1.1 PATIENT DATA AND METHODS

Patient data of anticonvulsant (CBZ, VPA, PHN, and PHB) monitoring were routinely collected in the Laboratory of Pharmacokinetics of Moscow Medical University (hereafter "the laboratory") since 1996. Usually adult and pediatric epileptic outpatients from different epilepsy clinics attended these consultations to evaluate potential reasons for lack or loss of efficacy and/or for toxicity of their antiepileptic therapy, as well as to establish or to check their baseline effective concentrations during a period of remission. Results of measurements and the suggested regimen were discussed with the patient's physician. Compliance was assessed by interview with the patients' families and the attending physicians. However, compliance cannot be absolutely guaranteed.

Patient records include visit data, age, gender, body weight, height, AEDs, dosing schedules, duration of therapy, sampling time in relation to the previous dose, serum levels, diagnosis, clinical data, and information on concomitant therapy.

The peak−trough sampling strategy is routine in this laboratory. After a valproate dose administration, time required to reach peak concentration is 1−2 h for conventional tablets and solutions, 3−6 h for enteric-coated (EC) forms, and 10−12 h for sustained-release (SR) dosage forms [32]. Following chronic oral administration of conventional CBZ tablets, plasma levels peak at approximately 4−5 h after administration and at 3−12 h after administration of CBZ-retard tablets. Because of prolonged T_{max} values of controlled-release CBZ and VPA dosage form, peak−trough sampling strategy is actually not convenient for outpatients. Such a peak−trough sampling strategy, furthermore, is actually not convenient for outpatients, as the visit becomes too prolonged. Simulation results show that serum levels measured 2.5−4 h after drug intake are close to 80−90% of the peak concentration, and such a quasi-peak−trough sampling strategy is a reasonable compromise between optimality and practicality.

Because of the great interindividual variability in CBZ PK parameter values, without knowledge of the individual parameter values, it is not possible to know when any particular patient's peak concentration is actually reached. However, when TDM is combined with a modelling approach, it is not important to measure a serum level at exactly the peak time (T_{max}) or at any other special times. To fit a PK model to data, it is only necessary to know accurately when each serum level was actually obtained in relation to the dose given.

Drug levels have been measured by high-performance liquid chromatography. The assay error polynomial equation (see Chapter 4: Optimizing Laboratory Assay Methods for Individualized Therapy) (usually of first or second order) was used in the pharmacokinetic analysis as a relationship between measured concentration and standard deviation of the method, to weight each concentration data point correctly by its Fisher information, the reciprocal of its variance. The standard deviation of the method was assessed by multiple measurements of various known concentrations covering the working range of the assay. These issues are discussed more fully in Chapter 4.

The population models for individualizing antiepileptic therapy were developed based on a relatively rich anticonvulsant TDM data (peak−trough sampling strategy for all patients, one to three additional samples in other dosing intervals for some patients, on multiple occasions in some patients) using the USC*PACK collection of PC programs for population pharmacokinetic modeling. All patients who were included in development of the population models had normal renal and hepatic function and no diseases that could influence drug plasma binding.

The rhythm of consultation was irregular, and repeated consultations of some patients after their dosage regimen corrections and adjustments helped to test and validate the procedure and the proposed population models in real clinical settings.

19.2 POPULATION MODELING: RESULTS

19.2.1 CARBAMAZEPINE

Carbamazepine (CBZ) was discovered in 1952 in connection with development of the antidepressant imipramine, to which it is structurally related. In Europe, CBZ has been used effectively for various types of epilepsy since 1962. In the United States, it was originally used successfully only for the treatment of trigeminal neuralgia because of a few cases of adverse effects reported in the early 1960s. It was later approved as an anticonvulsant [33,34]. Clinical trials and experience with it over the past 30 years have shown that CBZ is an effective anticonvulsive drug for partial and generalized seizures in both adults and children [10,11,13].

Much is now known about CBZ efficacy, safety, pharmacokinetics, adverse reactions, and drug interactions. Several investigators report different peak times and corresponding peak concentrations and different values of pharmacokinetic parameters [35−39]. Measurements of absolute bioavailability in humans are not available because CBZ has only been given orally and not intravenously.

Carbamazepine is poorly water soluble. Oral doses in tablet form are slowly and variably absorbed [38,40]. Estimates of bioavailability range from 75% to 85% [33]. Peak plasma concentrations of CBZ in tablet form generally are reached 3−8 h after drug intake [13]. In epileptic patients, the protein bound fraction was estimated as 75−85% of the total plasma concentration [39−41]. The apparent volume of distribution of CBZ varies from 0.8 to 2 L/kg in adults and older children [11,13,40,42]. Elimination is mostly by hepatic biotransformation, with only 1−3% of the dose excreted unchanged in the urine. The main pathway of CBZ biotransformation is epoxidation with an active metabolite CBZ-epoxide [33,39].

Carbamazepine markedly induces its own metabolism. The metabolic clearance of CBZ increases on continued administration until the microsomal enzymes are fully induced. It leads to a progressive decrease in CBZ serum levels. Autoinduction is usually complete within 20−30 days. CBZ behavior during this period is described by time-dependent kinetics [37,43−45]. The half-life of carbamazepine at steady state is reported to range from 5 to 27 h [13,42]. Children metabolize it more rapidly than adults ($T_{1/2} = 4−12$ h) [11].

19.2.1.1 Modeling of CBZ pharmacokinetics after completion of an autoinduction period

19.2.1.1.1 Methods

TDM data of 237 epileptic patients on chronic CBZ monotherapy were included to develop CBZ PK models for adults ($n = 99$), children ($n = 90$) and the elderly ($n = 48$) separately. The PK

Table 19.1 Demographic Characteristics of Patient Populations of various ages (Monotherapy With CBZ and CBZ Controlled-Release Dosage Form)

Patient Populations	Children CBZ	Adults CBZ	Elderly CBZ	Adults CBZ-Retard	Children CBZ-Retard
No. of patients	90	99	48	92	82
Female/male	42/48	53/46	23/25	40/52	39/43
Age, years	9.6 ± 6.8	27.4 ± 11.9	63.2 ± 6.3	24.2 ± 9.93	10.1 ± 2.8
CBZ dosage, mg/kg per day	16.5 ± 9.6	9.2 ± 5.0	5.94 ± 3.3	12.73 ± 5.9	20.2 ± 7.1

Age and CBZ dosage are mean ± standard deviation.

models for the CBZ controlled-release dosage form were based on data of 176 epileptic patients on chronic CBZ-retard monotherapy (adults, $n = 94$; children, $n = 82$). Descriptive statistics for demographic data are presented in Table 19.1.

The minimum time on oral CBZ dosing was 3 months, and the minimum time on an unchanged dosage regimen was at least 12 days, so for all patients, the steady state was probably reached, and autoinduction was probably complete. CBZ concentrations were measured by high-performance liquid chromatography. The population PK analysis was performed using the USC*PACK software (the NPEM program) based on *a linear one-compartment model with oral absorption* and routinely collected CBZ TDM data (peak−trough strategy). The assay error polynomial equation (SD = 0.1 + 0.1 C, where C is CBZ concentration, and SD is the standard deviation of the method) was incorporated into the program and used in the analysis. The NPEM program was used to find the most likely probability density function given the patients' data. The Wilcoxon-Mann-Whitney nonparametric test was used for group comparisons of the estimated PK parameters.

19.2.1.1.2 Results

In all patient populations, very poor correlation was found between serum concentrations and dose due to the large interindividual variability between patients (see typical relationships between dose and concentration in Fig. 19.1). The plot demonstrates the wide scattering of serum concentrations observed in different patients receiving the same daily dose adjusted for patient's body weight. It means that the relationship had essentially no predictive value. The results are in good agreement with those reported earlier in the literature [46].

Median PK parameter values of CBZ for age subgroups estimated by the NPEM program are given in Table 19.2. A statistically significant difference in the K_i values for the age subgroups ($p < 0.01$) and in the K_{abs} estimates for the compared dosage forms ($p < 0.001$) was found.

The results showed substantial interindividual variability in CBZ pharmacokinetics in the different age subgroups (CV values ranged up to 80−111%), as well as an age-related influence in CBZ clearance (Fig. 19.2). These findings should be considered in optimization of CBZ dosage regimens. For example, many elderly patients with epilepsy may need CBZ dosages lower than those estimated from the median population PK parameter values for younger patients. The results may have important practical consequences for the use of CBZ in the elderly as a growing sector of the population of patients with epilepsy.

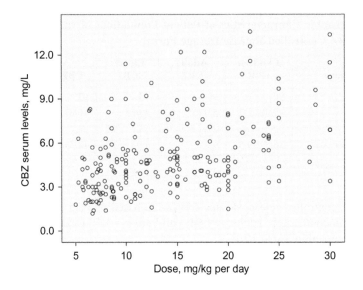

FIGURE 19.1

Relationship between CBZ serum level (mg/L) and daily dose (mg/kg per day) in the adult epileptic patients on chronic CBZ–monotherapy ($N = 218$).

Table 19.2 Median ± SD Pharmacokinetic Parameter Values for CBZ and CBZ Controlled-Release Dosage Form Estimated by the Nonparametric Expectation Maximization Algorithm, NPEM

Parameter/ Population	Children CBZ	Adults CBZ	Elderly Patients CBZ	Adults CBZ-Retard	Children CBZ-Retard
K_{abs}, 1/h	0.68 ± 0.42	0.67 ± 0.59	0.61 ± 0.5	0.2 ± 0.13	0.17 ± 0.19
	CV = 61.8%	CV = 88.1%	CV = 82.0%	CV = 65.0%	CV = 111.8%
K_i, 1/h	0.099 ± 0.08^a	0.07 ± 0.068	0.04 ± 0.016^a	0.062 ± 0.047	0.081 ± 0.037^a
	CV = 80.8%	CV = 97.1%	CV = 40.0%	CV = 75.8%	CV = 45.7%
VS1, L/kg	1.01 ± 0.72	0.94 ± 0.4	0.81 ± 0.5	0.92 ± 0.42	1.07 ± 0.76
	CV = 71.3%	CV = 42.6%	CV = 61.7%	CV = 45.7%	CV = 71.0%

[a]*Statistically significantly different from the corresponding value of the metabolic rate constant K_i in adults.*

19.2.1.2 Results for CBZ-polytherapy

Heteroinduction of CBZ metabolism often occurs during polytherapy with other anticonvulsants or enzyme inducers [13,33]. For example, heteroinduction of CBZ metabolism by PHT or PHB was demonstrated: serum CBZ level-to-dose ratios in patients on CBZ polytherapy were decreased, while CBZ-10,11-epoxide (CBZE) concentrations were increased as compared with those in patients receiving CBZ monotherapy.

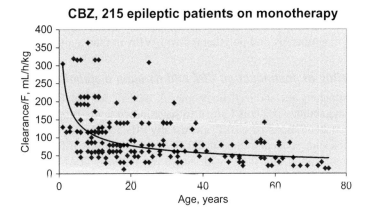

FIGURE 19.2

Relationship between age and postinduction CBZ apparent clearance for patients on chronic CBZ monotherapy.

Table 19.3 Median ± SD Pharmacokinetic Parameter Values for Models of Interactions Between CBZ and the other AEDs Estimated by the NPEM Program (Adult Chronically Treated Patients)

Parameter/Therapy	CBZ-Mono	CBZ + VPA	CBZ + PHN	CBZ + PHB
No. of patients	99	86	94	117
Age, years	27.4 ± 11.9	29.5 ± 11.8	28.4 ± 8.3	23.6 ± 8.7
Mean dose of CBZ, mg/kg per day	9.2 ± 4.96	9.9 ± 6.2	10.4 ± 4.9	10.3 ± 4.4
Mean dose of AEDs, mg/kg per day	–	16.9 ± 9.7	3.9 ± 2.6	2.9 ± 1.92
K_{abs}, 1/h	0.67 ± 0.59	0.75 ± 0.64	0.78 ± 0.56	0.75 ± 0.49
	CV = 88.1%	CV = 85.3%	CV = 71.8%	CV = 65.3%
K_i, 1/h metabolic rate constant	0.07 ± 0.068	0.073 ± 0.063	0.092 ± 0.06	0.089 ± 0.07
	CV = 97.1%	CV = 86.3%	CV = 65.2%	CV = 78.7%
			($p < 0.05$)	($p < 0.05$)
VS1, l/kg	0.94 ± 0.4	0.99 ± 0.61	1.07 ± 0.85	0.93 ± 0.6
	CV = 42.6%	CV = 61.6%	CV = 79.4%	CV = 64.5%

CBZ PK drug–drug interactions were estimated from data of 235 patients on chronic CBZ duotherapy (CBZ + VPA, $n = 86$; CBZ + PHN, $n = 94$; CBZ + PHB, $n = 117$). The estimated PK model parameters for CBZ monotherapy and duotherapy (Table 19.3) were in good agreement with theory of such PK drug–drug interactions [47,48]. Statistically significant ($p < 0.05$) differences in K_i estimates for CBZ monotherapy and its polytherapy with PHB and with PHN were found using the Wilcoxon-Mann-Whitney test. In most cases, more rapid metabolism of CBZ during antiepileptic co-medication with PHN and PHB was reported in various references [13,48]. Inhibition of CBZ-epoxide clearance by VPA was discovered several years ago and provided an explanation for the elevations in plasma concentrations of the main metabolite of carbamazepine [49]. That can be probably a reason for the lack of statistically significant differences ($p = 0.4$) in K_i estimates for CBZ levels between monotherapy and polytherapy with VPA in that study.

19.2.1.3 PK modeling of postinduction CBZ and its main metabolite

CBZ is virtually completely metabolized in people. A total of 33 metabolites of CBZ have been described. Its main metabolite CBZE is known to have antiepileptic properties similar to those of CBZ itself. Plasma concentrations of CBZE are usually 10–50% those of the parent drug during therapy. Clinically relevant concentrations of CBZE accumulate in CBZ-treated patients and may contribute to CBZ intoxication. For drugs with active metabolites, TDM can include measurement of the concentrations of both parent drug and its metabolites. A pharmacokinetic model of CBZ and its main metabolite during the postinduction period was developed, and the model parameters were estimated from TDM data of adult epileptic patients on chronic CBZ monotherapy (CBZ and CBZE levels were measured simultaneously). The nonparametric population PK analysis and simultaneous fitting technique was performed using the Pmetrics NPAG program based on a compartmental model with first-order absorption and linear elimination kinetics for both CBZ and CBZE.

The study included data of 52 adult patients (40.8 ± 14.3 years) for whom at least one pair of two measured serum levels of CBZ and CBZE (peak–trough strategy) was available. Data for this part were collected in the Department of Pharmacokinetics of the Research Center of Neurology, Russian Academy of Medical Science.

The results demonstrated wide interindividual variability in CBZ and CBZE pharmacokinetics and the need for individualizing of CBZ dosage regimens. The estimated CBZ and CBZE population PK parameter values were in good agreement with those obtained earlier for the steady-state CBZ population PK model for epileptic adult patients. Predictive performance showed a good fit of the individual models to both CBZ and CBZE data in all included patients (see examples in Fig. 19.3). Estimation of individual PK parameters of both drug and its active metabolite might help to optimize CBZ therapy in epileptic patients based on TDM data.

19.2.2 VALPROATE

Valproic acid (VPA) has been known as an organic solvent since 1881, but not until the early 1960s were its antiepileptic properties recognized [50]. It is now one of the most important AEDs and is an effective agent for the control of absence, myoclonic, tonic-clonic, and partial seizures [8,50]. VPA has a wide spectrum of activity against both generalized and partial seizures in adults and children [51].

All dosage forms of VPA for oral administration are absorbed rapidly, with peak serum concentrations reached within 1–3 h. EC VPA tablets were developed to decrease gastrointestinal discomfort by delaying absorption [50,52]. The EC formulation increases the latency period by 1–2 h [49,53]), and, as a result, peak concentration times (T_{max}) are delayed and are usually reached after about 3–5 h, although delays longer than 5 h are seen occasionally [49]. Once absorption begins with the EC formulation, the time course of the serum concentrations is similar to that seen with conventional formulations [50,52,54]. Despite differences in formulations, the absolute bioavailability of all valproate formulations is more than 90% [49,55].

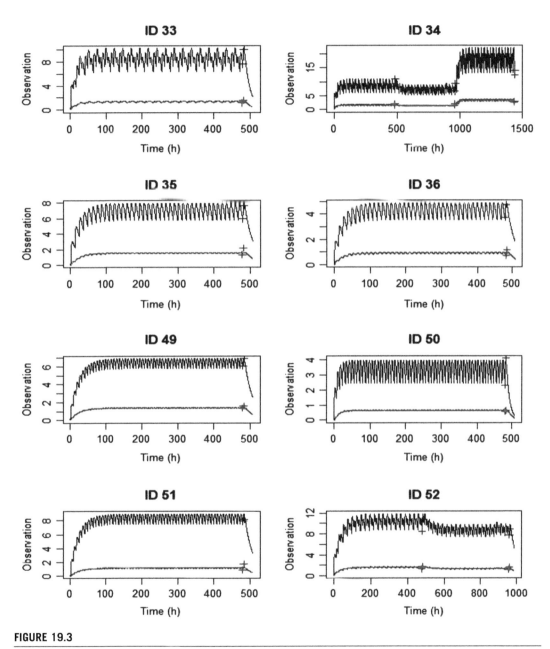

FIGURE 19.3

Visualization of individual time course of CBZ and CBZE serum concentrations simulated based on the individual PK parameter values estimated from the patient's TDM data. Crosses present measured CBZ and CBZE serum levels. Upper curve (higher levels) = CBZ. Lower curves (lower levels) = CBZE.

Valproate is 80−90% bound to plasma protein. This binding is saturable, nonlinear, and concentration-dependent [56]. Because the binding of valproate is so variable, the monitoring of unbound rather than of total serum VPA concentrations has been a subject of debate for many years [50,57].

The apparent volume of distribution of VPA varies widely, from 0.1 to 0.5 L/kg [50]. The drug is almost entirely eliminated by metabolism, with only 1−3% of the dose being excreted unchanged in the urine [58]. The half-life ranges from 4 to 17 h [42]. Children eliminate VPA more rapidly than do adults. Phenytoin, phenobarbital, primidone, and carbamazepine all significantly increase the clearance of VPA [48]. VPA has been associated with inhibition of hepatic enzymes that metabolize other drugs and with protein-binding displacement [48]. Enzyme inhibition typically occurs when two drugs compete for occupancy of the same enzyme site, each reducing the metabolism of the other drug. For example, phenobarbital clearance is markedly reduced in the presence of VPA [59]. The interaction between VPA and phenytoin is more complex. Protein-binding displacement leads to a decrease in the total phenytoin concentration, but the free fraction increases due to the combined effects of displacement and also of enzyme inhibition. Thus free phenytoin concentration may stay the same or may increase with VPA therapy [60]. Inhibition of CBZ-epoxide clearance by VPA was discovered several years ago and provided an explanation for the elevations in plasma concentrations of the main metabolite of CBZ caused by VPA [61].

The clinical pharmacokinetics and pharmacodynamics of VPA have been reviewed [51,53]. Therapeutic serum concentration ranges for VPA have been estimated as between 50 and 100 mg/L or 40 and 150 mg/L. Concentrations as high as 200 mg/L may be found in some patients, often without evidence of any adverse side effects [50].

The typical VPA pharmacokinetic profile has a rapid onset and a sharp peak of serum concentration, followed rapidly by a decline. For these reasons, VPA serum concentrations fluctuate significantly from peak to trough over a typical dosing interval [52,62]. In these conditions, the utility of monitoring only trough serum concentrations, as often proposed in the literature [42,63], appears open to question. To achieve more uniform VPA serum concentrations, frequent dosing or the use of a SR dosage form is useful.

19.2.2.1 Methods

Data of 89 adult and 110 pediatric epileptic patients who received chronic VPA monotherapy were examined. They received various dosage regimens of EC oral VPA tablets.

The wide spectrum of anticonvulsant activity against different seizure types as well as good tolerability makes VPA a useful drug for administration in a SR form. Absorption of the SR form begins soon after administration without any significant lag-time. Its absorption rate is clearly slower, with a later peak time and a lower peak concentration in comparison with the above EC formulation [50,52]. It produces smaller fluctuations in serum concentrations from peak to trough, fewer concentration-related side effects, and offers the possibility of more convenient once- or twice-daily dosage for many patients.

Data of 121 adult and 112 pediatric epileptic patients who received chronic VPA SR monotherapy were also examined. The patients were concurrently taking no other drug known to interfere or interact with VPA pharmacokinetics. Most patients had only two to three measured serum concentrations during one dosing interval. Some patients had four to eight serum levels related to being on different dosage regimens at different times.

Table 19.4 Descriptive Statistics for the Patient Populations

Patient Populations	Adults EC VPA Monotherapy	Children EC VPA Monotherapy	Adults VPA Sustained-Release Monotherapy	Children VPA Sustained-Release Monotherapy	Very Young Patients VPA Syrup Monotherapy
No. of patients	89	110	121	112	36
Female/male	49/40	58/52	56/65	59/53	17/19
Age, years	24.1 ± 8.5	9.53 ± 3.1	22 ± 8.8	9.15 ± 3.12	1.18 ± 0.52
VPA dosage, mg/kg per day	16 35 ± 6.7	32.7 ± 15.9	19.2 ± 8.3	33.26 ± 18.03	49.1 ± 22.0

Note: Age and VPA dosage are mean ± standard deviation.

Data files of 36 very young pediatric patients (aged only 3–26 months) who received chronic oral VPA monotherapy with VPA syrup were also included in the PK analysis.

Serum VPA concentrations were measured by high-performance liquid chromatography. The assay error pattern was found to be fitted by the following polynomial equation:

$$SD = 2.77 - 0.05 \times C + 0.0000821 \times C^2$$

where SD is standard deviation of the assay at a stated measured concentration C, and C^2 is the concentration squared.

A linear one-compartment model with first–order oral absorption was used to describe VPA pharmacokinetics. The sparsity of samples during the absorptive phase prevents estimation of the absorptive time delay of the EC tablet as a PK model parameter (Table 19.4).

19.2.2.2 Results

Median pharmacokinetic parameter values of VPA for the adult and children's populations are given in Table 19.5. The parameter estimates are in good agreement with those reported in the literature. A statistically significant ($p < 0.01$) difference in the elimination rate constant (K_{el}) estimates between adults and children was found using the Wilcoxon-Mann-Whitney test.

Several population studies [23,24,28,29] have studied age- or weight-related changes in VPA pharmacokinetics in adult and pediatric patients as well as in heterogeneous populations. In the present study (patients aged 0.25–53 years), VPA clearance declined with age, reaching adult values in patients over 10 years (see Fig. 19.4). These results are in agreement with those reported by other authors.

In the laboratory, only total AED concentrations were measured, and a traditional one-compartment linear model to describe VPA behavior and to predict individual total serum concentrations of VPA after dosage adjustments was used. This relatively simple PK model cannot take into consideration the absorptive time delay of the EC tablet or any apparent increase in the clearance of total VPA at high doses. However, the predictive performance results showed that, despite these limitations, the model used here can be useful for guiding initial VAL monotherapy when the

Table 19.5 Median ± SD Pharmacokinetic Parameter Values Estimated by the Nonparametric Expectation Maximization Algorithm NPEM

Parameter	Adults EC VPA Monotherapy	Children EC VPA Monotherapy	Adults VPA Sustained-Release Monotherapy	Children VPA Sustained-Release Monotherapy	Very Young Patients VPA Syrup Monotherapy
K_{abs}, 1/h	0.78 ± 0.67	0.66 ± 0.71	0.3 ± 0.36	0.24 ± 0.29	0.91 ± 0.78
	CV = 85.9%	CV = 107.6%	CV = 120.0%	CV = 120.8%	CV = 85.7%
K_{el}, 1/h	0.069 ± 0.04	0.096 ± 0.086	0.061 ± 0.059	0.087 ± 0.058	0.089 ± 0.07
	CV = 58.0%	CV = 89.6%	CV = 96.7%	CV = 66.7%	CV = 78.7%
VS1, L/kg	0.14 ± 0.084	0.13 ± 0.12	0.16 ± 0.12	0.18 ± 0.15	0.2 ± 0.12
	CV = 60%	CV = 92.3%	CV = 75.0%	CV = 83.3%	CV = 60.0%

Note: K_{el}, *elimination rate constant.*

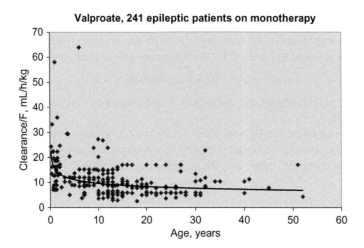

FIGURE 19.4

Relationship between age and VPA apparent clearance for patients on chronic VPA monotherapy.

patients are followed soon by TDM and Bayesian dosage individualization. Monitoring of free fraction might be useful if binding changes are suspected.

19.3 EXTERNAL VALIDATION

Carbamazepine and valproate have a broad spectrum of activity against both partial and generalized seizures and are widely used as monotherapy in the treatment of adult and pediatric patients [13,50]. When a sequence of monotherapies with AEDs is unsuccessful, combination therapy is usually tried in an attempt to improve effectiveness by improving efficacy, tolerability, or both [64]. Combination VPA + CBZ therapy is often used in the management of refractory epilepsy [65,66].

A traditional PK one-compartment linear model was used to describe postinduction CBZ and VPA behavior and to predict individual total serum concentrations after dosage adjustments [35,67,68]. Typical results of internal validation for VPA are presented in Fig. 19.5.

Results of the internal validation are shown in Fig. 19.5. Fig. 19.5A illustrates the wide interindividual variability in patient response from prediction of all patient serum concentrations based on the population median parameter values. For the same patients, their individual serum levels were predicted based on the median values of each patient's Bayesian posterior joint density, as shown in Fig. 19.5B. The regression line in Fig. 19.5B is not significantly different from the line of identity. The results show that the population model by itself gives poor prediction, while the individualized Bayesian posterior models give much improved prediction due to the removal of the interindividual variability.

External validation of a population PK model is a very important step in model development. The objective of external validation is to examine whether the model can describe equally well a new data set, which has not been used for model parameter estimation [69]. An important step is also to evaluate how well a Bayesian procedure of individualizing AED dosage regimens based on a proposed population PK model and the patient's sparse TDM data works and how helpful it is in real clinical settings.

The aim of the study [70] was to evaluate the predictability of individualized dosage regimens for monotherapy with either CBZ or VPA in the postinduction period or with CBZ and VPA given as combination therapy based on TDM data of epileptic patients and the population PK models developed earlier [35,67,68].

This study included adult epileptic patients for whom at least two pairs of measured serum levels related to different AED dosages were available. Some patients had long and rich TDM histories, with repeated measurements over 1- to 6-year periods on CBZ and/or VPA therapy.

Inclusion criteria for this retrospective statistical analysis were data of adult epileptic patients (age ≥ 18 years) who received chronic CBZ, VPA, or their combination, the availability of repeated serum concentration measurements on multiple occasions, and a detailed AED drug dosage history (drug formulation, dosage regimen, dosing intervals, duration of therapy, and verified compliance).

Exclusion criteria were data of patients used earlier to develop the original population models. In addition, as CBZ is an enzyme inducer, those time periods that might be related to CBZ autoinduction were also excluded, as were patients who were switched from one to another dosage form of CBZ or VPA. Patients with renal or hepatic disease or diseases that might influence drug plasma binding were also excluded.

Four groups of PK data were analyzed: 556 predictions for adult epileptic patients on CBZ monotherapy, 662 predictions for VPA monotherapy, 402 predictions of CBZ serum levels, and 430 predictions of VPA serum levels for adult epileptic patients on CBZ + VPA combination therapy. Demographic data for these four groups are presented in Table 19.6. Most patients were relatively young (only about 2–7% of patients were over 55 years) with normal BMI values (about 5–7% of patients were underweight). Obesity, with BMI = 30 or greater, was observed in approximately 10% of patients. Most patients had been given usual AED doses, and most observed AED serum concentrations were within the general therapeutic range. On the first occasion, about 90% of measured VPA serum levels ranged from 40 to 150 mg/L, and about 90% of measured CBZ

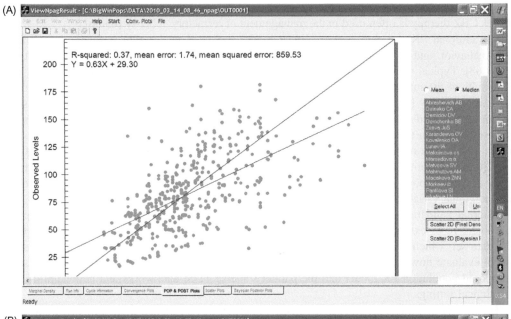

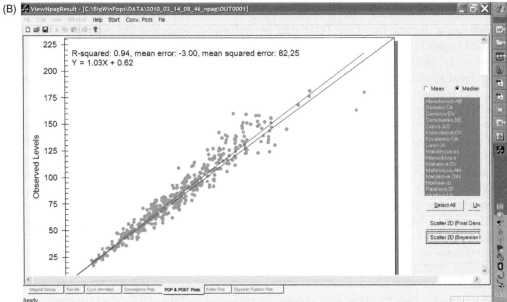

FIGURE 19.5

(A) Scatterplot of the predicted−found relationships based on the median values of the population parameter distributions for all patients in adult population. (B) Scatterplot of the predicted found relationships based on finding each subject's own Bayesian posterior joint density.

Table 19.6 Demographic Data for the Various Patient Groups

Demographic Parameter/ Therapy	CBZ Monotherapy	VPA Monotherapy	CBZ With VPA	VPA With CBZ
N	556	662	402	430
Age, years	25.4 ± 9.6	28.03 ± 11.7	23.9 ± 8.4	22.9 ± 7.1
	$(18-61)$	$(18-62)$	$(18-67)$	$(18-56)$
BMI, kg/m^2	24.6 ± 4.3	24.8 ± 4.3	25.3 ± 4.4	24.7 ± 4.5
	$(18-34)$	$(15-36.2)$	$(17.8-34)$	$(17.9-34.2)$
BW, kg	73.2 ± 16.9	72.7 ± 15.4	77.8 ± 20.4	73.7 ± 20.1
	$(48 \quad 122)$	$(42-125)$	$(50-120)$	$(49-120)$
$C_{observed}$, mg/L	CBZ: 6.9 ± 2.6	VPA. 88.1 ± 33.1	CBZ: 6.3 ± 2.1	VPA: 70.6 ± 23.5
	$(1.9-18.7)$	$(27-300)$	$(2-13.2)$	$(19-138)$
CBZ daily dose, mg/kg	14.2 ± 7.5	$-$	13.8 ± 7.3	12.9 ± 7.1
	$(3.8-40)$		$(3.6-38)$	$(2.3-38)$
VPA daily dose, mg/kg	$-$	18.02 ± 6.4	21.3 ± 8.5	22.1 ± 8.0
		$(5.45-41.7)$	$(4.6-50)$	$(4.62-50)$
Prediction time horizon, months	15.04 ± 16.3	17.15 ± 13.8	14.3 ± 11.5	14.7 ± 11.5
	$(0.24-84)$	$(0.25-68)$	$(0.5-54)$	$(0.4-54)$
	Median $= 9$	Median $= 13.2$	Median $= 11$	Median $= 12$

Note: Data are presented as mean ± standard deviation, minimum and maximum values are shown in the parentheses.
BMI, *Body mass index,* BW, *Body weight.*

serum levels ranged from 3 to 12 mg/L. The minimum time on oral CBZ dosing was 3 months and on an unchanged dosage regimen for at least 7 days, so for all patients, the steady state was probably reached, and CBZ autoinduction was probably complete.

19.3.1 PK ANALYSIS

The population PK analysis was performed using the USC*PACK software, which at the time employed maximum a posteriori probability (MAP) Bayesian analysis to make each patient's individual model. It used the earlier developed linear one-compartment model with oral absorption (body weight was the covariate for volume of distribution) and TDM data (peak−trough strategy).

The first pair of each patient's serum levels on a specific dosage regimen was used to estimate the patient's individual MAP Bayesian posterior PK parameter values and predict future serum levels according to the planned changes in the corresponding AED regimen. Then the observed serum levels on the new regimen (next occasions) were compared with those predicted using the patient-specific Bayesian posterior PK model (see Fig. 19.6, examples).

In general, validation of the procedure of individualizing AED dosage regimens for each included patient who had taken CBZ or/and VPA was based on the following scenario:

- Measurement of AEDs serum levels (peak−trough strategy) on the currently administered AEDs dosage regimen (the first occasion);

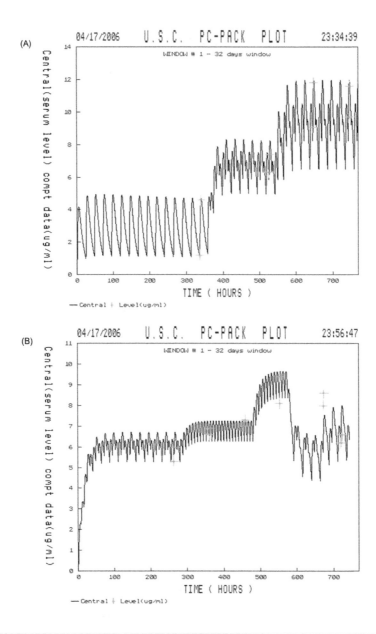

FIGURE 19.6

Visualization of individual time courses of CBZ serum concentrations simulated via the MB program in the USC*PACK collection based on the individual PK parameter values estimated from the patient's first pair of measured serum levels. Crosses—repeated measured CBZ serum levels. Plots B and especially plot C demonstrate fluctuations in the individual PK parameters of CBZ behavior in some treatment periods that cannot be described by the one-compartment linear model with the individual parameter values unchanged over observation period.

Note: The software is limited to a maximum of 99 doses in a dosing history. Because of this, only enough doses were used in the history to bring the patient to a steady state with regard to his serum concentrations. This helps to visualize on one screen the changes in serum concentrations over time for different dosage regimens received by the patient during long-term CBZ therapy.

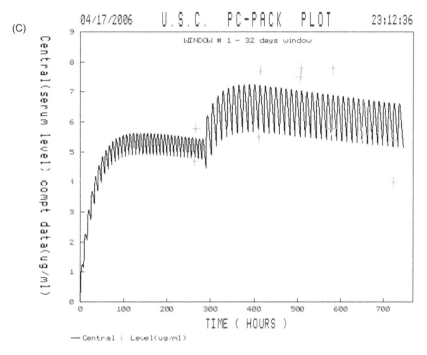

FIGURE 19.6

Continued

- Selection of the specific individualized therapeutic target serum concentration goal for each patient, and, if required, making a decision about adjustment of the dosage regimen by the physician;
- MAP Bayesian estimation of the individual PK parameter values based on the population PK model and the patient's TDM data measured on the first occasion and prediction of future serum levels according to the planned dosage regimen;
- Repeated TDM on repeated occasions, when requested by the patient's physician.

19.3.2 STATISTICAL ANALYSIS

The prediction error (PE) was estimated as the difference between observed and predicted levels, expressed as the percentage of the observed level (PE%). The mean prediction error (MPE, %) was used as a measure of bias, the percentage mean absolute deviation about MPE as well as the mean absolute prediction error (MAPE, %) (APE% = abs PE% values) were used as a measure of precision of predictions. To account for heteroscedasticity in the data, predictive performance was also assessed by calculation of weighted mean prediction error (WMPE). WMPE is the mean of the difference between the observed and predicted concentration divided by the estimate of the standard deviation of the assay, SD, on the observed concentration. This weighted procedure is usually used in the USC*PACK software. Distributions and statistical summary of the prediction errors as well as weighted prediction errors were analyzed to test normality (N(0, σ), via the Kolmogorov–Smirnov test) and bias (via the one-sample Student t-test). For predictions of AED concentrations, an absolute value of the individual PE% less or equal to 25% is generally considered by many clinicians as acceptable and even good from a practical point of view. The frequency distribution of the acceptable errors by category of the distance (months) of prediction into the future (future prediction time horizon) (cross tabulation) was also estimated. Intraindividual proportional errors were expressed as $C_{ij} = \hat{C}_{ij}(1 + e_{ij})$, where C_{ij} is the observed concentration in serum for the i-th individual at time j, $\hat{C}_{ij}$ is the estimated concentration in serum for the i-th individual at time j predicted by the model, and e_{ij} is the residual or intraindividual error with mean zero and variance s^2. Intraindividual variability was calculated as the square root of s^2. Interoccasional variability in predictions was estimated as intraindividual variability based on TDM data of patients who had repeatedly measured AED serum levels on unchanged dosage regimens within a 2-week period assuming unchanged individual pharmacokinetics (analogous to test–retest analysis).

In the context of prediction of unknown future serum concentration from previous measured data, a time horizon, or a prediction horizon, is a point of time in future at which point the next TDM occasion will be performed and a new portion of measured data will be available for comparison with the corresponding modeling results.

Linear regression was used to determine the relationship between the APE% values and the future prediction time horizon as an independent variable. For combination therapy, categorical variables of changed/unchanged CBZ or VPA dosage regimens were also used as independent predictors.

All statistical analyses were carried out at significance level of 0.05.

19.3.3 RESULTS AND DISCUSSION

Epilepsy is a chronic disease. Its treatment in most patients involves long-term therapy with one or more AEDs. During such long-term AED therapy, concentrations appear to vary due to inexplicable day-to-day or moment-to-moment kinetic variability due to errors in concentration measurement, changes in PK parameter values over time, possible drug–drug interactions, inaccurate dosage histories, and model misspecification. The low information content of traditional data on the random variability of PK parameters within a single occasion has precluded the estimation of the magnitude of differences in PK behavior between occasions [71]. Estimates of residual intrasubject and interoccasional variability are important for Bayesian individualization of dosage regimens based on TDM [72]. When intraindividual variability is relatively small (less than the acceptable variability in concentrations for safe and effective use of a drug), information on serum levels measured on only one occasion is often useful from a prediction standpoint.

Interoccasional variability was estimated from TDM data of patients who had repeatedly measured AED serum levels on unchanged dosage regimens within a 2-week period, assuming unchanged individual PK parameter values over this time. However, in most cases, measurements were repeated in a short time period as a retest due to unexpectedly high or low AED serum levels observed on the first occasion. This means that interoccasional variability (14.9% and 15.6% for CBZ and VPA monotherapy, correspondently, 18.7% for CBZ in the presence of VPA, and 19.4% for VPA in the presence of CBZ) might be slightly overestimated.

Table 19.7 Statistical Results of External Validation by Treatment Group

Statistical Parameter/Therapy	CBZ Monotherapy	VPA Monotherapy	CBZ With VPA	VPA With CBZ
N	556	662	402	430
MPE% bias	-1.7 ± 22.5	-0.19 ± 22.7	-2.7 ± 24.0	-4.6 ± 27.6
MAPE% precision	17.4 ± 14.2	17.7 ± 14.3	18.3 ± 15.7	21.7 ± 17.7
R^2	64.3	56.4	48.5	50.4
WMPE	-0.11 ± 1.9	-0.026 ± 2.47	-0.18 ± 2.04	0.08 ± 2.66
Kolmogorov−Smirnov test, p-value	0.28	0.18	0.06	0.26
One-sample t-test, H_0: the WMPE is equal to zero, p-value	0.16	0.8	0.074	0.55
Individual APE% $\leq 25\%$, n (%)	429 (77%)	504 (76.1%)	291 (72.4%)	275 (64%)
Individual APE% $\leq 35\%$, n (%)	496 (89.2%)	587 (88.7%)	338 (84.1%)	354 (82.3%)
Interoccasional variability of predictions, %	14.9%	15.6%	18.7%	19.4%
Intraindividual variability of predictions, %	24.4% (from 16%[a] to 32.4%[b])	25.7% (from 17.2%[a] to 31.1%[b])	27.1% (from 20.1%[a] to 29.6%[b])	27.7% (from 23.6%[a] to 31.8%[b])

Note: Data are presented as mean ± standard deviation.
[a]*For a 1-month prediction horizon.*
[b]*For prediction horizons longer than 2 years.*

The examples in Fig. 19.6 demonstrate typical cases of the individual course of serum AED concentrations over time during long-term epilepsy therapy: A: unchanged individual pharmacokinetics over a 1-year observation period; B: unexplained fluctuation of individual pharmacokinetics observed at only one occasion (the individual model underestimated the observed serum levels); C: unexplained fluctuations of individual pharmacokinetics observed at more than one occasion during a 2- to 3.5-year observation period.

The statistical results of prediction performance are summarized in Table 19.7.

This study demonstrated that in most cases of CBZ and VPA monotherapy and combination therapy, predictions of future AED concentrations (for each dosage form) based on the earlier developed population PK models, TDM data, and the patient-specific MAP Bayesian posterior parameter values provided clinically acceptable estimates. A plot of predicted versus observed concentrations for CBZ and VPA monotherapy gives an overall sense of the goodness of fit (see Fig. 19.7). The concentration−time points fell randomly (without bias) and relatively close to the line of identity Y = X throughout the concentration range.

The APE was less or equal to 25% and was considered as acceptable in 77.0% and 76.1% cases for CBZ and VPA monotherapy, respectively. The proportion of acceptable cases was slightly lower for CBZ in the presence of VPA (72.4%) and was significantly decreased for VPA in the presence of CBZ (64%). A similar tendency was seen in the MPAE values: $17.4 \pm 14.2\%$ and $17.7 \pm 14.3\%$ for CBZ and VPA monotherapy, respectively; slightly higher for CBZ in the presence

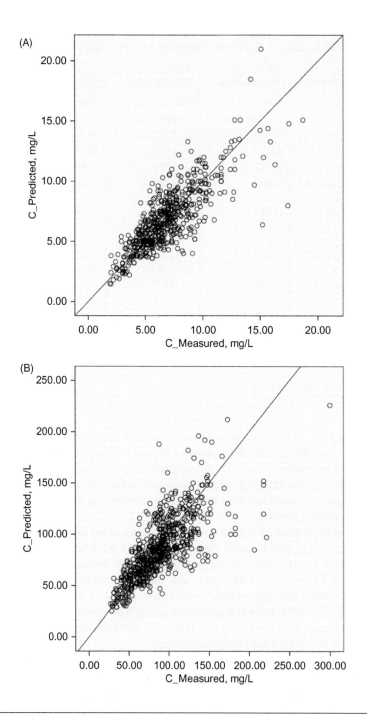

FIGURE 19.7

Predicted versus observed concentrations (mg/L) plot for (A) CBZ monotherapy; (B) VPA monotherapy. X = Y is line of identity.

of VPA ($18.3 \pm 15.7\%$); and significantly increased for VPA in the presence of CBZ ($21.7 \pm 17.7\%$). As the PE% versus observed concentrations plots demonstrate for all groups, visually the APE% was slightly higher at relatively low AED serum levels (see Fig. 19.8). In some cases (the circled points in Fig. 19.8A and B), it might be explained by poor compliance.

Statistical analysis of the residuals demonstrated that the distributions of residuals (PE%) and weighted residuals were close to a normal distribution (Kolmogorov−Smirnov test, $p > 0.05$), and their mean values did not differ statistically significantly from zero (no statistically significant bias, $p > 0.05$) for all groups of predictions. Plots of weighted residuals versus predicted concentrations had no bias or no trend and had equal and random distribution throughout the prediction range (see Fig. 19.9 as an example).

The decreased quality of predictions of VPA concentrations during CBZ + VPA combination therapy, especially when CBZ dosages were changed, might well be explained by their PK interactions. The observed tendency to overestimate predicted VPA concentrations during CBZ + VPA combination therapy when CBZ dosages were increased (versus unchanged CBZ dosages, CBZ dosages were decreased only in 10% of cases) supported this conclusion. It is well known that CBZ is a potent enzyme inducer, and CBZ can increase the clearance of VPA and lead to a reduction in VPA serum concentrations [13,73]. This clinically significant drug interaction at a metabolic level can result in the need to adjust dosage regimens [74]. This conclusion can be also supported by another part of the results. In the linear regression analysis, the APE% of VPA serum levels was relatively higher when the predictions were based on changed versus unchanged CBZ dosages ($p = 0.021$), and higher CBZ doses were associated with an increased APE% ($p = 0.03$) (see Fig. 19.10B). The absolute PE was less or equal to 25% in 67.5% versus 57.7% of cases when based on unchanged and changed CBZ dosages, respectively ($p = 0.041$). WMPE was estimated at 0.21 ± 2.44 ($N = 304$, $p = 0.14$) versus -0.75 ± 3.09 ($N = 98$, overestimation, $p = 0.019$) for subgroups with unchanged and increased CBZ dosages, respectively (see Fig. 19.10A and B).

There was no apparent influence of VPA in changed or unchanged dosages on the APE% and the proportions of acceptable predictions of CBZ serum levels. These results correspond well to those reported in the literature: VPA had no significant effect on total free CBZ concentration, but it increased CBZ-epoxide levels [74,75]. These results are also in good agreement with those obtained for population models of CBZ behavior in the presence of VPA versus CBZ monotherapy. From TDM data of other patients, the population median metabolic rate constant value was estimated at 0.078 for CBZ in the presence of VPA versus 0.07 for CBZ monotherapy, respectively ($p = 0.4$).

A unique feature of VPA binding to plasma proteins is its dependence on the concentration over the therapeutic range (50−150 mg/L) [49,52]. The variation in the free fraction of VPA is considered to become significant at a total drug concentration above 100 mg/L [2,76]. Nevertheless, in the results presented here, no statistically significant bias or decrease in precision of predictions was associated with measured VPA levels higher than 100 mg/L or with significant changes in VPA dosages either for VPA monotherapy or for VPA in the presence of CBZ. No dependence of percentage PEs on VPA serum levels (lower or higher than 100 mg/L) ($p = 0.3$) or on increased/unchanged VPA daily dose ($p = 0.7$) was found in regression analysis for the VPA monotherapy group. For combination VPA + CBZ, the APE% of VPA serum levels was less or equal to 25% in 65.5% and 61.3% of cases for patients on unchanged and changed VPA dosage, respectively ($p = 0.38$).

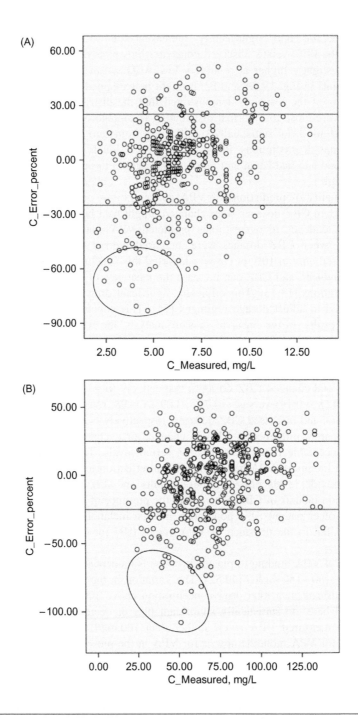

FIGURE 19.8

Percentage prediction error values versus observed concentrations (mg/L) for (A) CBZ in the presence of VPA; (B) VPA in the presence of CBZ. Horizontal lines demonstrate acceptable ranges of 25% for individual PE% values. Circled regions represent probable poor compliance.

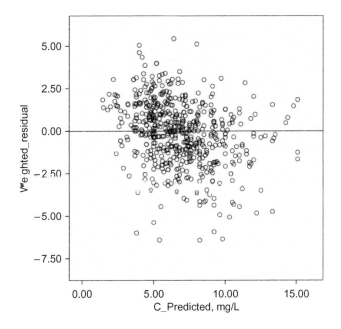

FIGURE 19.9

Weighted prediction errors (weighted residuals) versus predicted concentrations (mg/L) plot for CBZ monotherapy.

These results show that the linear one-compartment model had no tendency to either overestimate or underestimate the measured total concentration levels of VPA found with increases in dosage or at high VPA concentrations. Thus, there was no statistically significant influence of concentration–dependent VPA binding by plasma proteins on the predictability of total valproate serum levels.

For all groups in linear regression analysis, the observed trend of increasing of the APE% over future time horizons was considered statistically significant (regression coefficients ranged 0.15 to 0.26, $p < 0.05$) (see Fig. 19.11 as an example).

With CBZ monotherapy and with multiple repeated measurements, the precision of predictions decreased, on average, with increasing prediction horizon into the future. The absolute PE was less or equal to 25% in 88% of cases within a 1-month prediction horizon compared to 69.1% of predictions for time horizons longer than 2 years ($p < 0.001$). Intraindividual variability was estimated as 24.4% (from 16% for predictions within 1 month, up to 32.4% of predictions for horizons longer than 2 years).

Using linear regression analysis with the APE% as the dependent variable, the time horizon was not considered to be a statistically significant variable ($p = 0.42$) for repeated measurements in the epileptic patients on chronic VPA monotherapy. However, it was statistically significant for the majority of predictions from 0.25 up to 30 months ($p = 0.003$). Absolute PE was less or equal to 25% in 85.9% of cases within 2 months compared to 72% for prediction times longer than 1.5 years. Intraindividual variability was estimated as 25.7% (from 17.2% within a 1-month horizon up to 31.1% for prediction horizon longer than 2 years).

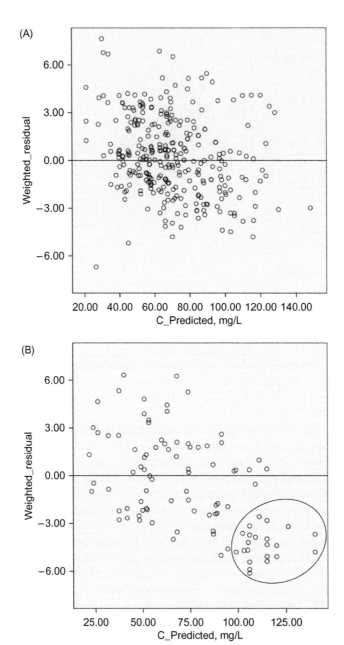

FIGURE 19.10

Weighted prediction errors (weighted residuals) versus predicted concentrations (mg/L) plot for VPA in the presence of CBZ: (A) unchanged CBZ dosage; (B) increased CBZ dosage. Circled regions represent probable poor compliance.

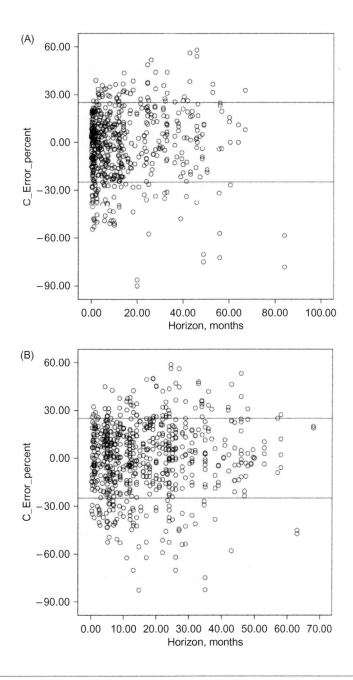

FIGURE 19.11

Scatterplots for PE% and time horizon (months) for (A) CBZ monotherapy; (B) VPA monotherapy. Horizontal lines demonstrate acceptable ranges of 25% for individual PE% values.

For CBZ given in combination with VPA in linear regression analysis of the APE%, the prediction horizon was considered as a statistically significant variable ($p = 0.01$), but categorical variables of changed versus unchanged CBZ and VPA dosage were not ($p = 0.2$ and 0.6, respectively). The absolute PE was less or equal to 25% in 78.1% cases within a 2-month horizon compared to 64.5% for prediction times longer than 2 years. The absolute value of the PE was less or equal to 25% in 74.2% and 69.9% of cases for patients on unchanged or changed VPA dosage, respectively ($p = 0.34$). Intraindividual variability was estimated as 27.1% (from 20.1% within 1-month horizon up to 29.6% for prediction periods longer than 2 years).

For TDM data of patients on CBZ + VPA combination therapy with repeated VPA measurements in linear regression analysis of the APE%, the prediction horizon was considered as a statistically significant variable ($p < 0.001$). A categorical variable of changed/unchanged CBZ dosage was also statistically significant ($p = 0.021$), but the variable of changed/unchanged VPA dosage was not ($p = 0.68$). The absolute PE was less or equal to 25% in 71.1% of cases within a 2-month horizon compared to 59.5% for prediction periods longer than 2 years. While the rate of absolute PE less or equal to 25% was not statistically significantly different in patients on unchanged versus changed VPA dosage ($p = 0.38$), this proportion was estimated at 67.5% and 57.7% of cases for patients on unchanged versus changed CBZ dosage, respectively ($p = 0.041$). Intraindividual variability was estimated as 27.7% (from 23.6% within a 1-month horizon, up to 31.8% for prediction horizons longer than 2 years).

Although the proportions of acceptable predictions also demonstrated a decrease of prediction quality over time, even for time horizons longer than 2 years, the precision of the predictions (especially for monotherapy) was acceptable in the majority of cases (absolute value of PE was less or equal to 25% in 69.1% and 72% of cases for CBZ and VPA, respectively). No bias in predictions was associated with the time horizon.

To demonstrate the advantage of this manner of individualizing AED therapy, for relatively homogeneous subgroups aged from 18 up to 50 years old, all patients' concentrations were also predicted based on the median population parameter values adjusted only for BW for volume of distribution. For example, MAPE% were $43.4 \pm 34.3\%$ ($N = 584$) and $78.2 \pm 65.1\%$ ($N = 348$) for VPA monotherapy and for CBZ with VPA combination therapy, respectively. Absolute PE was less or equal to 25% only in 34.8% of cases and 28.3% of cases for VPA monotherapy and CBZ with VPA combination therapy, respectively. In most patients included in this statistical analysis, the reasons for TDM were lack of efficacy and/or signs of toxicity observed at recommended AED daily doses, probably due to unusual individual pharmacokinetics. This means that the mean errors of predictions based only on the population models might be slightly overestimated. Fig. 19.12 and the corresponding statistical characteristics illustrate higher variability and decreasing quality of predictions based on the median population parameter values compared to predictions based on the patient-specific Bayesian posterior parameter values. These results support the opinion that goal-oriented, model-based Bayesian adaptive control based on at least two feedback AED concentrations measured as a part of TDM can provide quite useful help in the management of epileptic patients.

These results may also help physicians and clinical pharmacists make dosage adjustments for long-term AED therapy. Individualizing AED therapy can help estimate individual patient Bayesian posterior model pharmacokinetic parameters as baseline values when the patient has achieved the goal of therapy, can identify individuals who are slow and fast metabolizers, and can

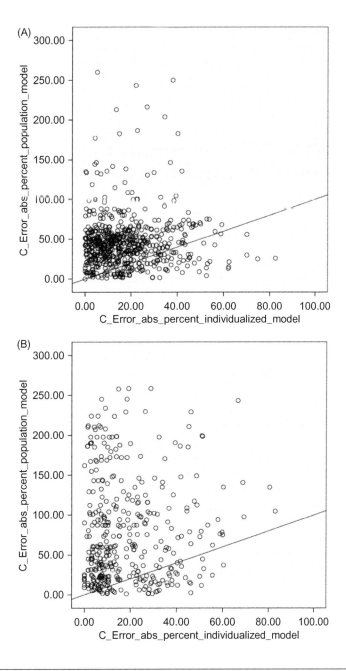

FIGURE 19.12

Scatterplots for APE% estimated on the base of the median population parameter values versus APE% estimated on the base of the patient-specific Bayesian posterior parameter values for (A) VPA monotherapy; (B) CBZ with VPA combination therapy. X = Y is line of identity.

help the clinician assess whether breakthrough seizures may be due to changing AED pharmacokinetics resulting from a physiologic condition, a pathologic condition, a change in formulation, or a drug—drug interaction. This technique can also help estimate more precisely the "room to move" or when to change AEDs.

19.4 MORE COMPLEX NONLINEAR PK MODELS

19.4.1 TIME-DEPENDENT CBZ PHARMACOKINETICS DURING AUTOINDUCTION

The literature results for CBZ are consistent with self-induction of microsomal enzymes [37,43—45]. The occurrence of such autoinduction has been established based on pharmacokinetic and stable isotope-labeled studies of CBZ and its metabolites. If a drug is subject to autoinduction, total clearance is higher after multiple doses than following the first dose, and the Css cannot be predicted well from TDM data obtained after first few doses of the drug. The metabolic clearance of CBZ increases with continued administration until the microsomal enzymes are fully induced. Studies with laboratory animals show that the decline in CBZ Csss begins after a lag time and during a continuous infusion at a constant rate appeared to be an exponentially asymptotic process. In patients, the process is completed in about 3—5 weeks of CBZ oral daily intake. Apparent total clearance increases by a factor of approximately 2.5 [42,77]. The PK model with an exponentially asymptotic increasing metabolic clearance during induction has been tested earlier with CBZ as inducer and clonazepam as the drug affected [78].

19.4.1.1 Patient data and PK analysis

The objective of the study was to develop a nonlinear model of CBZ time-dependent pharmacokinetic behavior during its autoinduction period and to estimate the model parameters from TDM data of drug-naïve adult epileptic patients who started on CBZ monotherapy.

This study included 19 drug-naïve adult epileptic patients for whom measured CBZ serum levels (peak—trough strategy) were available on at least at four occasions from 1 to 2 days to up to 1.5 to 2 months of CBZ monotherapy (mean = 9.5 CBZ serum levels per patient, 180 serum levels total). No medicines taken concurrently with carbamazepine were known to interfere with CBZ pharmacokinetics. CBZ concentrations were measured by high-performance liquid chromatography. The assay error pattern was used as: $SD = 0.1 + 0.01\ C$ (where SD is the standard deviation of the assay at a measured CBZ concentration C). The population PK analysis was performed using the USC*PACK software based on a nonlinear one-compartment model with linear absorption. The data of the 19 outpatients who were closely monitored at the beginning of CBZ monotherapy were analyzed by the NPEM program (Table 19.8).

CBZ time-dependent behavior during the autoinduction period was described here using a one-compartmental model with linear absorption. The main feature of this model is an increase in the metabolic rate constant value during autoinduction, starting from a preinduction value (D) before

Table 19.8 Demographic and Other Characteristics

Parameter	Patient Group
N patients on CBZ monotherapy	19
Age, years	40.6 ± 13.5 (18–60)
Gender: female/male	16(84.2%)/3(15.8%)
BMI, kg/m^2	26.8 ± 4.9 (17.6–36.2)
Body weight, kg	82.9 ± 19.8 (52–120)
N levels per patient	9.5 ± 2.0 (6–13)
N occasions per patients	4.5 ± 0.6 (4–6)
Days under observation	33.3 ± 10.4 (20–49)
Started CBZ daily dose, mg	180 ± 72 (100–300)
End-of-observation CBZ daily dose, mg	300 ± 122 (200–500)

Note: Data are presented as mean $\pm$ standard deviation (minimum–maximum value).
BMI, *Body mass index.*

the time (λ) at which induction begins and increasing asymptotically to a maximum ($D + A$) value after autoinduction is completed. The following equations were used:

$$\dot{X}_1 = -K_{abs} \cdot X_1$$
$$\dot{X}_2 = K_{abs} \cdot X_1 - K_{el} \cdot X_2,$$
$$K_{el} = \begin{cases} D, t \le \lambda; \\ D + A[1 - \exp\{-B \cdot (t - \lambda)\}], t > \lambda, \end{cases}$$
$$Y = \frac{X_2}{V},$$

where $\dot{X}_1$ is rate of change of CBZ amount in the absorption compartment (mg/h), $\dot{X}_2$ is the rate of change of CBZ amount in the serum compartment (mg/h), K_{abs} is the absorption rate constant (1/h), V is the volume of distribution (L), λ is the time at which induction begins (h), D is the preinduction elimination rate value (1/h), B is the first-order autoinduction rate constant (1/h), and Y is the CBZ serum concentration (mg/L).

A similar model might be used to describe heteroinduction as result of a drug–drug interaction. The model should be fitted to the multiple PK data of patients for whom measured serum levels relate to both monotherapy and polytherapy.

19.4.1.2 Results

Table 19.9 gives descriptive statistics for the estimated PK parameters of the CBZ autoinduction model.

Preinduction CBZ pharmacokinetics were also analyzed. That study examined data sets of 16 adult healthy volunteers, who took 200 mg of carbamazepine in tablet form as a single dose. Median PK parameter values for the one-compartment linear model of preinduction CBZ behavior estimated by the NPEM program were compared with those for CBZ postinduction pharmacokinetics. The

Table 19.9 Estimated Population PK Parameters (Median ± SD) for the CBZ Autoinduction Model

Parameter	Results
K_{abs}, 1/h	0.9 ± 0.85; CV = 94.4%
D, 1/h	0.023 ± 0.012; CV = 52.2%
A, 1/h	0.029 ± 0.026; CV = 89.7%
B, 1/h	0.009 ± 0.007; CV = 77.8%
Lambda (λ), h	165.4 ± 70.6; CV = 42.7%
V, L	64.5 ± 25.7; CV = 39.8%

Table 19.10 Estimated Population (Median ± SD) PK Parameters for the Steady-State CBZ Data and the Single-Dose CBZ Data

PK Parameter/ Study	Data Set for CBZ Steady State N = 99	Data Set for CBZ Single Dose N = 16
K_{abs}, 1/h	0.67 ± 0.59	0.62 ± 0.22
K_{el}, 1/h	0.07 ± 0.068	0.018 ± 0.0039
V_d, L/kg	0.94 ± 0.4	0.93 ± 0.16
$T_{1/2}$, h	$3.2 - 50.6$	$26 - 63$

mean metabolic rate constant found before induction was three to four times smaller than the one observed after the induction period. The $T_{1/2}$ values just after a single dose ranged from 26 to 63 h, and these values decreased to 3.2—50.6 h (with a median value of 10 h) for the postinduction period in the adult epileptic patients studied. Thus, CBZ markedly induces its own metabolism. This leads to a progressive decrease in CBZ serum levels during chronic drug dosing.

The estimated pharmacokinetic parameter values of the preinduction elimination rate value (D) and the maximum postinduction elimination rate value ($D + A$) are in good agreement with those estimated in the population studies of preinduction (0.018 ± 0.004 1/h) and postinduction CBZ metabolism (0.07 ± 0.068 1/h) (see Table 19.10). The data indicate that carbamazepine autoinduction after initiating CBZ monotherapy started within the first week. After 3—4 weeks on monotherapy, the individual half-lives approach the postinduction values. Initial half-life values range from 15 to 69 h (median = 29 h), decreasing to 7—26 h (median = 14.8 h) on repeated doses. Wide interindividual variability in serum CBZ concentrations to dose ratios, as well as in ratios of postinduction to preinduction rate constant of CBZ metabolism, was observed.

The PK profile calculated for an individual patient on the basis of his TDM data related to the first days of therapy and the assumption of linear kinetics demonstrates 1.3 (11 vs 8.6 mg/L) and 1.45 (16 vs 11 mg/L) times the difference between the predicted and observed peak serum levels at 22 days and 28 days of CBZ dosing, respectively.

This PE is not random, and its level is not acceptable for a drug with a narrow therapeutic range as for CBZ (the therapeutic range for serum CBZ is 3—12 mg/L). It means that traditional methods of predicting CBZ steady-state serum concentrations based on a linear PK model as well as a population model with estimated PK parameters from steady-state data are not useful during the autoinduction period. When CBZ is started and the patient is titrated to a reasonable target goal, TDM and Bayesian adaptive estimation of the individual parameter values may be helpful to determine the next step and avoid CBZ toxicity or lack of clinical effect.

19.4.2 PHENYTOIN CONCENTRATION-DEPENDENT, OR SATURABLE, PHARMACOKINETICS

Phenytoin has been widely used in the treatment of epilepsy for a long time. Clinical trials and experience over the past years have shown phenytoin effective for the chronic treatment of tonic-clonic (grand mal) or partial seizures and the acute treatment of generalized status epilepticus. Phenytoin is still one of the most commonly used anticonvulsant agents. The pharmacokinetic characteristics of PHN increase the risk for toxicity: saturable concentration-dependent metabolism, relatively narrow therapeutic index, wide interindividual PK variability, and clinically significant drug–drug interactions.

Phenytoin is eliminated predominantly by metabolism, with less than 2–5% of an administered dose being excreted unchanged in the urine [79]. The clearance of PHN is concentration-dependent within the usual therapeutic concentration ranges 3–20 mg/L [42], as a result of saturable biotransformation [60,79,80] (Table 19.11).

It is well documented that the decline in serum PHN concentration after a dose could be fitted to the integrated form of the Michaelis–Menten equation and that the elimination kinetics of PHN are concentration-dependent [81]:

$$v = \frac{V_{\max} \cdot C}{K_{\mathrm{m}} + C}$$

where v—the rate of metabolism, C—PHN serum concentration, $V_{\max}$—maximal elimination velocity, and K_{m}—Michaelis constant.

Phenytoin exhibits nonlinear kinetics in clinical practice because the K_{m} value (equivalent to the serum concentration at which the elimination rate is one-half of the maximal rate) is usually in the same range as clinically effective concentrations (10–30 mg/L [56,77,82]), and the $V_{\max}$ value

Table 19.11 Demographic Characteristics

Parameter	Patient Group
N patients on chronic PHN	42
Age, years	28.66 ± 10.7 (18–58)
Gender: female/male	17(40.5%)/25(59.5%)
BMI, kg/m^2	24.2 ± 4.2 (18–32)
Body weight, kg	69.78 ± 12.6 (42–90)
N levels per patient	4.34 ± 0.69 (4–6) (at least 2 PHN dosage)
PHN daily dose, mg/kg	4.9 ± 1.51 (maximum dose)

Note: Data are presented as mean ± standard deviation (minimum–maximum value).
BMI, *Body mass index.*

Table 19.12 Estimated Population PK Parameters

Parameter	Results
K_m, mg/L	8.12 ± 3.27 (7.5), CV = 40.3%
V_{max}, mg/kg per h	0.37 ± 0.14 (0.35), CV = 37.8%
V_d, L/kg	0.6 ± 0.32 (0.59), CV = 53.3%
K_{abs}, 1/h	2.02 ± 1.33 (1.72), CV = 65.8%

Note: Data are presented as mean ± standard deviation (median value).

(the maximal rate of PHN elimination) is not much greater than usual daily dose required to achieve therapeutic Css [42,77,80]. The maximum reaction velocity concept can be expressed in mg/day or mg/kg per day for comparison with the PHN dosing rate. The estimated median value for V_{max} in adult population is about 8.9 mg/kg per day (see Table 19.12). This means that the liver of a normal 70-kg patient cannot metabolize more than about 623 mg of PHN per 24 h. If this patient's daily PHN intake should exceed the individual maximum elimination rate, extra drug will accumulate and lead to increasing PHN serum concentrations. This relatively small daily increase in patient's serum concentrations may result in toxic levels after a week or a month of such therapy. That is why to prescribe an effective and safe maintenance PHN dose it may be especially important to know the individual V_{max} and K_m values.

If the small amount of the drug excreted unchanged can be ignored, an open one-compartment pharmacokinetic model with a capacity-limited route of elimination (Michaelis–Menten kinetics) can be used for a model of PHN pharmacokinetics [77,79,82]. At rates of administration approaching the maximum metabolic rate (V_{max}), renal elimination of unchanged phenytoin can significantly influence the steady-state serum phenytoin concentration. A population pharmacokinetic model with the parallel Michaelis–Menten and first-order elimination (MM + FO) has been also reported [83].

It has been found that the pharmacokinetic parameters such as the maximum rate of elimination (V_{max}) and the serum PHN concentration at which the rate of elimination is one-half the maximum (K_m) are highly variable between patients [79,80,82,84,85]. For phenytoin, V_{max} values range between 100 and 1000 mg per day and K_m values between 1 and 15 mg/L [77]. Several studies have reported the pharmacokinetic parameters (V_{max} and K_m) in various ethnic populations [82,84,86,87]. The apparent volume of distribution of PHN is approximately 0.6–0.8 L/kg [42,88].

For PK analysis, the majority of these studies have used only one pair of steady-state PHN concentration related to an actual PHN dosage regimen for each included patient. The presented results were limited and controversial. The usual therapeutic range of PHN is about 10–20 mg/L [60]. However, seizure control has been obtained with concentrations less than 10 mg/L. Often concentrations more than 20 mg/L have been needed and have been observed in patients without signs of toxicity [80,89]. Due to the saturable metabolism of PHN, the higher the Css is in any given patient, the greater the probability that PK nonlinearity will lead to extreme increases in patient's serum PHN concentration. For PK analysis, the majority of the published studies have used one pair of steady-state PHN concentration related to an actual PHN dosage regimen for each included patient. Those results are limited and controversial.

A number of pharmacokinetic methods for individualizing PHN dosing have been developed, most of which assume Michaelis–Menten elimination kinetics and predict the individual V_{max} and K_m values from 0 (without TDM) or more Csss. Most of them have used the following relationship between PHN C_{ss}'s and dosing rate:

$$Css = \frac{K_m \cdot D}{V_{max} - D}$$

or its different linearized forms.

Without TDM (no feedback), the PHN dose (D) to reach the target Css can be calculated on the basis of the mean population parameter values (K_m and V_{max}) from the previous equation. From two or more sets of steady-state dosage regimens and Css measurements, an individual patient's V_{max} and K_m values can be estimated either graphically [82,90] or by direct computation from the previous equation. With only a single pair of dose-Css measurements, only one individual parameter value can be estimated when another one is fixed [91], or a maximum a posterior probability Bayesian estimate of the most likely individual V_{max} and K_m values can be obtained [79,92–94].

Many studies have compared the accuracy of the various methods of PHN concentration predictions [80,90,95,96]. All feedback methods improve the predictability of steady-state PHN serum concentrations in comparison with predictions based on the population parameter values. However, a reliable Css value for PHN often can be obtained only after about 3 weeks on an unchanged dosage regimen. Changes in concentration can occur up to 2–3 weeks after a dosage change. Besides, the time required to achieve any fraction of steady state also changes with the dosing rate and also depends on the individual PK parameter values, so it cannot be predicted without TDM data [80,97]. Therefore, Bayesian approaches for phenytoin concentration prediction based on minimum sampling steady-state or nonsteady-state TDM measurements appear to be preferable [80,96].

19.4.2.1 Patient data and PK analysis

A nonlinear model of PHN pharmacokinetics was developed and its parameters from steady-state and/or nonsteady-state TDM data of adult epileptic patients on chronic PHN monotherapy were estimated. This study included 42 adult epileptic patients for whom at least two pairs of measured serum levels (peak–trough strategy) related to different PHN dosages were available (182 PHN serum levels totally were collected in our laboratory). The patients had received different treatment schedules of oral PHN dosing. All studied patients were relatively young and had normal renal and hepatic function and no diseases that could influence drug plasma binding to a clinically significant degree. No medicines taken concurrently with phenytoin were known to interfere with PHN pharmacokinetics. PHN concentrations were measured by high-performance liquid chromatography. The assay error pattern was used as: $SD = 0.1 + 0.011C + 0.003C^2$ (where SD is standard deviation of the assay at measured PHN concentration C). The population PK analysis was performed using the NPEM program (USC*PACK software) based on a one-compartment model with first-order absorption and Michaelis–Menten elimination kinetics. The pharmacokinetic model of PHN was developed as a system of differential equations with model parametrization by the rate constant of absorption (K_{abs}), the apparent volume of distribution (V_d), the maximum elimination rate constant (V_{max}), and the Michaelis–Menten constant (K_m):

$$\dot{X}_1 = -K_{abs} \cdot X_1$$

$$\dot{X}_2 = K_{abs} \cdot X_1 - \frac{V_{max} \cdot W \cdot X_2}{K_m \cdot W \cdot V_d + X_2},$$

$$Y = \frac{X_2}{V_d \cdot W},$$

where W is body weight (kg), the elimination parameters are V_{max} (mg/kg per h) and K_m (mg/L), $\dot{X}_1$ is the rate of change of the amount of PHN in the absorption site (mg/h), $\dot{X}_2$ is the rate of change of the amount of PHN in the serum compartment (mg/h), K_{abs} is the absorption rate constant (1/h), V_d is the apparent volume of distribution (L/kg), and Y is the serum PHN concentration (mg/L).

19.4.2.2 Results

Assuming 100% bioavailability of orally administered PHN, estimated median population PK parameter values for the rate constant of absorption ($K_{abs} = 1.72$ hr^{-1}, CV $= 65.8\%$), for the apparent volume of distribution ($V_d = 0.6$ L/kg, CV $= 53.3\%$), for the maximum elimination rate constant ($V_{max} = 0.35$ mg/kg per h, CV $= 37.8\%$), and for the Michaelis–Menten constant ($K_m = 7.5$ mg/L, CV $= 40.3\%$) are in good agreement with those reported in the literature.

The predictive performance evaluation illustrates the wide interindividual variability in patient response when all patient serum concentrations were predicted based on the population mean (or median) parameter values (see Fig. 19.13A). This is especially clear for relatively high PHN concentrations (higher than 10 mg/L) where phenytoin nonlinear elimination is more close to saturation. In contrast, the individual serum levels predicted on the basis of the mean (or median) values of each patient's Bayesian posterior joint density gave good prediction for all subjects in the population (Fig. 19.13B).

The most widely used methods of AED dosage adjustment have been based on the measured serum concentrations at steady state. When a steady state is achieved, the rate of drug administration (D) is equal the rate of elimination. For Michaelis–Menten kinetics, when D is less than $0.1 V_{max}$, the Css is proportional to D (linear kinetics). As D approaches V_{max}, the Css increases exponentially. When D is equal to or larger than V_{max}, a steady state is not achieved. In addition, the time to reach a fraction of the steady state increases with D [77,97]. This nonlinear relationship between PHN dose (D) to reach the target Css depends on two parameter values: V_{max} and K_m.

Very few patients have parameter values corresponding to the population averages. For example, in the present population, the median V_{max} parameter value was estimated by the NPEM program as 8.9 mg/kg per day with interindividual CV about 40%. The majority of individual V_{max} values ranged from 4.6 to 16 mg/kg per day, but a few patients had very high V_{max} parameter values, up to 24 mg/kg per day. The nonlinear relationship between phenytoin dose and steady-state levels is such that minimal changes of dose can often cause major concentration changes. For example, for a normal 70-kg patient with individual parameter values $V_{max} = 8$ mg/kg per day and $K_m = 8$ mg/L, a daily phenytoin dose of 400 mg (about 5.7 mg/kg per day) leads to average steady-state serum concentrations of about 20 mg/L. Changing the daily dose to 450 mg (6.4 mg/kg per

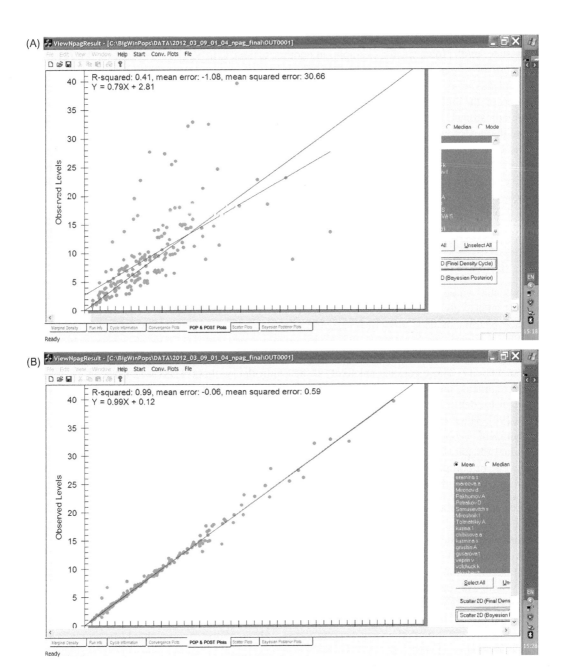

FIGURE 19.13

(A) Scatterplot of the predicted–found relationships based on the mean population parameter values for all patients in the adult population on PHN monotherapy. (B) Scatterplot of the predicted–found relationships based on finding each subject's own mean value of his Bayesian posterior joint parameter density. Horizontal axis — predicted levels. Vertical axis — observed levels.

day) means a 12.5% increase and achieves a Css of 32 mg/L, a 60% increase over the previous steady-state level. However, for example, in another patient with V_{max} value of 12 mg/kg per day, a daily dose of 400 mg may correspond to a level of 7.2 mg/L. Adding 50 mg to that daily dose (12.5%) leads to a Css of 9.1 mg/L, a 27% increase over the previous steady-state level. Only identification of the individual parameter values can improve concentration predictions for phenytoin dosage adjustment. In addition, without knowledge of the individual parameter values, one cannot be sure that a steady state is really reached.

The USC*PACK programs permit one to estimate the individual parameter values and to make dosage adjustments without having to wait for a steady state before sampling. Bayesian feedback adaptive control and the proposed population model can improve PHN dosage adjustment and identify how close a patient is to the more saturated part of the PK curve.

19.5 INDICATIONS FOR TDM AND INDIVIDUALIZING AED DOSAGE

The potential value of TDM for old and newer AEDs performed on blood (serum/plasma) or on saliva is intensively discussed in the literature in relation to their mode of action, drug interactions, and their pharmacokinetic properties [2,5,7,56,98].

Clinical experience has shown that many epileptic patients who take an average dose of an acceptable formulation of an appropriate medication have acceptable efficacy without significant signs of toxicity. These patients are likely to be controlled without TDM when placed on standard dosage regimens, but even in such average patients with average AED pharmacokinetics, TDM can be useful to identify the causes of unwanted or unexpected responses and to improve clinical outcomes [99]. Thus, one of the important indications for TDM of AEDs is assessment of an individual therapeutic concentration related to attainment of that patient's desired clinical response. The individual PK parameter values estimated from these data might be used then as the baseline effective levels for comparison in case of an unexpected change in the patient's response.

Among others, there are the following indications for TDM of AEDs:

- Lack (uncontrolled seizures) or loss (breakthrough seizures) of clinical response;
- Signs of clinical toxicity;
- Dosage adjustments for drugs with nonlinear pharmacokinetics;
- Overdosing and underdosing (compliance);
- Patients in whom potentially important pharmacokinetic change is anticipated due to physiological (eg, age or pregnancy) or pathological conditions (eg, renal and hepatic insufficiency, concomitant diseases, obesity);
- Potential drug–drug interactions;
- Change in drug formulation/switching to generic formulations, if there should be an unexpected change in clinical response.

There are situations when identification of the patient's individualized Bayesian posterior PK model from TDM data might be especially useful.

For example, patient N, female, 15 years old, body weight = 59 kg, on CBZ monotherapy about 4 months. For this patient, a regimen 300 mg 3 times a day was ineffective. CBZ daily dose was increased, and over one month, the current daily dosage regimen of 400−300−400 mg, with an approximately equal 8-h interval between the three doses resulted in improvement of seizure control. However, the dosing intervals were then changed, and at the same dosage regimen of 400−300−400 mg but with real dosing intervals of 5.5, 7, and 11.5 h, the patient reported occurrence of seizures in a regular manner before the morning dose. The modeling from TDM data measured on the unsuccessful therapy showed that the time period when her seizures usually appeared was related to serum CBZ levels lower than 9 mg/L. The measured peak−trough serum levels 11−8.3 mg/L were close to the upper limit of the general therapeutic range for CBZ (3−12 mg/L). The comparison of the patient-specific pharmacokinetic profile with information on the patient's response helped us to plan future successful CBZ monotherapy with serum concentrations exceeding 9 mg/L during all her dosing intervals. The new dosage regimen was calculated as 400 mg 3 times a day, adding only 100 mg (about 10%) to the previous daily dose. This approach helped the patient to be controlled satisfactorily on the new regimen of CBZ monotherapy and avoid switching to polytherapy.

A similar approach might be applied if a patient reports adverse events in a regular manner, for example, in a few hours after drug intake. Simulation with the patient's individualized Bayesian posterior PK model estimated from the TDM data can help identify the probable toxic serum levels for such a patient and adjust the dosage regimen accordingly.

In most patients who visited the laboratory, the reasons for TDM were the following: newly initiated or reinitiated AED therapy, lack or loss of efficacy, signs of toxicity, potential drug−drug interactions, potential risk of change in pharmacokinetics, and a retest in case of unexpected AED serum level values. Monitoring also helped the physicians establish and then check the optimal therapeutic concentration range for each individual patient, so they could be given the most effective and best tolerated individualized doses of AEDs.

19.6 CONCLUSION

AEDs have a relatively narrow therapeutic index, and the optimal dosing, especially in special patient subgroups such as elderly and pediatric patients, pregnant women, as well as in pathological conditions (eg, renal and hepatic insufficiency, concomitant diseases) depends on the understanding of the corresponding changes in their pharmacokinetics.

Serum AED concentrations correlated poorly with daily doses in both the adult and child populations. Because of the diversity within the population, use of the mean population model without knowledge of an individual patient's pharmacokinetic characteristics gives poor prediction. In contrast, the individual Bayesian posterior models gave good prediction for all subjects in the population due to removal of the interindividual variability.

Moreover, seizure control improves when the physician utilizes measured PK data in conjunction with information on individual data: seizure control, toxicity, patient compliance, and other clinical data. A modelling approach for planning, monitoring, and adjusting dosage appropriately, based on a population PK/PD model as the prior and using Bayes' theorem to fit the serum concentration data, can help develop an individualized model that best describes the behavior of the drug in a particular individual patient.

In most cases, predictions of future AED concentrations based on these population PK models, supplemented by TDM data and patient-specific MAP Bayesian posterior parameter modeling, provided clinically acceptable predictions of serum levels. Taking into consideration possible changes in individual pharmacokinetics between occasions during long-term treatment as well as unpredictable fluctuations of CBZ and VPA serum levels, the external validation results obtained suggest good predictive performance of the proposed population models even with simplified structure and of the MAP Bayesian individualized dosage regimens for CBZ and VPA therapy. This means that the proposed population models can be used to plan individualized dosage regimens in epileptic patients on AED therapy. This approach is also especially well suited for use with the multiple model design of dosage regimens (see Chapter 3) to achieve desired therapeutic target goals.

With the approach of Bayesian adaptive control, the serum AED concentrations are used not only to note if they are within some general therapeutic range, but most importantly, to make a specific Bayesian individualized model of the behavior of the drug in that particular individual patient. One can then reconstruct and see graphically what the patient's probable serum concentrations were at all other times when they were not measured. An important task is to compare the behavior of the patient-specific pharmacokinetic model with the clinical response of each patient. This comparison can be done by the USC*PACK programs via the fitted pharmacokinetic model and the plot of its serum concentration profile. Visualization of the individual concentration time course can also help in selection of each patient's individualized therapeutic target goal.

The patient's individualized model permits one to make dosage adjustments without having to wait for a steady state before sampling serum concentrations. This is especially important when individual half-life values may be prolonged. The patient's individualized Bayesian posterior PK model can help clinicians establish an effective target concentration goal for each patient, identify individuals who are fast or slow metabolizers, evaluate potential PK causes for alteration of drug utilization as a consequence of pathologic and/or physiological conditions as well as drug—drug interactions or change in drug formulation, and develop the optimal individualized dosage regimen for the patient.

In our laboratory, only total AED concentrations were measured, and the proposed population models do not take into consideration protein binding. When binding is altered, the total concentration no longer reflects the amount of pharmacologically active drug in the plasma. The potential discordance between total and free AED levels determines the value of TDM of the free concentration. Many pathophysiologic states or drug—drug interactions may influence plasma binding dramatically [100—102], and monitoring of free fraction might be useful if such binding changes are suspected.

ACKNOWLEDGMENTS

I wish to express my sincere gratitude to all who in different ways have contributed to this work, especially:

- Director of Research Institute of Physical-Chemical Medicine, Full Member of the Russian Academy of Medical Sciences, professor Valerii Sergienko, my boss, who led and supported this work for many years.
- Professor Roger Jelliffe, a great tutor, for brilliant explanations of crucial points in the concept of individualizing pharmacotherapy, for giving me access to his methods and software, for help during our long collaboration, and for many valuable discussions and comments.

- All personnel working in the pharmacokinetic laboratories who collected medical records, samples, and performed drug analysis, especially professor Sokolov A., Tischenkova I., Professor Sariev A., Abaimov D.
- All physicians who use TDM of AEDs and the presented models and results in clinical settings, especially Russian key opinion leaders in neurology, professor Alla Guekht and professor Vladimir Karlov for their work with the clinical interpretation of the results and help with application of the individualizing AED dosage based on TDM data and population modeling in clinical practice in Russia.

REFERENCES

[1] Perucca E. An introduction to antiepileptic drugs. Epilepsia 2005;46(Suppl. 4):31–7.

[2] Affolter N, Krähenbühl S, Schlienger RG. Appropriateness of serum level determinations of antiepileptic drugs. Swiss Med Wkly 2003;133:591–7.

[3] Battino D, Bossi L, Croci D, et al. Carbamazepine plasma levels in children and adults: influence of age, dose and associated therapy. Ther Drug Monit 1980;2:315–27.

[4] Brodie MJ, Dichter MA. Drug therapy—antiepileptic drugs. N Engl J Med 1996;334:168–75.

[5] Neels HM, Sierens AC, Naelaerts K. Therapeutic drug monitoring of old and newer antiepileptic drugs. Clin Chem Lab Med 2004;42(11):1228–55.

[6] Patsalos PN. New antiepileptic drugs. Ann Clin Biochem 1999;36:10–19.

[7] Patsalos PN, Berry DJ, Bourgeois BFD, et al. Antiepileptic drugs—best practice guidelines for therapeutic drug monitoring: a position paper by the subcommission on therapeutic drug monitoring, ILAE commission on therapeutic strategies. Epilepsia 2008;49:1239–76.

[8] Walson PD. Role of therapeutic drug monitoring (TDM) in pediatric anti-convulsant drug dosing. Brain Dev 1994;16:23–6.

[9] Bartels H. Rational usage of therapeutic drug monitoring in antiepileptic treatment. Eur J Pediatr 1980;133:193–9.

[10] Choonara IA, Rane A. Therapeutic drug monitoring of anticonvulsants. State of the art. Clin Pharmacokinet 1990;18(4):318–28.

[11] Cloyd JC, Birnbaum AK, Kreil RL. Pharmacokinetics in infancy, childhood, and adolescence. In: Wyllie E, editor. The treatment of epilepsy: principles and practice. 2nd ed. Baltimore: Williams & Wilkins; 1997. p. 737–47.

[12] Larkin JG, Herric AL, McGuire GM, et al. Antiepileptic drug monitoring at the epilepsy clinic: a prospective evaluation. Epilepsia 1991;32(1):89–95.

[13] Sillampaa M, Carbamazepine. In: Wyllie E, editor. The treatment of epilepsy: principles and practice. 2nd ed. Baltimore: Williams & Wilkins; 1997. p. 802–24.

[14] Strandjord RE, Johannessen SI. Single-drug therapy with carbamazepine in patients with epilepsy: serum levels and clinical effect. Epilepsia 1980;21:655–62.

[15] Gerber N, Wagner JG. Explanation of dose dependent decline of diphenylhydantoin plasma levels by fitting to the integrated form of the Michaelis–Menten equation. Res Commun Chem Pathol Pharmacol 1972;3:455–66.

[16] Jannuzzi G, Cian P, Fattore C, et al. A multicenter randomized controlled trial on the clinical impact of therapeutic drug monitoring in patients with newly diagnosed epilepsy. Epilepsia 2000;41:222–30.

[17] Tomson T, Dahl ML, Kimland E. Cochrane review, prepared and maintained by The Cochrane Collaboration and published in *The Cochrane Library* 2010, (5): 1–16.

[18] Dodge WF, Jelliffe RW, Richardson CJ, et al. Population pharmacokinetic models. Measures of central tendency. Drug Investig 1993;5(4):206–11.

[19] Sheiner LB. Population pharmacokinetics/dynamics. Ann Rev Pharmacol Toxicol 1992;32:185−209.

[20] Sheiner LB, Rosenberg B, Marathe VV. Estimation of population characteristics of pharmacokinetic parameters from routine clinical data. J Pharmacokinet Biopharm 1977;5:445−79.

[21] Vozeh S, Maitre PO, Stanski DR. Evaluation of population (NONMEM) pharmacokinetic parameter estimates. J Pharmacokinet Biopharm 1989;18(2):161−73.

[22] Jerling M. Population kinetics of antidepressant and neuroleptic drugs. Studies of therapeutic drug monitoring data to evaluate kinetic variability, drug interactions, nonlinear kinetics, and the influence of genetic factors. PhD Thesis, Karolinska Institute at Huddinge University Hospital, Stockholm, Sweden: 1995.

[23] Blanco-Serrano B, Garsia-Sanchez MJ, Otero MJ, et al. Valproate population pharmacokinetics in children. J Clin Pharm Ther 1999;24:73−80.

[24] Blanco-Serrano B, Otero MJ, Santos-Buelga D, Garsia-Sanchez MJ, Serrano J, Dominguez-Gil A. Population estimation of valproic acid clearance in adult patients using routine clinical pharmacokinetic data. Biopharm Drug Dispos 1999;20:233−40.

[25] Graves NM, Brundage RC, Yandong W, et al. Population pharmacokinetics of carbamazepine in adults with epilepsy. Pharmacotherapy 1998;18(2):273−81.

[26] Jiao Z, Shi XJ, Zhao ZG, Zhong MK. Population pharmacokinetic modeling of steady state clearance of carbamazepine and its epoxide metabolite from sparse routine clinical data. J Clin Pharm Ther 2004;29 (3):247−56.

[27] Milovanovic JR, Jankovic SM. Population pharmacokinetic of antiepileptic drugs in different populations. Cent Eur J Med 2013;8(4):383−91.

[28] Yukawa E, Honda T, Ohdo S, Higuchi S, Aoyama T. Detection of carbamazepine-induced changes in valproic acid relative clearance in man by simple pharmacokinetic screening. J Pharm Pharmacol 1997;49:751−6.

[29] Yukawa E, To H, Ohdo S, Higuchi S, Aoyama T. Population-based investigation of valproic acid relative clearance using nonlinear mixed effects modeling: influence of drug−drug interaction and patient characteristics. J Clin Pharmacol 1997;37:1160−7.

[30] Yukawa E, To H, Ohdo S, et al. Detection of a drug−drug interaction on population-based phenobarbitone clearance using nonlinear mixed-effects modeling. Eur J Clin Pharmacol 1998;54:69−74.

[31] Yukawa E, Nonaka T, Yukawa M, Higuchi S, Kuroda T, Goto Y. Pharmacoepidemiologic investigation of a clonazepam-valproic acid interaction by mixed effect modeling using routine clinical pharmacokinetic data in Japanese patients. J Clin Pharm Ther 2003;28(6):497−504.

[32] Puentes E, Puzantian T, Lum BL. Prediction of valproate serum concentrations in adult psychiatric patients using Bayesian model estimations with NPEM2 population pharmacokinetic parameters. Ther Drug Monit 1999;21:351−4.

[33] Faigle JW, Feldman KF. Pharmacokinetic data of carbamazepine and its major metabolites in man. In: Schneider H, Janz D, Gardner-Thorpe C, et al., editors. Clinical pharmacology of antiepileptic drugs. Berlin, Germany: Springer-Verlag; 1975. p. 159−65.

[34] Troupin AS, Green JR, Levy RH. Carbamazepine as an anticonvulsant. Neurology 1974;24:863−9.

[35] Bondareva IB, Jelliffe RW, Gusev EI, Guekht AB, Melikyan EG, Belousov YB. Population pharmacokinetic modeling of carbamazepine in epileptic elderly patients. J Clin Pharmacol Ther 2006; 31:1−11.

[36] Cereghino JJ, Brock JT, Van Meter JC, et al. Preliminary observations of serum carbamazepine concentration in epileptic patients. Neurology 1973;23:357−66.

[37] Eichelbaum M, Ekbom K, Bertilsson VA. Plasma kinetics of carbamazepine and its epoxide metabolite in man after single and multiple doses. Eur J Clin Pharmacol 1975;8:337−41.

[38] Levy RH, Pitlick WH, Troupin AS, et al. Pharmacokinetics of carbamazepine in normal man. Clin Pharmacol Ther 1975;17(6):657−68.

[39] Morselli PL, Frigerio A. Metabolism and pharmacokinetics of carbamazepine. Drug Metab Rev 1975;4:97−113.

[40] Rawlins M, Collste P, Bertilsson L, Palmer L. Distribution and elimination kinetics of carbamazepine in man. Eur J Clin Pharmacol 1975;8:91−6.

[41] DiSalle E, Pacific GM, Morselli PL. Studies on plasma protein binding of carbamazepine. Pharmacol Res Commun 1974;6:193−202.

[42] Bourgeois BFD. Pharmacokinetics and pharmacodynamics in clinical practice. In: Wyllie E, editor. The Treatment of epilepsy: principles and practice. 2nd ed. Baltimore: Williams & Wilkins; 1997. p. 728−37.

[43] Bernus I, Dickinson RG, Hooper WD, Eadie MJ. Early-stage autoinduction of carbamazepine metabolism in humans. Eur J Clin Pharmacol 1994;47:355−60.

[44] Bertilsson L, Hojer B, Tybring G, et al. Autoinduction of carbamazepine metabolism in children examined by a stable isotope technique. Clin Pharmacol Ther 1980;27:83−8.

[45] Pitlick WH, Levy RII. Pharmacokinetical model to describe self-induced decreases in steady-state concentrations of carbamazepine. J Pharm Sci 1976;65(3):462−3.

[46] Gonzalez ACA, Sanchez MJG, Hurle AD. Intra- and Interindividual relationship between serum level and dose in epileptic patients treated with carbamazepine monotherapy. Ther Drug Monit 1988;10:501−3.

[47] Browne TR. Pharmacokinetics of antiepileptic drugs. Neurology 1998;51(Suppl. 4):S2−7.

[48] French JA, Gidal BE. Antiepileptic drug interactions. Epilepsia 2000;41(Suppl. 8):S30−6.

[49] Shen DD. Absorption, distribution, and excretion. In: Loscher W, editor. Valproate. Basel-Boston-Berlin: Birkhauser Verlag; 1999. p. 77−90.

[50] Dean JC. Valproate. In: Wyllie E, editor. The treatment of epilepsy: principles and practice. 2nd ed. Baltimore: Williams & Wilkins; 1997. p. 824−32.

[51] Loscher W. Valproate: a reappraisal of its pharmacodynamic properties and mechanisms of action. Prog Neurobiol 1999;58:31−59.

[52] Loiseau P. Sustained release valproate—a review. A sanofi winthrop sattelite symposium presented at the Bethel-Cleveland Epilepsy Symposium, Bielefeld, Germany, March 10, 1993.

[53] Gugler R, von Unruh GE. Clinical pharmacokinetics of valproic acid. Clin Pharmacokinet 1980;5:67−72.

[54] Gulder R, Schell A, Eichelbaum M, Froscher W, Schulz H-U. Disposition of valproic acid in man. Eur J Clin Pharmacol 1977;12:125−32.

[55] Perucca E. Pharmacological and therapeutic properties of valproate. A summary after 35 years of clinical experience. CNS Drugs 2002;16:695−714.

[56] Glauser TA, Pippenger CE. Controversies in blood-level monitoring: reexamining its role in the treatment of epilepsy. Epilepsia 2000;41(Suppl. 8):S6−15.

[57] Froscher W, Burr W, Penin H, Vohl J, Bulau P, Kreiten K. Free level monitoring of carbamazepine and valproic acid: clinical significance. Clin Neuropharmacol 1985;8:362−6.

[58] Boggs J, Waterhouse E, DeLorenzo RJ. The use of antiepileptic medications in renal and liver disease. In: Wyllie E, editor. The treatment of epilepsy: principles and practice. 2nd ed. Baltimore: Williams & Wilkins; 1997. p. 753−63.

[59] Clancy RR. Valproate: an update—the challenge of modern pediatric seizures management. Curr Probl Pediatr 1990;2:161−233.

[60] Graves NH, Ramsay RE. Phenytoin and fosphenytoin. In: Wyllie E, editor. The treatment of epilepsy: principles and practice. 2nd ed. Baltimore: Williams & Wilkins; 1997. p. 833−44.

[61] Mc Kauge L, Tyrer JH, Eadie MJ. Factors influencing simultaneous concentrations of CBZ and its epoxide in plasma. Ther Drug Monit 1981;3:63−70.

[62] Rowan AJ, Binnie CD, de Beer-Pawlikowski NKB, et al. Sodium valproate: serial monitoring of EEG and serum levels. Neurology 1979;29:1450−9.

[63] Levy RH, Wilensky AJ, Anderson GD. Carbamazepine, valproic acid, phenobarbital, and ethosuximide. In: Evans WE, Schentag JJ, Jusko WJ, editors. Applied pharmacokinetics: principles of TDM. Vancouver, WA: Applied Therapeutics, Inc.; 1992 chapter 26

[64] Deckers CLP, Czuczwar SJ, Hekster YA, et al. Selection of antiepileptic drug polytherapy based on mechanisms of action: the evidence reviewed. Epilepsia 2000;41(11):1364−74.

[65] Gram L, Flachs H, Wurtz-Jorgensen A, et al. Sodium valproate, serum level and clinical effect in epilepsy: a controlled study. Epilepsia 1979;20:303−11.

[66] Harden CL, Zisfein J, Atos-Radzion EC, Tuchman AJ. Combination valproate-carbamazepine therapy in partial epilepsies resistant to carbamazepine monotherapy. J Epilepsy 1993;6:91−4.

[67] Bondareva IB, Jelliffe RW, Sokolov AV, Tischenkova IF. Nonparametric population modeling of valproate pharmacokinetics in epileptic patients using routine serum monitoring data: implications for dosage. J Clin Pharm Ther 2004;29:1−16.

[68] Bondareva IB, Sokolov AV, Tischenkova IF, Jelliffe RW. Population pharmacokinetic modeling of carbamazepine by using the iterative Bayesian (IT2B) and the nonparametric EM (NPEM) algorithms: implications for dosage. J Clin Pharm Ther 2001;26:213−23.

[69] U.S. Department of Health and Human Services, Food and Drug Administration, Center for Drug Evaluation and Research (CDER), Center for Biologics Evaluation and Research (CBER) Population Pharmacokinetics Guidance for Industry. Rockville: 1999.

[70] Bondareva IB, Jelliffe RW, Andreeva OV, Bondareva KI. Predictability of individualized dosage regimens of carbamazepine and valproate mono- and combination therapy. J Clin Pharm Ther 2010;36(5):625−36.

[71] Karlsson MO, Sheiner LB. The importance of modeling interoccasion variability in population pharmacokinetic analyses. J Pharmacokinet Biopharm 1993;21(6):735−50.

[72] Holford NHG. Target concentration intervention: beyond Y2K. Br J Clin Pharmacol 1999;48:9−13.

[73] Kondo T, Otani K, Hirano T, et al. The effects of phenytoin and carbamazepine on serum concentrations of monounsaturated metabolites of valproic acid. Br J Clin Pharmacol 1990;29:116−19.

[74] Patsalos PN, Froscher W, Pisani F, et al. The importance of drug interactions in epilepsy therapy. Epilepsia 2002;43:365−85.

[75] McKee PJW, Blacklaw J, Butler RA, et al. Variability and clinical relevance of the interaction between sodium valproate and carbamazepine in epileptic patients. Epilepsy Res 1992;11:193−8.

[76] Gomez Bellver MJ, Garcia Sanchez MJ, Alonso Gonzalez AC, et al. Plasma protein binding kinetics of valproic acid over a broad dosage range: therapeutic implications. J Clin Pharm Ther 1993;18:191−7.

[77] Levy RH, Thummel KE. Basic principles of drug absorption, distribution, and elimination. In: Wyllie E, editor. Treatment of epilepsy: principles and practice. 2nd ed. Baltimore: Williams & Wilkins; 1997. p. 712−28.

[78] Lai AA, Levy RH, Culter RE. Time-course of interaction between carbamazepine and clonazepam in normal man. Clin Pharmacol Ther 1978;24(3):316−23.

[79] Martin E, Tozer TN, Sheiner LB, Riegelman S. The clinical pharmacokinetics of phenytoin. J Pharmacokinet Biopharm 1977;5(6):579−97.

[80] Levine M, Chang T. Therapeutic drug monitoring of phenytoin. Rationale and current status. Clin Pharmacokinet 1990;19(5):341−58.

[81] Froscher W, Keller F, Vogt H, Krämer G. Prospective study on concentrations-efficacy and concentration-toxicity correlations with lamotrigine serum levels. Epileptic Disord 2002;4:49−56.

[82] Ludden TM, Allen JP, Valutsky WA, et al. Individualization of phenytion dosage regimens. Clin Pharmacol Ther 1976;21(3):287−93.

[83] Valodia PN, Seymour MA, McFadyen ML, et al. Validation of population pharmacokinetic parameters of phenytoin using the parallel Michaelis−Menten and first-order elimination model. Ther Drug Monit 2000;22(3):313−19.

[84] Jusko WJ, Koup JR, Alvan G. Nonlinear assessment of phenytoin bioavailability. J Pharmacokinet Biopharm 1976;4(4):327−36.

[85] Ludden TM, Allen JP, Schneider LW, Stavchansky SA. Rate of phenytoin accumulation in man: a simulation study. J Pharmacokinet Biopharm 1978;6(5):399−415.

[86] Chan E, Ti TY, Lee HS. Population pharmacokinetics of phenytoin in Singapore Chinese. Eur J Clin Pharmacol 1990;39:177−81.

[87] Grasela TH, Sheiner LB, Rambeck B, et al. Steady-state pharmacokinetics of phenytoin from routinely collected patient data. Clin Pharmacokinet 1983;16:254−60.

[88] Nation RL, Evans AM, Milne RW. Pharmacokinetic drug interactions with phenytoin (Part I). Clin Pharmacokinet 1990;18(1):37−60; (Part II). Clin Pharmacokinet. 1990;18(2):131−50.

[89] Hayes G, Kootsikas ME. Reassessing the lower end of the phenytoin therapeutic range: a review of the literature. Ann Pharmacother 1993;27:1389−92.

[90] Mullen PW, Foster RW. Comparative evaluation of six techniques for determining the Michaelis−Menten parameters relating phenytoin dose and steady-state serum concentration. J Pharm Pharmacol 1979;31:100−4.

[91] Richens A, Dunlop A. Nomogram for adjusting phenytoin dosage. Lancet 1975;27:1305−6.

[92] Gaulier JM, Boulieu R, Fischer C, et al. Evaluation of a Bayesian pharmacokinetic program for phenytoin concentration predictions in outpatient population. Eur J Drug Metab Pharmacokinet 1998;23 (2):295−300.

[93] Sheiner LB, Beal SL. Evaluation of methods for estimating population pharmacokinetic parameters. I. Michaelis−Menten model: routine clinical pharmacokinetic data. J Pharmacokinet Biopharm 1980;8 (6):553−71.

[94] Vozeh S, Muir KT, Sheiner LB, Follath F. Predicting individual phenytoin dosage. J Pharmacokinet Biopharm 1981;9(2):131−46.

[95] Murphy JE, Bruni J, Stewart B. Clinical utility of six methods of predicting phenytoin doses and plasma concentrations. Am J Hosp Pharm 1981;38:348−54.

[96] Yukawa E, Higuchi S, Aoyama T. Evaluation of single-point phenytoin dosage prediction methods in pediatric patients. J Pharmacobiodyn 1988;11:736−43.

[97] Tozer TN, Winter ME. Phenytoin. In: Evans WE, Schentag JJ, Jusko WJL, editors. Applied pharmacokinetics: principles of therapeutic drug monitoring. Vancouver: Applied Therapeutics; 1992. chapter 25.

[98] Patsalos PN, Berry DJ. Therapeutic drug monitoring of antiepileptic drugs by use of saliva. Ther Drug Monit 2013;35:4−29.

[99] Walson PD. Therapeutic drug monitoring in special populations. Clin Chem 1998;44(2):415−19.

[100] Zini R, Riant P, Barre J, Tillement J-P. Disease-induced variations in plasma protein levels. Implications for drug dosage regimens (Part I). Clin Pharmacokinet 1990;19(2):147−59; (Part II). Clin Pharmacokinet. 1990;19(3):218−29.

[101] Davis R, Peters DH, McTavish D. Valproic acid: a reappraisal of its pharmacological properties and clinical efficacy in epilepsy. Drugs 1994;47:332−72.

[102] Rimmer EM, Buss DC, Routledge PA, Richens A. Should we routinely measure free plasma phenytoin concentration. Br J Clin Pharmacol 1984;17:99−102.

INDIVIDUALIZING DRUG THERAPY IN THE ELDERLY

20

P. Maire, L. Bourguignon, S. Goutelle, M. Ducher and R. Jelliffe

CHAPTER OUTLINE

20.1 INTRODUCTION

Currently, elderly patients are defined as aged from about age 65 years on, based on arbitrary societal norms resulting from policies beginning with the retirement criteria of Bismarck to actuarial data from insurance companies. It is difficult to define scientifically the beginning of the aging process for any individual. It generally begins at about the onset of maturity, and is accelerated at the end of the reproductive period [1]. Aging is a set of nonaccidental processes that not only alters the composition of cells, organs, and bodies, but which also affects major physiological functions and ultimately the ability to restore normal functions following environmental changes [2]. The changing physiological processes affect various pharmacokinetic and pharmacodynamic processes. They change due to different aging processes at work, and with varying intensities depending on the individual. The iatrogenic risk of under- or overdosing a drug is greater in the elderly, eg, with benzodiazepine use and falls [3]. Polytherapy, as a result of polypathology, in the form of multiple chronic diseases, explains part of this.

The goal of this chapter is to offer a *way of thinking* that the reader can apply to many drugs and clinical situations for the optimal care of each elderly patient. First, some examples from the literature will illustrate the need for individualization of therapy, case by case, related to pharmacodynamic variability. In a second part, an illustrative clinical situation will show the possibility of developing a reasoned approach based on the consequences of the aging kidney affecting the pharmacokinetic elimination process.

Individualized Drug Therapy for Patients. DOI: http://dx.doi.org/10.1016/B978-0-12-803348-7.00020-4

20.2 HIGHLIGHTS OF SOME BIOLOGICAL ASPECTS OF AGING

For all animal species, including humans, aging requires a protected environment to permit aging to take place. Aging reduces one's ability to respond appropriately to the demands of the environment due to reduced capacity for physiological adaptation to it. The processes of decline vary widely among individuals, but all tend to become frail or very frail. Because of these changes, elderly patients are more susceptible to diseases, polypathology, iatrogenic problems, and greater morbidity.

The overall mechanism of aging is still unknown. Two general theories have been proposed. One is called genetic and developmental. The other is called stochastic or accidental. For the former, aging is genetically predetermined and favorable environmental conditions help to achieve maximum longevity for the species, related perhaps to internal clocks. For the latter, accidental events either suddenly or gradually alter physiological adaptation capacities, with an inexorable cumulative aspect [1].

All phases of pharmacokinetic processes—the fate of the drug in the body—can be affected by the aging process. Catalogs of variations of pharmacokinetic processes and parameters have been developed over many years, such as the book *Gerontokinetics*, published at the end of the 1980s [4]. Reduced renal elimination, having been the largest and most studied process, will be discussed in the second part of this chapter.

The effect of the drug depends not only on the pharmacokinetic processes and the amount of drug placed in contact with the site of action, but also on the number of receptors and the overall response capacity. All of these can be altered by aging. Examples will be discussed in the next section.

20.3 PHARMACODYNAMIC CHANGES IN THE ELDERLY AND THEIR THERAPEUTIC IMPLICATIONS

For the cardiovascular system, there are structural changes in the heart and vascular system such as the reduction in the number of pacemaker cells in the sinoatrial node, increasing left atrial size, and decreased ventricular and vascular compliance, which can increase afterload. At the cellular level, the number of myocytes decreases with age, as does the recapture of intracellular calcium back into the sarcoplasmic reticulum during diastole. Added to this are the decreased sensitivity of chemoreceptors and baroreceptors, increased activity of the sympathetic nervous system, desensitization of beta-adrenergic receptors, and a decrease in the number of these receptors [5].

Ultimately, such disturbances linked to aging may help to explain variations in response to certain treatments of the cardiovascular system, independent of pharmacokinetic variability. Thus, beta-blockers do not show the same effectiveness in elderly patients. In younger patients, beta-blocker administration before exercise produced a greater decrease in heart rate in the young than in the elderly [6]. Vasodilation produced by the same beta-blockers is reduced in elderly patients [7].

Similarly, the response to beta-adrenergic agonists is less pronounced in elderly patients. The dose of isoproterenol required to increase the heart rate by 25 beats per min is greater in the elderly compared to young subjects. Blocking of the positive chronotropic effect of isoprenaline by propranolol is also reduced [8].

Another example can be seen with drugs that affect the renin-angiotensin system. The clinical benefit of angiotensin converting enzyme inhibitors, which is very good for heart failure in young patients, appears to be less so in patients over 75 years [9].

The same discussion can be had concerning central nervous system drugs. Many disturbances of neurotransmitters have been described in connection with aging, such as disruption of the dopaminergic system with fewer D2 receptors in the striatum, the decreased activity of acetylcholine transferase, or the GABA system [10]. To illustrate, the response of older patients to benzodiazepines seems changed, regardless of any pharmacokinetic changes. Short-acting benzodiazepines cause a greater reduction of psychomotor performance in elderly patients compared to younger ones, which is not explained by blood concentrations of the parent compound or by active metabolites [11]. Similarly, drug concentrations required for sedation are reduced in patients up to 80 years compared to 20-year-old patients [11].

Through these illustrations, it seems clear that a significant part of the variability in response to drugs in elderly patients is due to greater pharmacodynamic variability in addition to pharmacokinetic variability. Without a means to explore it—to describe, predict and control it—the clinician is often forced simply to observe and take into account empirically, through the often stated rules of practice: "Start low, go up slow!"

However, with pharmacokinetic software, the clinician can compare the behavior of each patient with that of her individualized pharmacokinetic model, to better evaluate each patient's clinical sensitivity to the drug. One can then select a specific target goal for that patient based on her always unique clinical situation. Then one can develop an individualized dosage regimen, using multiple model (MM) dosage design, to hit that target goal specifically with maximum precision.

20.4 THE RENAL AGING PROCESS AND ITS PHARMACOKINETIC CONSEQUENCES

Many drugs are eliminated by the kidney, at least partially.

Aminoglycosides, excreted essentially entirely by the kidneys, can be a danger in geriatric patients if dosed as for younger adults, because of their three major pharmacokinetic characteristics: high renal clearance, low protein binding, and a distribution volume overlapping that of extracellular fluid volume.

Rowe's work showed that glomerular filtration decreased with age, by an average of 0.8 mL/min per year after age 40 [12]. Similar results were found for aminoglycosides by population pharmacokinetic modeling. However, the reduction in the average value clearance of amikacin from 6 L/h at age 20 to 3 L/h at age 80 is also accompanied by an increase in the dispersion (standard deviation) from 1.0 at age 20 to 1.7 L/h at age 85. These results complement those obtained for gentamicin in the elderly [13] (Fig. 20.1).

According to this first point of view, based on averages, it is necessary to reduce the dosages of drugs for reduced renal clearance. However, simultaneously, parametric population pharmacokinetic studies show us that an attempt to properly handle this population, based on average values, makes the treatment of a specific individual less precise than in the case of young adults, since the dispersion around the mean values is greater.

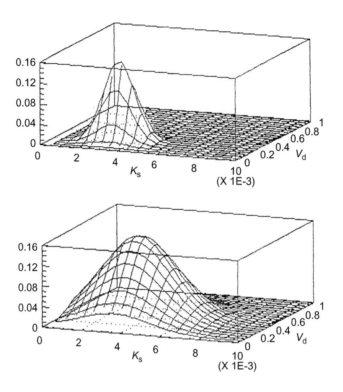

FIGURE 20.1

Parametric descriptions of aging. Compared to that of the young adult reference clinical trials (top), the distribution curve of the renal elimination constant (K_s) of gentamicin in the elderly (bottom) is not Gaussian. It has skewness and kurtosis, and it is wider and shifted.

A parametric population pharmacokinetic study of 50 elderly patients treated with amikacin (mean age 79 years (range = 59–92), average weight: 57 ± 12 kg, creatinine clearance (CCr) estimated at 41 ± 17 mL/min per 1.73m²), showed a wide dispersion, with mean clearance of amikacin of 3.3 ± 1.7 L/h, volume of distribution of 22.2 ± 7.4 L, or 0.39 ± 0.19 L/kg, and a renal elimination rate constant of 0.0034 ± 0.0018 per h. The use of covariates (weight and CCr) decreased the variability around the initial mean pharmacokinetic parameters from 50% to 25% [14].

Moreover, in parallel with the results of Lindeman's longitudinal study [15] that showed differential renal aging with age in general, nonparametric population modeling has independently documented the existence of an elderly subpopulation unaffected by glomerular aging, including clearance of amikacin remaining at the value for young adult patients [15,16].

Furthermore, nonparametric model parameter distributions are often multimodal. While about two-thirds of an elderly population had a lowered clearance of about 2.5 L/h, fully one-third of the population still had a clearance preserved at about 6 L/h [17]. This cross-sectional study of the renal elimination of aminoglycosides corresponds to a "slice" of a longitudinal study such as that of Baltimore, as shown in Fig. 20.2. It confirms that differential renal aging occurs, and that it is necessary to adjust dosages to take into account these subpopulations, and the location of each

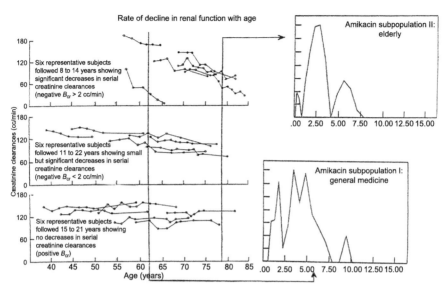

FIGURE 20.2

Effect of aging and renal function according to the study of Baltimore [15]. With advancing age, subpopulations appear. Some subjects with impaired renal function decline more strongly (top), others decline less strongly (middle), and still others retain renal function much better (bottom), whether for clearance of creatinine, left, or for that of an antibiotic mainly excreted by the kidney, amikacin, right.

individual patient's renal function within the subpopulation, in order to achieve the desired target goal with the greatest possible precision.

Given such results, it seems wise for the clinician to decrease the average doses in elderly patients. However, with this model of differential aging, existing also for ofloxacin [18], no simple formula exists to identify which subpopulation an elderly patient belongs to. Using dosage based on average values of CCr, we risk a 1 in 3 chance of underdosing.

Maximum a posterior probability (MAP) Bayesian methods have been used for decades for the adaptive control of possibly long-term therapy in the elderly [19] for treatment of endocarditis [20] (Fig. 20.3). These methods have significantly improved the probability of achieving desired therapeutic targets, while reducing the risk of nephrotoxicity [21], and also by estimation of the diffusion of the antibiotic in endocardial vegetations [22]. They have also helped to highlight the role of circadian variations in antibiotic therapy [23].

MM design of dosage regimens, developed by the USC Laboratory of Applied Pharmacokinetics [24] to achieve maximally precise achievement of target goals using unconstrained nonparametric population model parameter distributions, has been implemented in the Bestdose clinical software geared to everyday practice in geriatrics [available at www.lapk.org]. Incidentally, the plots generated by this new software illustrate well the greater variability resulting from the differential aging process. The set of the different possible trajectories becomes more diverse with age. Fig. 20.4 is an example of the greater variability in the elderly illustrated by the diverse set of possible trajectories for one specific individual patient.

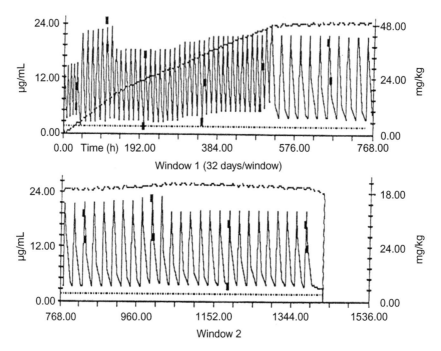

FIGURE 20.3

Example of monitoring of amikacin in an old patient treated for infective endocarditis. Therapeutic drug monitoring with periodic measurements of blood concentrations keep serum concentrations under control over 60 days (dots: weekly measured serum concentrations (μg/mL); solid line: central (serum level) computed data (μg/mL); dotted line: peripheral computed data (mg/kg)). Approaches such as this can prevent accumulation or nephrotoxicity in very frail elderly patients.

20.5 A SPECIAL CASE: INTRAINDIVIDUAL VARIABILITY IN THE ELDERLY

Over a span of about 30 years in our hospital, we have had some patients treated several times with therapeutic monitoring and dose adjustment, often in connection with different hospitalizations. The study by S. Vincent [25] analyzed possible changes in estimated pharmacokinetic parameters in patients who had at least two treatments with amikacin. Furthermore, should we consider a patient who returns again as a new patient or as a continuation of his state during previous therapy?

The pharmacokinetic parameters examined in that study were total distribution volume, volume of distribution per kg, total elimination rate constant, and elimination rate constant per unit of CCr. They considered parameter values that did not differ by more than 10% between two courses of therapy that were at least 2 months apart. Two hundred seventy files were reviewed, 18 patients were selected, of which 4 patients also met criteria for 3 successive treatments.

In six patients (33%), the pharmacokinetic parameters were essentially unchanged from one admission to another. Of the 12 others, changes in the pharmacokinetics of 5 subjects (42% of the courses of therapy) were explained by changes in covariates: a change in weight for 2 cases, a change in estimated CCr for 3 cases. For the other seven subjects, the pharmacokinetic

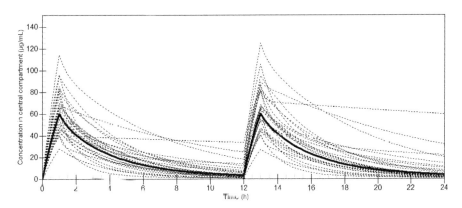

FIGURE 20.4

An example of greater variability in the elderly, illustrated by the set of probable trajectories for one specific individual patient. Possible pharmacokinetic profiles predicted by the initial population pharmacokinetic model in adult subjects receiving a single dose of amikacin. The solid line represents the weighted average of all trajectories. The dotted lines are generated by the multiple predicted trajectories from each model support point, each weighted by the probability of each support point generating that trajectory. X-axis, time (h); Y-axis, plasma concentration of amikacin.

parameters varied significantly, despite adjustments made for the changes in the covariates of interest. At this level, two clinical situations were distinguished in their medical records. The patients showed either changes in their fluid and electrolyte balance and nutritional input (mostly related to the introduction or removal of total parenteral nutrition (four patients)), or dramatic changes in their clinical status.

In practice, a patient who returns may appear unchanged, and it may then be possible to use the estimated values of his individual pharmacokinetic parameters from the first admission. However, if the patient's clinical status appears different, it is probably better then to plan therapy as though a new patient is being treated.

In addition, a sudden worsening of a patient's condition, with a significant change in clinical status such as with septic shock or a neutropenic state, eg, are difficult to track, even during a single treatment, using conventional Bayesian software, even that based on nonparametric models. It is in such situations where the patient is acutely unstable, that the interacting multiple model (IMM) sequential Bayesian software can be especially useful to track drug behavior optimally, showing the changing model pharmacokinetic parameter distributions with each new data point and to develop maximally precise dosage regimens for the very near future in such patients. This software should also permit maximally precise tracking of drug behavior during treatment with long-term teicoplanin [26].

20.6 **CONCLUSIONS AND PERSPECTIVES**

In the elderly patient, pharmacological variability is greater than in young subjects, with both initial genomic and phenotypic variability, plus further variability resulting from individual human life experiences in interaction with changing customs, techniques, and habits, plus the random acquisition of various diseases [27]. Cultural evolution, which until recently led to an increase in longevity, now with accelerating environmental changes and the acquisition of diseases that affect living conditions from embryogenesis to aging, plays an increasing role. Drug therapy in the elderly must prepare to cope with rapid changes in the physiological pharmacokinetics and pharmacodynamics in these specific patients.

Simple adaptation of dosage following regulatory recommendations based on weight, estimated CCr, or both, may induce a false sense of security. The link between these covariates and pharmacological parameters can be of varying intensity, depending on the particular age groups under consideration, especially for patients between 60 and 105 years old. Other characteristics associated with aging and concomitant diseases and treatments may act as hidden variables. In any case, tracking drug behavior best will permit maximum understanding of the clinical situation and optimal dosage for the very near future, at least.

After administration of the drug in the current clinical situation, a nonparametric population model and an MM dosage regimen, along with optimally timed plasma concentration measurements, are the best techniques guaranteeing maximal reduction of individual variability in geriatric therapy. The IMM software can be used as needed.

In addition, it is the responsibility of the geriatrician to use his general experience to compare the behavior of the individual patient's individual drug model with the patient's clinical behavior, to select the target that is considered best suited to each patient's need for, and especially sensitivity to, the drug under consideration. Just as bacteria have their individual sensitivities to antibiotics, so does each patient have a similar individual sensitivity to any drug. This fact has not received nearly the attention it deserves, especially as the practice of therapeutic drug monitoring, with its so-called therapeutic ranges, specifically ignores any real consideration of individual variation in sensitivity of patients to any drug. As in other situations with individualized therapy, it has also been shown that significant economic benefit of therapeutic monitoring can be obtained [28].

It is necessary, in geriatrics at least as much as elsewhere, above all to do only minimal harm. It is necessary to be at least as active in this regard as it is with young adults, especially in cases of acute pathology.

ACKNOWLEDGMENTS

To all members of ADCAPT (Association pour le Développement du Contrôle Adaptatif en Pharmacocinétique et Thérapeutique) who have been with us for more than 30 years, including especially PhDs, interns, and students.

REFERENCES

[1] Turnheim K. When drug therapy gets old: pharmacokinetics and pharmacodynamics in the elderly. Exp Gerontol 2003;38:843–53.
[2] Canguilhem G. Le normal et le pathologique. PUF – Paris. 1966: 224p.

[3] Uhart M, Odouard E, Carlier C, Maire P, Ducher M, Bourguignon L. Relationship between benzodiazepines use and falls in the elderly: a multicenter study in three geriatric centers of a university hospital.
Ann Pharm Fr 2012;70(1):46−52.

[4] Ritchel WA. Gerontokinetics, the pharmacokinetics of drugs in the elderly. Caldwell, NJ: The Telford
Press; 1988. p. 114.

[5] Raza JA, Movahed A. Use of cardiovascular medications in the elderly. Int J Cardiol 2002;85
(2):203−15.

[6] Fleg JL, Schulman S, O'Connor F, Becker LC, Gerstenblith G, Clulow JF, et al. Effects of acute beta-
adrenergic receptor blockade on age-associated changes in cardiovascular performance during dynamic
exercise. Circulation 1994;90(5):2333−41.

[7] van Brummelen P, Bühler FR, Kiowski W, Amann FW. Age-related decrease in cardiac and peripheral
vascular responsiveness to isoprenaline: studies in normal subjects. Clin Sci 1981;60(5):571−7.

[8] Vestal RE, Wood AJ, Shand DG. Reduced beta adrenoceptor sensitivity in the elderly. Clin Pharmacol
Ther 1979;26(2):181−6.

[9] McLean AJ, Le Couteur DG. Aging biology and geriatric clinical pharmacology. Pharmacol Rev
2004;56(2):163−84.

[10] Catterson ML, Preskorn SH, Martin RL. Pharmacodynamic and pharmacokinetic considerations in
geriatric psychopharmacology. Psychiatr Clin North Am 1997;20(1):205−18.

[11] Hämmerlein A, Derendorf H, Lowenthal DT. Pharmacokinetic and pharmacodynamic changes in the
elderly. Clin Pharmacokinet 1998;35(1):49−64.

[12] Rowe J, Andres R, Tobin J. The effect of age on creatinine clearance in man: a cross-section and
longitudinal study. J Gerontol 1976;31:155−63.

[13] Maire P, Roux D, Vermeulen E, Dumarest C, Chauvet C, Courpron P, et al. Choix d'une méthode de
simulation pour adapter les posologies de gentamicine chez des patients très âgés. In: Brès J, Panis G,
editors. Intérêts et limites de la pharmacocinétique en recherche et développement. Paris: Sauramps
Médical - Diffusion Vigot; 1988. p. 301−10.

[14] Maire P, Barbaut X, Girard P, Mallet A, Jelliffe RW, Berod T. Preliminary results of three methods for
population pharmacokinetic analysis (NONMEM, NPML, NPEM) of amikacin in geriatric and general
medicine patients. Int J Biomed Comput 1994;36:139−41.

[15] Lindeman R, Tobin J, Shock N. Longitudinal studies on the rate of decline of renal function with age.
J Am Geriatr Soc 1985;33:278−83.

[16] Jelliffe R, Laffont A, Barbaut X, Girard P, Chapelle G, Pobel C, et al. Pharmacokinetics of amikacin in
a large population using the NPEM algorithm. Clin Pharmacol Therap 1994;160 PII-30.

[17] Maire PH, Jelliffe RW, Schumitzky A, Berod T. Estimation de la variabilité des paramètres pharmacocinétiques de l'amikacine en pratique clinique gériatrique par un programme non paramétrique EM de
modélisation en pharmacocinétique de population. In: Brès J, Panis G, editors. Pharmacocinétique: de la
recherche à la clinique. Paris: John Libbey Eurotext; 1992. p. 262−7.

[18] Corvaisier S, Bleyzac N, De Montclos M, Druguet M, Albrand G, Carret G, et al. Renal differential
aging processes and ofloxacin pharmacokinetics in the elderly. Thérapie 1999;54(2):223−31.

[19] Maire PH, Bleyzac N, Jelliffe RW, Thalabard JC. Théorie de l'adaptation de posologie chez le sujet âgé.
Act Pharm Biol Clin 1995;8:171−82.

[20] Foltz F, Ducher M, Rougier F, Coudray S, Bourhis Y, Druguet M, et al. Efficacy and toxicity of aminoglycoside therapy in the elderly: combined effect of both once-daily regimen and therapeutic drug monitoring. Pathol Biol (Paris) 2002;50(4):227−32.

[21] Rougier F, Claude D, Maurin M, Sedoglavic A, Ducher M, Corvaisier S, et al. Aminoglycoside
nephrotoxicity: modeling, simulation, and control. Antimicrob Agents Chemother 2003;47(3):
1010−16.

[22] Maire P, Barbaut X, Vergnaud JM, el Brouzi M, Confesson MA, Pivot C, et al. Computation of drug concentrations in endocardial vegetations in patients during antibiotic therapy. Int J Biomed Comput 1994;36(1−2):77−85.

[23] Bleyzac N, Allard-Latour B, Laffont A, Mouret J, Jelliffe R, Maire P. Diurnal changes in the pharmacokinetic behavior of amikacin. Ther Drug Monit 2000;22(3):307−12.

[24] Jelliffe RW, Schumitzky A, Bayard D, Milman M, Van Guilder M, Wang X, et al. Model-based, goal-oriented, individualised drug therapy. Linkage of population modelling, new 'multiple model' dosage design, bayesian feedback and individualised target goals. Clin Pharmacokinet 1998;34(1):57−77.

[25] Vincent S, Maire PH, Bataillard T, Denjean E, Ducrozet P, Laffont A, et al. Variabilité intra-individuelle des paramètres pharmacocinétiques de l'amikacine chez le sujet âgé: investigations rétrospectives. Pathol Biol 1996;44(7):667−74.

[26] Uhart M, Leroy B, Michaud A, Maire P, Bourguignon L. Inter-individual and intra-individual pharmacokinetic variability during teicoplanin therapy in geriatric patients. Med Mal Infect 2013;43(7):295−8.

[27] Lieberman ED. L'histoire du corps humain: évolution, dysévolution et nouvelles maladies. Paris: JC Lattès; 2015. p. 541.

[28] Leon-Djian CB, Bourguignon L, Späth HM, Maire P. Cost-effectiveness analysis of active TDM in elderly patients treated with aminoglycosides. Therapie 2011;66(5):445−52.

THE PRESENT AND FUTURE STATE OF INDIVIDUALIZED THERAPY

21

R. Jelliffe and M. Neely

CHAPTER OUTLINE

21.1 MODELS OF LARGE, NONLINEAR SYSTEMS OF MULTIPLE INTERACTING DRUGS

MN has now upgraded the Pmetrics modeling software, in which the nonparametric adaptive grid population modeling software has been embedded in the R language. This much improved, more capable and flexible software is freely available over our laboratory's website (www.lapk.org). It has grown from being able to model the behavior of a single drug to now being capable of modeling the behavior of multiple drugs acting together, with combined effects resulting from synergy, additivity, or antagonism between the drugs and their shared effects such as bacterial kill or any other effects. Multiple drug-drug interactions can be modeled, and combination dosage regimens optimized. This software is now being used to model the effects of combination antiepileptic drug therapy, for example. Not only drugs, but any model system or collection of systems that can be described with ordinary differential equations can be analyzed with this software.

Individualized Drug Therapy for Patients. DOI: http://dx.doi.org/10.1016/B978-0-12-803348-7.00021-6

21.1.1 OPTIMIZING COMBINATION DRUG THERAPY

Our laboratory has also developed multiple model dosage design for nonlinear drug models in addition to the earlier linear models used in the current BestDose clinical software. A new clinical version of BestDose is in development where the large nonlinear, multidrug models can be used and where one can optimize combination drug therapy in which each of several drugs can be dosed to achieve and maintain its own target goal, even in the presence of multiple drug — drug interactions. The relative clinical importance of each goal can also be given its appropriate clinical weight, if desired. This software should be directly useful in optimizing maximally precise combination chemotherapy for patients with transplants, cancer, solid tumors, leukemia, and infectious diseases such as multiple drug resistant TB, for example. For all who are interested, you might consider starting to get your data now.

Laptop computers with such software can easily be used in all parts of the world. Assay methods may well be improved to measure drug concentrations in dried blood spots that may well not require refrigeration and can be transported more easily to nearby laboratories for analysis. The Internet will greatly facilitate communication of results of assays and patient data, to the software and from it as well, to remote areas wherever the patients may be.

21.2 EQUATIONS WITHOUT CONSTANT COEFFICIENTS

All current equations describing pharmacokinetic/pharmacodynamic (PK/PD) systems use constant or piecewise constant coefficients. Even the changing model parameters seen with the interacting multiple model software still assume piecewise constant coefficients (parameters) until new data appear, with an update, but still with constant coefficients afterward until the next data point is encountered.

In contrast, satellites orbiting the Earth cannot use these equations. As a satellite or spacecraft approaches the equator, the gravitational pull of the Earth is increasing due to its greater radius and mass there. As it approaches the poles, the pull is decreasing. At each instant in time the behavior of the system is changing. Use of such equations with changing coefficients may well help us develop much more flexible descriptions of drug behavior in patients and also of creatinine clearance. For example, modeling the effects of the patient's fluid therapy upon the continuously changing volumes of the vascular, extracellular, and intracellular compartments may permit better assessment of the effects of administered fluids to dilute serum creatinine, with CCr appearing to be better than it actually is and vice versa with hypovolemia.

21.2.1 OBSTACLES TO PROGRESS: INSTITUTIONALIZED RITUALISTIC BEHAVIOR, IN WHICH THE PATIENT IS NOTHING AND RITUAL IS EVERYTHING

One of the main obstacles to progress is the current mindset of the medical, pharmacy, and nursing professions to organize all behavior into a set of socially and legalistically approved rituals. Classification takes precedence over everything else, and quantitative relationships are usually ignored.

This mindset is very strong and is, we believe, almost totally unconscious. We believe it comes from the work and thought patterns of those at the time of Linnaeus, who classified the various plants and animals he and those in his profession found around them. In the same way, the medical community still classifies diseases, even though they may be quantitative disturbances from the normal, such as hypertension, diabetes, hyperthyroidism, and hypothyroidism, to name only a very few. Usually when the quantitative disturbance becomes significant enough that something must be done about it, the problem is then given a name, such as one of the above, and criteria such as certain blood pressure values are developed for it. Below these values, there is no problem. Above them, the problem exists, and something must be done to treat it.

We are also taught, for example, to remember the fact that hypokalemia aggravates digitalis toxicity, but to our knowledge, only one attempt has ever been made to quantify this relationship [1]. Similarly, there have been many different criteria developed to recognize left ventricular hypertrophy on the electrocardiogram (EKG) but little or no effort actually to relate what is seen on the EKG directly to estimate heart weight in a given patient except in categorical ways. We categorize almost all our clinical and scientific experience even when it reflects quantitative relationships. We then store this altered version of experience as a "fact" to be remembered, and we seem to be almost totally unaware of what we have done. It all just seems so natural to do things this way.

In a community hospital we know, if a patient needs to be anticoagulated, the physician writes the order, and the pharmacist takes over. The patient is dosed with Coumadin to keep the international normalized ratio (INR) in the range of 2 to 3.5, for example, regardless of the patient's clinical situation that led to the decision to anticoagulate the patient in the first place. This might be regarded as individualized therapy in that hospital, as the dose was adjusted to be in the stated range. However, no thought at all was given to anticoagulation using a gentle, moderate, or aggressive individualized approach.

I know a patient whose INR on the day of hospital discharge was 1.88. At home before admission, the patient had been on Coumadin for years and had been dosed to achieve a gentle INR of 2.0. The patient had been on Coumadin 2 mg 5 days per week at home and 1 mg on Mondays and Fridays, and the INR always had been close to 2.0, as was the 1.88 value above.

Nevertheless, on the afternoon of discharge, since the INR was less than 2.0, a dose of 3.5 mg of Coumadin was ordered for her and also 80 mg of Lovenox. This illustrates the dangers of such ritualistic approaches to dosing. There was no apparent thought of communication between physician, pharmacist, the patient, or the family. Each one performed the ritual he had been carefully trained to do by his various school without any thought of the patient as an individual, only of carrying out the prescribed robotic ritual. Nobody communicated with anybody.

Nurses are actually taught that it is permissible to actually falsify their records and to record a dose of drug as "given when ordered" if it was given within half an hour of when it was ordered. Actually, if a dose was ordered to be given at 8 am, for example, hardly any patient ever gets a dose at exactly 8 am. The staff go around to the various patients with the drugs to be given on that run, starting before it and ending after it. It is so easy for them simply to replace the check mark with the military time, 0000 to 2359, when the drug was actually given. Then it is known not only that the dose *was* given but also exactly *when* it was given. Taking good care of such information is something to be taken quite seriously. Bar codes for the drug and the patient help, and the information can all go in the electronic medical record (EMR), but the act must be carried out when recorded. The lack of such information about when doses are given is the single greatest source of uncertainty in the precise management of drug dosage [2,3].

RJ had been at a hospital where there was a well-functioning EMR. He and his colleagues there looked up data on a patient who had been given vancomycin. They pulled up his EMR data of the doses and serum concentrations to analyze them with the BestDose software. It was only at this time that it became apparent that almost all the supposed trough serum concentrations actually appeared to have been drawn about half an hour into the next vancomycin infusion of 1-hour duration. It was a very instructive time for all of us that day, as it was painfully apparent that none of the patient's data could be trusted.

When garbage is entered into the EMR, it becomes a garbage can. What then happens to all the big data mining studies? When, how, and by whom can data be entered and trusted? This is a big problem for the "big data" community. Physicians, pharmacists, and nurses all very much need to pay close attention to the data they enter. The deadening effect of ritual and the small regard for careful attention to data greatly limit what can be done to optimize the precision of drug therapy with potentially toxic drugs. Such ritualistic behavior, which is currently so firmly institutionalized, apparently without any conscious thought of what is actually being done in the medical, pharmacy, and nursing communities, badly needs the equivalent of a new Flexner Report and a real social revolution. So many opportunities are missed today because of such ritualistic behavior.

The International Association for Therapeutic Drug Monitoring and Clinical Toxicology (IATDM-CT) is a most useful society in this area. Of all the many pharmacokinetic and pharmacometric societies that have developed in recent years, the IATDM-CT has been the one, in our opinion, that is most oriented to the patient as an individual and the least dominated by the pharmaceutical industry and its continuing resistance to anything other than one-size-fits-all ritualistic approaches to dosing.

21.3 THE PHARMACEUTICAL INDUSTRY, DOSES, PATIENTS, AND MISSED OPPORTUNITIES

At present, the pharmaceutical industry appears to see its job as finding the dose to put in the package insert. Its job appears to them to be done at this point. Physicians blindly take this dose and give it to the patient. That is all they have been taught to do in their poor medical education today.

Each drug has two lives. Its first life begins as it is developed by the pharmaceutical industry. As it is codified into the dose and enters the marketplace, its first life ends. Its second life begins when it is given to a patient. What might be so easily done to help this transition into its second life is for the pharmaceutical industry to supply the medical community with a population PK/PD model of its behavior (they have to have all the data—see, [4−6]), best in a nonparametric format as advocated in earlier chapters in this book, to permit maximally precise dosing. However, the pharmaceutical industry appears to have given no thought to the subsequent life of the drug with the patients to whom it is given, except to note adverse reactions. This could easily be remedied by using nonparametric models that permit maximally precise dosing, presenting the dose as the starting point for subsequent optimal individualization for each patient according to his needs and his covariates such as age, gender, height, weight, and renal function.

Rituals of this type are also formulated so that if one does things by the book, one supposedly cannot be sued if anything goes wrong. Our software first began to be used in 1967. Since that time we have not had, nor have we heard of, any lawsuit or any other kind of legal problem stemming from the use of our software, or any other similar software, to individualize drug therapy for patients in the manner described in this book. Indeed, we think that just the opposite is happening.

Careful analysis and management of each patient's problem as described in this book provide good documentation of exactly what is happening with each patient and of the transparent clinical decision making involved in setting an individualized target goal for each patient. Using the best tools available at the time actually provides the best substantiation of individualized drug therapy as the standard of care to be employed whenever possible.

Follow the patient closely. We all have been taught to do this, but now let us seek to do it with a view to quantitative control of a therapeutic process, which is described in the form of controlling the pharmacokinetic model of the drug's behavior in each individual patient, so we hit a desired target goal set specifically for that patient according to his own special needs. The physician can set a specific therapeutic target, (not a range), and the pharmacist can then dose to achieve that specific target with maximal precision. Think what a total revolution that would bring about for each patient, right now!

21.4 THE PHARMACEUTICAL INDUSTRY AND CLINICAL TRIALS

Many clinical trials done by the pharmaceutical industry might be rather irreverently paraphrased as follows. One might begin a flight from Los Angeles to New York and decide on the most appropriate compass course to fly. One could study the results of using several different courses and report the percent of successful arrivals in New York. No instruments or other navigational aids except the compass can be employed in the study. One must be blind to everything except the outcome. Only the outcome—the endpoint—can be observed. One would need a large study involving many flights in order to obtain enough statistical power to conclude that one compass course was significantly more successful than another in the incidence of successful arrivals.

This is a provocative but nevertheless basically similar design to those employed in many clinical trials of drugs in which only a certain outcome is selected to be observed (the primary or secondary endpoints of the study) and the lack of concern with the actual performance of each aircraft (think patient) as could be observed by the radar and controlled by the pilot and the flight control system (think individualized therapy) that guides it. Only the arrival is noted and whether it is successful or not. Based on the results of such a fashionably randomized double-blind trial, the optimal course is selected for all flights, with no pilot knowing what his actual course is, just as one dose fits all, and the single most successful compass course would then be prescribed for all flights going from Los Angeles to New York.

21.4.1 TEACHING PHARMACOKINETICS

Pharmacokinetics needs to be taught to medical students, not as a dry basic science discipline but as a highly useful clinical tool, using appropriate clinical software to enable us to do our best for each individual patient. Such courses have been taught, but have been dropped by curriculum committees after student complaints that "it's too hard", "more work than it's worth", and "more appropriate for pharmacists". The curriculum committees have dropped the courses, sacrificing quality training for student popularity.

21.4.2 TEACHING DECISION ANALYSIS

Another subject that badly needs to be taught to medical students is decision analysis. Physicians have to make extremely important decisions but are never trained to do this as well as they can be. RJ was at a conference recently. There were highly important decisions to be made about giving tissue plasmino-gen activator to a patient with a pulmonary embolus. After much discussion, it was decided to give it. The standard dose was stated and was given. There was no thought at all of a gentle, moderate, or aggressive approach to its administration. The dose was the dose. There was also no thought of monitoring the effect of the drug on various clotting factors in the patient after it was given. Later on, after the patient had developed a hematoma with spinal cord compression, there was similarly no thought of the best method (gentle, moderate, or aggressive) of undoing this move. Everything was described in a yes-no, this-or-that manner, with no thought of any quantitative approach to the patient's extremely serious and ultimately lethal problems. Such categorical approaches to the patient's problems were a key factor in the totally categorical approach to decision making seen at this conference.

There was much talk about weighing risks and benefits for the patient in coming to decisions of this type. However, those thought processes were exactly the same as those RJ had heard 60 years ago. There was much discussion about the frequency of various therapeutic outcomes but none of the quantitative significance or importance of these outcomes to that patient.

It is not uncommon now to multiply the probability of an outcome by a numerical index of its relative importance and arrive at a calculated expected value for a certain outcome or course of action, which then can be compared with that of others. This is a very useful way to compare a frequent outcome of moderate significance with a rare one having great significance. Multiplying probability times significance is a most useful way to calculate and compare the expected value of various outcomes to be seen with various therapeutic approaches.

As to the problem of assigning a number or index to reflect the significance quantitatively, this can be quite painful. Physicians are not taught how to weigh risks and benefits, but as an example, RJ has arbitrarily taken death to be minus 100 and uses clinical judgment to scale the significance of other outcomes, positive or negative, relative to this number.

Physicians have so many decisions to make that are of the utmost importance, but the subject of medical decision making, of calculating, and even the basic idea of comparing the expected value (probability times significance) of various courses of action is, to my knowledge, not taught to students-think of the conference above-, though it has been possible to go to Tufts University and take a 2-year postgraduate fellowship in medical decision making. Good for Tufts!

21.4.3 GENOMICS

Genomics is a popular subject today, and many different variants have clearly documented effects on drug behavior. There are many new facts to memorize. Sometimes it is highly important to know if a patient has a certain gene variant or not before starting therapy (see the chapter on solid tumors). However, there has been a tendency to look for these variants, most of which have only modest effects on drug behavior, and predict such behavior without seeking to confirm its magnitude in each patient by looking at the direct behavior of the drug itself. A good example of looking at the drug itself is the paper by Asberg et al. on tacrolimus [7], in which a modest genetic effect is seen. However, after as few as three or four serum concentrations are obtained, they showed that one has learned everything contained in the genetic information and, in addition, all the effects of all the many genotypes and phenotypes (and all interactions and other effects) that have not yet been discovered.! This is a good example of why it is so useful to continue to monitor the behavior of the drug itself.

21.5 **BAYES' THEOREM AND MEDICAL DECISIONS**

Let us consider a physician in practice in a small town, actually a closed social system. Our physician has just reviewed his records and found that he had seen 1000 women, obtained Papanicolau (Pap) smears on them, and found that in his office, 1 of the 1000 patients had cancer of the cervix.

Let us call the Pap smears either positive or negative, with no grades of positivity, for the sake of simplicity. Let us also say that the smears are extremely reliable and that quality control tests by a proper board of certification had found that of 1000 surgically proven cases of cervical cancer, 999 smears were correctly positive, and only one was falsely negative. Similarly, of 1000 autopsy specimens where cervical cancer was not present, the Pap smear was correctly negative 999 times and was only falsely positive once. It is highly unlikely that any test might be more sensitive (sensitivity = 0.999) or specific (specificity = 0.999) than that.

The next day our physician is having lunch with Joe, who does all the surgery in the area, and George, the only pathologist for the area. Our physician mentions to them what he has just found about the incidence of cervical cancer in his patients. Joe, the surgeon, recalls that he just did a similar audit of his surgical experiences, and of the last 1000 patients he had operated on who had proven cervical cancer in the surgical specimen, George's Pap smears were of similar quality, meaning 999 of the Pap smears were correctly positive, and only one was falsely negative. George also adds that the smears are also very reliable in the opposite direction. He said that he also had just examined 1000 autopsy specimens in which the cervix was free of any cancer. They all had had Pap smears done beforehand, and 999 of those smears were correctly negative. Only one was falsely positive.

The next day, our physician is back in his office. He sees a female patient, does a pelvic examination that is grossly negative, and gets a Pap smear done. The smear comes back positive for cervical cancer.

What should our physician do now? Should he tell the patient she has cancer? Should he call Joe? The real answer depends on the probability that the positive Pap smear actually means that she has cancer. Remember that the Pap was falsely negative in 1 of 1000 patients with cervical cancer. What is her probability of having cancer? Should our physician consult the literature to see what the latest news is about cervical cancer?

Consider now the probability of her having cancer. Do not bother looking at the literature. We are talking about this particular situation, and the data has all been presented to calculate her probability of having cervical cancer. Do not read on until you have her probability in your mind.

Table 21.1 shows how this calculation can be made.

Table 21.1 Incidence Times Pap Results (FTP, FFN, FTN, or FFP) generate the Number of TPs, FNs, TNs, and FPs. See text below for explanations of these letters

Incidence	Pap Results	P's and N's
Positive = 1	FTP = 0.999	TP's = 0.999
	FFN = 0.001	FN's = 0.001
Negative = 999	FTN = 0.999	TN's = 998.001
	FFP = 0.001	FP's = 0.999

As shown in Table 21.1, of the number of patients tested, FTP, the fraction true positive, generates $1 \times 0.999 = 0.999$ TPs. The fraction false negative (FFN) similarly generates $1 \times 0.001 = 0.001$ false negatives (FNs). FTN, the fraction true negative, generates $999 \times 0.999 = 998.001$ true negatives (TNs), and FFP, the fraction false positive, generates 1×0.999 FPs.

The Bayesian posterior probability of being positive given a positive result is $TP/(TP + FP) = 0.999/(0.999 + 0.999) = 0.5$. Similarly, the Bayesian posterior probability of being negative given a negative result is $TN/(TN + FN) = 998.001/(998.001 + 0.001) = 998.001/998.002 = 0.999998998$.

What is happening here? The test is so good, but the patient has only a 50% probability of being positive. You could flip a coin and do just as well as the Pap smear! Now what do you think of the Pap smear? Is it really a good test or not? Has it actually done anything useful at all?

The answer is that the Pap smear has been highly useful. It has raised the patient from a very small Bayesian prior probability of 0.001 to a very significant Bayesian posterior probability of 0.5. What should our physician tell the patient?

Perhaps another test of a different type (to perceive the problem with a different type of data) such as a cervical biopsy might be useful. Let our physician do this. Let us also suppose that the cervical biopsy has sensitivity and specificity equally as good as the Pap smear: also 99.9% sensitive (99.9% true positives and 0.1% false negatives) and 99.9% specific (99.9% true negatives and 0.1% false positives).

The patient gets her biopsy, and it too is positive. Now what is the Bayesian posterior probability that she has cervical cancer under these circumstances? Let us look at Table 21.2.

The Bayesian posterior probability of being positive given a positive result is $TP/(TP + FP) = 0.999/(0.999 + 0.001) = 0.999/1 = 0.999$. Similarly, the Bayesian posterior probability of being negative given a negative result is $TN/(TN + FN) = 0.999/(0.999 + 0.001) = 0.999/1 = 0.999$.

Note that the old Bayesian posterior probability of 0.5 becomes the new prior probability with regard to her cervical biopsy. The probability of having cervical cancer has now become extremely high at 99.9%. Now is the time to call Joe.

Bayes theorem runs throughout the process of decision analysis. Here we see it applied to qualitative data, whereas in the other chapters, it was applied to quantitative PK/PD data. The scenario here is just one example of its importance and the need to teach proper quantitative approaches to decision making to medical students.

Table 21.2 Incidence Times Biopsy Results (FTP, FFN, FTN, or FFP) Generate the Number of TPs, FNs, TNs, and FPs

Incidence	Biopsy Results	P's and N's
Positive = 1	FTP = 0.999	TP's = 0.999
	FFN = 0.001	FN's = 0.001
Negative = 1	FTN = 0.999	TN's = 0.999
	FFP = 0.001	FP's = 0.001

21.6 **THE TWO-ARMED BANDIT**

We seek to control the PK/PD model of a drug in an individual patient optimally. A famous example of the process of learning about the behavior of a system while having to control it at the same time is called the problem of the two-armed bandit.

The scenario is that you are in Las Vegas and have 1000 silver dollars to spend. There are two different dollar slot machines in front of you, and you are told that one of them will pay off better than the other. Your job is to test the machines, find out as soon as possible which machine is the one you truly want, and put all the dollars you can in the good machine.

However, one machine or the other may also have a run of good (or bad) luck for you. You never know with statistical things like this. That means that you must find out as soon as possible which machine appears to be the best, but you must be sure to recheck this from time to time so that you do not put your money in the wrong machine. It turns out that the optimal procedure to deal with this problem is formulated but still remains unsolved in its implementation.

We want to do a similar thing with each patient. We have a therapeutic target goal (serum concentration or effect) in mind. We want to achieve (hit) this target goal as soon and as precisely as possible and keep it there throughout the planned course of therapy. That is why we use nonparametric models of the drug so we can use multiple model dosage design and hit our target most precisely. This is close to truly optimal dosage.

At the same time, we also plan in advance to monitor the patient's serum concentrations and other effect responses in the most informative and cost-effective way to learn as soon as possible how the drug is really behaving in that individual patient, so we can adjust the dose to again hit our target (or perhaps a different target we now think might be better for the patient) most precisely. The process is one of optimizing learning about the patient while treating him at the same time. That is what this book is about. This process is being improved upon each year, by us and many others.

21.7 **CONCLUSION—MONITOR EACH PATIENT OPTIMALLY AND CONTROL THE SYSTEM OPTIMALLY**

How can the current ritualistic point of view be improved? Something to consider as a template is a piano concerto we recently heard. The piano soloist could easily be seen as the patient, the conductor as the physician, and the orchestra as the entire medical care industry. The conductor obviously knew his business, and he masterfully directed the orchestra to do what was required of it.

However, the conductor, the soloist, and the orchestra were not separately doing their own separate rituals as do the physicians, the pharmacists, and the nurses in the hospital today. They were a closely coordinated whole. In addition, the conductor carefully watched and followed the soloist and made sure everything was in synchrony with the performance of the soloist. That is what we need and what we can achieve for the patient, now, today, in medicine.

Another example we like is the flamenco guitarist (the ideal physician) who ever so carefully follows the dancer (the patient) as they perform the beautiful music and the dance together. They are truly one, just as in the magical relationship that can exist between each physician and each individual patient!

REFERENCES

[1] Jelliffe R. Effect of serum potassium level upon risk of digitalis toxicity. Ann Int Med 1973;78:821.

[2] Charpiat B, Breant V, Dumarest C, Maire P, Jelliffe RW. Prediction of future serum concentrations with Bayesian fitted pharmacokinetic models: results with data collected by nurses versus trained pharmacy residents. Ther Drug Monit 1994;16:166—73.

[3] Jelliffe RW, Schumitzky A, Van Guilder M. Nonpharmacokinetic clinical factors affecting aminoglycoside therapeutic precision. A simulation study. Drug Invest 1992;4:20—9.

[4] Miglioriri A, Valenti R, Parodi G, et al. Comparison of the degree of platelet aggregation inhibition with prasugrel versus clopidogrel and clinical outcomes in patients with unprotected left main disease treated with everolimus-eluting stents. Am J Cadriol 2013;112:1843—8.

[5] Jelliffe R. Concerning antiplatelet therapy — a letter to the editor. Am J Carrdiol 2014;113:2086—7.

[6] Antoniucci D, Migliorini A, Valenti R. Reply. Am J Cardiol 2014;113:2087.

[7] Aasberg A, Midtvedt K, van Guilder M, Storset E, Bremer S, Bergan S, et al. Inclusion of CYP3A5 genotyping in a nonparametric population model improves dosing of tacrolimus early after transplantation. Transpl Int 2013;26:1198—207 ISSN 0934-0874.

Index

Note: Page numbers followed by "*f*" and "*t*" refer to figures and tables, respectively.